AF763586

CYBERBULLYING IN SCHOOLS, WORKPLACES, AND ROMANTIC RELATIONSHIPS

This volume brings together research on cyberbullying across contexts, age groups, and cultures to gain a fuller perspective of the prevalence and impact of electronic mistreatment on individual, group, and organizational outcomes. This is the first book to integrate research on cyberbullying across three contexts: schools, workplaces, and romantic relationships, providing a unique synthesis of lifespan contexts.

For each context, the expert chapter authors bring together three different 'lenses': existing research on the predictors and outcomes of cyberbullying within that context; a cross-cultural review across national borders and cultural boundaries; and a developmental perspective that examines age-related differences in cyberbullying within that context. The book closes by drawing commonalities across these different contexts leading to a richer understanding of cyberbullying as a whole and some possible avenues for future research and practice.

This is fascinating reading for researchers and upper-level students in social psychology, counseling, school psychology, industrial-organizational psychology, and developmental psychology, as well as educators and administrators.

Gary W. Giumetti is associate professor of psychology at Quinnipiac University in Hamden, CT. Gary holds Bachelor's and Master's degrees in Psychology from Villanova University and a PhD in Industrial-Organizational Psychology from Clemson University. His research focuses on fairness and employee well-being in the 21st century workplace.

Robin M. Kowalski is a Trevillian professor of psychology at Clemson University. She obtained her PhD in social psychology from the University of North Carolina at Greensboro. Her research interests focus primarily on aversive interpersonal behaviors, most notably complaining, teasing, and bullying, with a particular focus on cyberbullying.

CYBERBULLYING IN SCHOOLS, WORKPLACES, AND ROMANTIC RELATIONSHIPS

The Many Lenses and Perspectives of Electronic Mistreatment

Edited by Gary W. Giumetti and Robin M. Kowalski

Routledge
Taylor & Francis Group
NEW YORK AND LONDON

First published 2019
by Routledge
52 Vanderbilt Avenue, New York, NY 10017

and by Routledge
2 Park Square, Milton Park, Abingdon, Oxon OX14 4RN

Routledge is an imprint of the Taylor & Francis Group, an informa business

© 2019 Taylor & Francis

The right of Gary W. Giumetti and Robin M. Kowalski to be identified as the authors of the editorial material, and of the authors for their individual chapters, has been asserted in accordance with sections 77 and 78 of the Copyright, Designs and Patents Act 1988.

All rights reserved. No part of this book may be reprinted or reproduced or utilised in any form or by any electronic, mechanical, or other means, now known or hereafter invented, including photocopying and recording, or in any information storage or retrieval system, without permission in writing from the publishers.

Trademark notice: Product or corporate names may be trademarks or registered trademarks, and are used only for identification and explanation without intent to infringe.

Library of Congress Cataloging-in-Publication Data
A catalog record for this title has been requested

ISBN: 978-1-138-08715-6 (hbk)
ISBN: 978-1-138-08716-3 (pbk)
ISBN: 978-1-315-11055-4 (ebk)

Typeset in Bembo
by Taylor & Francis Books

This book is dedicated to my sons, Gavin and Maxwell, and to my parents, Judy and Hector. Thank you for giving my life meaning and direction.

GWG

I dedicate this book to my sons, Noah and Jordan. I'm so proud of the young men you have become, and excited to see what the future holds for you.

RMK

ILLUSTRATIONS

Figures

Tables

1

INTRODUCTION

Cyberbullying Across Contexts, Age Groups, and Cultures

Robin M. Kowalski and Gary W. Giumetti

Research on cyberbullying has been growing steadily over the last 15 years as the Internet and Internet-connected devices take an ever-more prominent place in our lives. Cyberbullying takes place using the Internet or cell phones, and involves multiple acts of aggressive behavior against an individual who cannot easily defend him/herself (Kowalski, Limber, & Agatston, 2012). The majority of this research on cyberbullying has focused on children and adolescents in middle school or high school and has demonstrated strong links with both internalizing problems (such as anxiety, depression, or suicidal ideation; Bonanno & Hymel, 2013; Kowalski, Giumetti, Schroeder, & Lattanner, 2014; Tsitsika et al., 2015) and externalizing problems (such as aggression, suspensions from school, and drug and alcohol use; Kowalski et al., 2014; Tsitsika et al., 2015). Whereas less research has been conducted on cyberbullying among working adults or romantic partners, the existing findings seem to indicate that electronic mistreatment is also prevalent in these other contexts, and it is associated with a host of negative outcomes for individuals and organizations. For example, recent workplace research has found a link between cyberbullying and increased emotional exhaustion and decreased perceptions of fairness for employees (Farley, Coyne, Axtell, & Sprigg, 2016). Additionally, research on cyberbullying among romantic partners indicates that such mistreatment is associated with perceived stress among college students (Leisring & Giumetti, 2014) as well as depressive symptoms and delinquency among teens (Zweig, Lachman, Yahner, & Dank, 2014).

To date, however, no efforts have been made to bring together this research across contexts, age groups, and cultures to gain a fuller perspective of the impact of cyberbullying and similar forms of electronic mistreatment. Social-ecological analyses have been proposed for understanding cyberbullying by taking into account individual, peer, family, school, and cultural factors. However, as noted by Görzig, Milosevic, and Staksrud (2017, p. 1199),

> the evidence to date is limited in terms of understanding the contexts in which cyberbullying takes place … Most research in this tradition [social ecological] has investigated cyberbullying in the context of schools, families, and peers; research looking at the wider cultural context, however, is scarce …

As will be seen in the pages that follow, the field of cyberbullying research, as is often the case with relatively new fields of investigation, has been fraught with a lack of clarity. Even defining cyberbullying remains unclear as definitions depend upon the type of cyberbullying being investigated (e.g., verbal, visual; Nocentini et al., 2010), the country in which the research is being conducted, and, within-country, the setting in which researchers are focusing their efforts (e.g., school, work, relationships). The purpose of the current book is to provide some unity to the disunity currently characterizing the field by examining the different contexts in which cyberbullying may occur, and the different lenses through which we can understand the phenomenon of cyberbullying.

Cyberbullying Defined

Over the last 15 years, researchers have failed to reach a consensus on exactly how cyberbullying should be defined (Kowalski et al., 2014; Slonje, Smith, & Friesen, 2013). This lack of consensus in conceptualizing cyberbullying has had implications for how cyberbullying is measured, leading to variations, for example, in prevalence rates across studies. One conceptual sticking point is the extent to which cyberbullying is both similar to and different from traditional bullying (e.g., Cassidy, Faucher, & Jackson, 2013). Traditional bullying has been defined as an act of aggression that is intended to cause harm or distress, that is typically repeated over time, and that occurs among individuals whose relationship is characterized by a power imbalance (Olweus, 1993; 2013). Building upon this definition, Smith et al. (2008, p. 376) defined cyberbullying as "an aggressive, intentional act carried out by a group or individual, using electronic forms of contact, repeatedly and over time against a victim who cannot easily defend him or herself."

Support for building a conceptual foundation for cyberbullying out of the traditional bullying model can be found in the relationships between involvement in the two types of behavior across many studies. For example, in their meta-analysis, Kowalski et al. (2014) found correlations of 0.40 between traditional bullying victimization and cybervictimization. Similarly, they found correlations of 0.45 between being a perpetrator of traditional bullying and perpetrating cyberbullying. In addition, Olweus (2013) stated that only 10% of individuals are cyberbullied independently of also being involved in traditional bullying. Together, these findings suggest that if an individual is involved with traditional bullying, he or she also tends to be involved with cyberbullying.

However, although most researchers agree that cyberbullying, like traditional bullying, is an act of aggression whose intent is to harm the victim (see, however, Coyne et al., 2017 and Farley et al., 2016 who note that intent is difficult to establish in workplace cyberbullying, and, therefore, it is left out of their definition), some researchers perceive that cyberbullying differs from traditional bullying in the extent to which cyberbullying is repetitive and the degree to which the relationship between the cyberbullying victim and perpetrator is characterized by a power imbalance (Slonje et al., 2013). Minimally, the concepts of repetition and power imbalance do not necessarily mean the same thing for cyberbullying that they mean for traditional bullying (Vranjes, Baillien, Vandebosch, Erreygers, & de Witte, 2017). Repetition in cyberbullying may mean a single email being disseminated to hundreds of recipients (e.g., Cassidy et al., 2013) or an individual reading a bullying text message over and over again. Whereas in traditional bullying, power imbalance typically refers to differences in physical strength or social status, in the online world, power differentials may take the form of technological expertise or stem from anonymity (e.g., Cassidy et al., 2013; Kowalski et al., 2014).

In addition, not all researchers agree that all three components of intentionality, repetition, and power imbalance are even necessary for cyberbullying to occur (e.g., Nocentini et al., 2010). More specifically, several investigators have suggested that repetition is not essential for a situation to be defined as cyberbullying (Dooley, Pyzalski, & Cross, 2009; Nocentini et al., 2010; Slonje & Smith, 2008). Furthermore, the importance of the components of intentionality, repetition, and power imbalance for defining cyberbullying appear to vary cross-culturally (Menesini et al., 2012; Nocentini et al., 2010; Palladino et al., 2017). Palladino et al. (2017) and Menesini et al. (2012), in their studies of several countries, found that the imbalance of power was the most important component for identifying behavior as cyberbullying. However, Nocentini et al. (2010), in a focus group study with participants from Italy, Germany, and Spain, found intentionality to play a critical role in determinations of cyberbullying.

In addition, the appropriateness of each of these components appears to depend on the context in which cyberbullying is being examined. For example, workplace bullying has been defined as "instances where an employee is repeatedly and over a period of time exposed to negative acts (i.e., constant abuse, offensive remarks or teasing, ridicule, or social exclusion) from co-workers, supervisors, or subordinates" (Hershcovis, 2011, p. 501; see also Einarsen, 2000). Workplace cyberbullying would be the occurrence of these behaviors online. Defined in this way, the power imbalance factor appears less critical as subordinates as well as superiors could perpetrate cyberbullying. Relatedly, Coyne et al. (2017, p. 947), who defined workplace cyberbullying as "repeated and enduring negative behavior in the workplace that occurs via technology," suggested that intent should not be included within a definition of workplace cyberbullying as workers will often disguise their true intent or attempt to rationalize their actions. Definitional issues surrounding these three components of intentionality, repetition, and power imbalance highlight the need for a book that examines the contextual and cultural lenses through which cyberbullying can be viewed.

Prevalence Rates of Cyberbullying

As noted at the beginning of this chapter, the majority of the research on cyberbullying to date has been conducted with middle school students in North American and Europe (see Chapter 4, this volume; Brochado, Soares, & Fraga, 2017). Not only has this largely ignored the international nature of the behavior, but it has also failed to account for other age demographics for whom cyberbullying is an issue and other settings in which cyberbullying might occur (e.g., the workplace).

As technology has become increasingly available, younger and younger children are using it in some form (see Chapter 2, this volume), increasing the likelihood that they, too, will become involved with cyberbullying (Çelik, Atak, & Erguzen, 2012). While data are limited on victimization and perpetration prevalence rates among very young children, existing data suggest that the rates are highly variable across studies and across countries. In one study, 18% of children in 3rd, 4th, and 5th grade in a US sample reported being victims of cyberbullying (DePaolis & Williford, 2014). Monks and colleagues conducted two studies with elementary school aged youth in the United Kingdom (Monks, Robinson, & Worlidge, 2009; Monks, Worlidge, Robinson, & Ortega, 2012). In the first study (2009), 23% of the youth ages 7 to 11 reported cyberbullying victimization and 5% reported cyberbullying perpetration. In a second study, Monks et al. (2012) found prevalence rates of victimization and perpetration of 21% and 5%, respectively, among youth of the same age. Similarly, among Italian youth, also 7 to 11 years of age, 21% said they had been victims of cyberbullying (Livingstone & Haddad, 2009). Among Turkish youth, however, between the ages of 8 and 11, rates were higher, with the children reporting a victimization rate of 27% and a perpetration rate of 18% (Arslan, Savaser, Hallett, & Balci, 2012). The most common venue by which cyberbullying seems to occur among elementary school aged youth appears to be online gaming (Englander, 2012).

While the venue by which cyberbullying occurs changes as children enter middle and high school, shifting more to social media and text messaging, prevalence rates of cyberbullying victimization and perpetration remain stable or increase, depending on the study (Kowalski et al., 2012). Kowalski and Limber (2007), in a study of over 3600 middle school youth, found that 18% reported being a victim of cyberbullying and 11% reported perpetrating cyberbullying during the preceding two months. Mishna and colleagues, in their study of middle and high school students, reported victimization and perpetration rates of

50% and 33%, respectively (Mishna, Cook, Gadella, Daciuk, & Solomon, 2010). Meta-analyses of cyberbullying victimization rates among middle school students place the prevalence rate at around 15% (Modecki, Minchin, Harbaugh, Guerra, & Runions, 2014). (For more detailed coverage of cyberbullying prevalence rates among youth, see Chapter 2 and Chapter 5, this volume.)

Similar to traditional bullying (Chapell et al., 2006), involvement in cyberbullying in college as victim, perpetrator, or bully/victim seems to reflect the continuation of a behavior that started in elementary school and continued through middle and high school (Beran, Rinaldi, Bickham, & Rich, 2012; Selkie, Kota, Chen, & Moreno, 2015; Watts, Wagner, Velasquez, & Behrens, 2017). In a review of the literature of prevalence rates of bullying and cyberbullying victimization and perpetration among college students, Lund and Ross (2017) observed rates of cyberbullying victimization between 10 and 15% and a rate of cyberbullying perpetration of 5%. They found that college males were more likely than college females to report perpetrating cyberbullying, but no differences between males and females were observed for victimization. Another study reported cyberbullying victimization rates of 27.9% and cyberbullying perpetration rates of 8% among college students (Francisco, Simao, Ferreiro, & Martins, 2015; see also Kowalski, Morgan, Drake-Lavelle, & Allison, 2016; Selkie, Kota, & Moreno, 2016).

Cyberbullying is certainly not limited to individuals in school, although research on cyberbullying among adults is much more limited and much of it focuses on college students (Jenaro, Flores, & Frias, 2018). Outside the university setting, increasing attention is being directed toward cyberbullying as it occurs in the workplace and in romantic relationships. Kowalski, Toth, and Morgan (2018) found that 20% of the 3,699 participants in their sample reported that the majority of the cyberbullying victimization they had experienced occurred in adulthood, much of this at work. Privitera and Campbell (2009) found that 11% of Australian male workers reported having been cyberbullied. Gardner et al. (2016) found that 2.8% of the workers in their study had similarly been cyberbullied. Cyberabuse in romantic relationships can occur through any of a number of different channels, including text messages, emails, and social media platforms. Individuals who abuse their partners can use electronic forms of communication to harass, stalk, humiliate, or threaten their romantic partner, to name just a few forms the abuse can take (Bennett, Guran, Ramos, & Margolin, 2011; Leisring & Giumetti, 2014).

In examining the considerable variability in prevalence estimates across studies, it is important to keep in mind a number of variables. First, as noted earlier, researchers have yet to reach a consensus on how cyberbullying should be defined (Slonje et al., 2013). Thus, in any study, participants are being asked whether they have experienced cyberbullying as victim, perpetrator, or both based on definitions provided by the researchers themselves. Differences in these definitions across studies likely yield differences in prevalence rates of the behavior. Furthermore, depending on the context, different terms may be used to refer to the same or similar behavior. For example, particularly among adults, a variety of terms are used somewhat loosely to refer to cyberbullying, including cyber incivility (Giumetti, McKibben, Hatfield, Schroeder, & Kowalski, 2012; Lim & Teo, 2009), virtual harassment (Ford, 2013), and cyberaggression (Coyne et al., 2017; Weatherbee & Kelloway, 2006), to name a few. Questions remain regarding the extent to which cyber incivility, for example, is the same as cyberbullying (see, e.g., Kowalski et al., 2018).

Second, the definitions of cyberbullying provided by researchers to participants inform the measures and methodology used in a particular study. Whereas some studies may simply ask participants a single question ("Have you ever been cyberbullied?"), others may ask multiple questions regarding the venue by which cyberbullying may have occurred (e.g., "Have you ever been cyberbullied via social media?"), and still others may ask about specific cyberbullying behaviors (e.g., "How often have you had negative rumors or gossip spread about you online?"). Depending on the type of measure used, prevalence estimates will vary. The time parameter used in these questions will also determine prevalence. Brochado et al. (2017) observed in their scoping review that the most common time period across studies was one year; however, participants could be asked if they had been cyberbullied or cyberbullied others in the past two months, six months, lifetime, etc., yielding varying rates of cyberbullying victimization and perpetration.

Prevalence rates will also vary with the liberal versus conservative criteria used to determine whether cyberbullying occurred, for example, including participants who report the behavior having occurred at least once versus two to three times a month or more. Characteristics of the sample, such as age, gender, and race/ethnicity, also influence prevalence statistics, and these demographic characteristics may interact with other features of the measurement setting. For example, in one study of traditional bullying, African American youth presented with a definition-based question about their bullying victimization underreported their experiences relative to White participants compared to when they were asked more specific behavior-based questions about their bullying experiences (Sawyer, Bradshaw, & O'Brennan, 2008).

Finally, as discussed above, prevalence statistics vary with the context (e.g., school, workplace, relationships) and country of origin in which the data are collected. However, even meta-analyses and scoping reviews may not tell the complete picture regarding prevalence statistics as most of those published to date have relied on studies published in English, omitting many cyberbullying studies that have been conducted in other countries but that were written in languages other than English (Brochado et al., 2017). Importantly, even when certain of these parameters are held constant, such as comparing studies within the same country or for a given time parameter, considerable variability in prevalence estimates has been found (Brochado et al. 2017).

In summary, the existing research suggests that there is wide variability in prevalence rates for cyberbullying victimization (ranging from 2.8 to 50%) and cyberbullying perpetration (ranging from 5% to 33%). The variability in these prevalence rates is likely due to a number of factors, including differences in the cyberbullying definition adopted, the type of measure used, the time parameter used in the measure, the frequency criterion adopted by the researchers (once vs. two or more times), and the context (e.g., school, workplace, and romantic relationships). Whereas there is wide variability in prevalence rates across studies, researchers have tended to report similar findings regarding the correlates or outcomes of cyberbullying. We turn to this next.

Outcomes of Cyberbullying

The outcomes associated with cyberbullying for both victims and perpetrators are perhaps the most consistent aspect of the behavior across contexts, ages, and cultures. School-aged youth, emerging adults, as well as members of the workforce who are victims and perpetrators of cyberbullying report negative physical and psychological effects. Among youth, victims and perpetrators of cyberbullying report higher levels of anxiety, depression, loneliness, and suicidal ideation (e.g., Didden et al., 2009; Hinduja, & Patchin, 2010; Kowalski et al., 2014). Compared to individuals who are not involved in cyberbullying, they also report lower levels of self-esteem, disinterest in school, and poor academic performance (Gardella, Fisher, & Teurbe-Tolon, 2017; Kowalski & Limber, 2013).

Although research regarding the effects of cyberbullying on adults, specifically adults in the workplace, is much more limited, available evidence suggests that the outcomes are very similar to those experienced by youth. Among the negative effects of cyberbullying victimization reported among employees are increased anxiety, emotional exhaustion and mental strain, and lower job satisfaction (Baruch, 2005; Coyne et al., 2017; Farley et al., 2016; Snyman & Loh, 2015; Staude-Müller, Hansen, & Voss, 2012; Vranjes et al., 2017). In addition to these individual costs, higher absenteeism and turnover intentions, reduced job performance, and counterproductive work behaviors also result in costs to the organization (Baruch, 2005; Coyne et al., 2017; Farley et al., 2016; Gardner et al., 2016).

The experience of cyberbullying depends, in part, on the frequency with which the cyberbullying occurs and the perceived severity of the cyberbullying (Cassidy et al., 2013). Importantly, however, just as there are individual differences in perceived severity, there also appear to be country differences in perceptions of cyberbullying severity. In one study with over 1900 adolescents in middle and high schools in Italy, Germany, Turkey, and Estonia, Italian students perceived anonymous online attacks as less severe than participants from the other three countries (Palladino et al., 2017).

Overview of the Book

An examination of the definition, prevalence, and outcomes associated with cyberbullying highlights both the great strides that have been made in the field in the last 15 years, but also the work that remains to be done. A strong foundation has been laid, but the literature is filled with gaps and questions that remain to be addressed. To address some of these gaps in the literature that were outlined at the beginning of this chapter, we bring together cyberbullying researchers who examine cyberbullying within three contexts: school (from grade school to college), the workplace, and romantic relationships. Within each of these three contexts, we aim to provide readers with three different lenses through which to view cyberbullying. First, experts will provide a review of existing research on cyberbullying within the particular context (i.e., in school, in the workplace, or among romantic partners) and outline the possible predictors and outcomes of cyberbullying within that context. Second, experts will provide a review of cross-cultural issues within the school, workplace, and relationships, to help us understand how these problematic behaviors may be similar and different across national borders and cultural boundaries. Third, experts will take a developmental perspective to look at how the predictors and outcomes of cyberbullying and electronic mistreatment may be similar and different at various age points in one's life.

In Chapter 2, we provide an overview of the increasing use of Information and Communication Technologies (ICTs). While ICTs have made much of our communication more fluid, they have also been fraught with negative outcomes, including cyberbullying. The chapter examines the variable use of ICTs and cyberbullying involvement by age, race/ethnicity, and gender. The demographic correlates of ICT use are important as the means by which cyberbullying occurs for a particular demographic reflect the most common type of technology used by that group.

The following three chapters focus on cyberbullying in schools. The first chapter in this group, Chapter 3 by Sheri Bauman and Diana Meter, provides a review of cyberbullying research conducted on school-aged youth within the United States. Their chapter examines both risk factors and outcomes associated with cyberbullying involvement. In addition, they examine the relationship between involvement in traditional bullying and cyberbullying as victim and perpetrator. Before turning their attention to policies and laws, Bauman and Meter devote particular attention to online gaming, an understudied area within the cyberbullying community that has particular relevance for younger children involved in cyberbullying. In the second chapter in the "Cyberbullying in Schools" section of the book (Chapter 4), Peter Smith, Susanne Robinson, and Anke Görzig focus on cross-cultural issues. In spite of the fact that much of the research on cyberbullying has been conducted in Western countries, cyberbullying occurs throughout the world. It is, therefore, important to examine similarities and differences in cyberbullying across countries. Smith and colleagues compare the data from two large scale surveys: the EUKO (EU Kids Online) survey which compared cyberbullying across 25 European countries, and the HBSC (Health Behavior of School-Aged Children) survey, which examined cyberbullying across 42 European and North American countries. Variations in cyberbullying across countries are explained using the five factors of the EU Kids Online Model—cultural values, education system, technological infrastructure, regulatory framework, and socio-economic stratification. The "Cyberbullying in Schools" section is rounded out with a chapter by Elizabeth Englander (Chapter 5), who adopts a developmental perspective as she discusses variability in prevalence estimates of cyberbullying across the school years from elementary school through high school. She examines some of the causes for differences in prevalence between younger and older youth including differential access to technology, cognitive limitations in younger children, and less education about cyberbullying and uses of technology among younger children. She also discusses the importance of examining prevalence rates of cyberbullying across developmental stages. This examination provides information about relationship dynamics at each developmental period.

The next section of the book examines cyberbullying in the context of the workplace, a relatively understudied area of investigation. In Chapter 6 (Cyberbullying in the Workplace: A Review of the Research), Jenna Scisco reviews the literature on workplace cyberbullying. You will note the relatively recent publication date of much of this literature, reflecting the recent attention of cyberbullying researchers to cyberbullying as it occurs outside the realm of school-aged youth. Erin Richard, Julianna Walsh, and Zhiqing Zhou focus on cross-cultural issues related to workplace cyberbullying in Chapter 7 (Cyberbullying in the Workplace—Cross-Cultural Issues). Because of the paucity of research on not only workplace cyberbullying but more specifically culture and workplace cyberbullying, they begin their chapter by reviewing the literature on workplace bullying and culture, turning their attention to culture and computer-mediated communication. In their discussion of computer-mediated communication, Richard and colleagues focus specifically on the role of high-context versus low-context cultures as well as the concept of face. They then advance a model of workplace cyberbullying and its possible predictors based on the sender-message-receiver model of communication. Nicole Mowry and Gary Giumetti address "Cyberbullying in the Workplace—Developmental Perspectives" in Chapter 8. In their chapter, Mowry and Giumetti begin by providing an overview of age differences in workplace technology use. Then, they describe research on age differences in cyberbullying among adults in the general population and employed adults more specifically. They also discuss some possible ways in which age may interact with cyberbullying in predicting outcomes for employees. They conclude the chapter with a number of future research directions related to age and workplace cyberbullying.

The final context in which cyberbullying is viewed in this volume is the context of romantic relationships. Chapter 9 (Cyberbullying in Romantic Relationships: A Review of US Research) by Penny Leisring begins with a look at different forms of cyber abuse in romantic relationships, namely emotional/psychological abuse, intrusion/monitoring behaviors, exclusionary acts, and sexual coercion. Dr. Leisring then examines correlates of cyber abuse for both victims and perpetrators, noting the relationship of many of these correlates to those that accompany traditional partner abuse. She concludes her chapter with suggestions for individuals, parents, and clinicians, and provides suggestions for cyber abuse prevention programs. As with the other lenses through which cyberbullying can be examined, cyber abuse in dating relationships can also be examined cross-culturally, which Esther Calvete, Manuel Gámez-Guadix, and Erika Borrajo do in Chapter 10 (Cyberbullying in Romantic Relationships—Cross-Cultural Issues). In their discussion of cyber abuse in romantic relationships (CARR), Calvete and colleagues highlight the measurement issues that have plagued not only the field of cyberbullying in general, but the study of CARR more specifically. After examining a multitude of measures that have been used across studies to examine CARR, Calvete et al. identified five common modalities that they describe in their chapter—direct verbal aggression, control/monitoring, relational abuse, excessive communication, and cyber sexual abuse. They also discuss the varying prevalence estimates of CARR, which, they note, likely stem from the myriad instruments used to measure the construct. Following an examination of the reciprocal relationship between cyber abuse victimization and perpetration and cultural influences on this relationship, Calvete et al. conclude the chapter with recommendations for individuals and practitioners. The final chapter viewing cyberbullying in the context of romantic relationships is Chapter 11 (Cyberbullying in Romantic Relationships—Developmental Perspectives) by Diana Bennett and Michelle Ramos. Using the term Electronic Dating Aggression (EDA), Bennett and Ramos examine the prevalence rates and correlates of EDA in adolescence and emerging adulthood. They include in their chapter a discussion of the transitions that accompany these developmental stages, and the use of electronic media to accomplish developmental tasks such as the development of identity, autonomy, and romantic relationships.

We conclude the book in Chapter 12 with a look at common themes that emerge across the different cyberbullying lenses. We also discuss the similarities and differences in the research findings across contexts, age groups, and cultures. Then, we outline a series of future research directions related to cyberbullying in schools, in the workplace, and in romantic relationships.

References

Arslan, S., Savaser, S., Hallett, V., & Balci, S. (2012). Cyberbullying among primary school students in Turkey: Self-reported prevalence and associations with home and school life. *Cyberpsychology, Behavior, and Social Networking*, 15(10), 527–533. doi:10.1089/cyber.2012.0207

Baruch, Y. (2005). Bullying on the net: Adverse behavior on e-mail and its impact. *Information & Management*, 42(2), 361–371. doi:10.1016/j.im.2004.02.001

Bennett, D. C., Guran, E. L., Ramos, M. C., & Margolin, G. (2011). College students' electronic victimization in friendships and dating relationships: Anticipated distress and associations with risky behaviors. *Violence and Victims*, 26(4), 410–429.

Beran, T. N., Rinaldi, C., Bickham, D. S., & Rich, M. (2012). Evidence for the need to support adolescents dealing with harassment and cyber-harassment: Prevalence, progression, and impact. *School Psychology International*, 33(5), 562–576. doi:10.1177/0143034312446976

Bonanno, R. A., & Hymel, S. (2013). Cyber bullying and internalizing difficulties: Above and beyond the impact of traditional forms of bullying. *Journal of Youth and Adolescence, 42*(5), 685–697. doi:10.1007/s10964-013-9937-1

Brochado, S., Soares, S., & Fraga, S. (2017). A scoping review on studies of cyberbullying: Prevalence among adolescents. *Trauma, Violence, and Abuse, 18*, 523–531. doi:10.1177/1524838016641668

Cassidy, W., Faucher, C., & Jackson, M. (2013). Cyberbullying among youth: A comprehensive review of current international research and its implications and application to policy and practice. *School Psychology International, 34*, 575–612. doi:10.1177/0143034313479697

Çelik, S., Atak, H., & Erguzen, A. (2012). The effect of personality on cyberbullying among university students in Turkey. *Eurasian Journal of Educational Research, 49*, 129–150.

Chapell, M. S., Hasselman, S. L., Kitchin, T., Lomon, S. N., MacIver, K. W., & Sarullo, P. L. (2006). Bullying in elementary school, high school, and college. *Adolescence, 41* (164), 633–648.

Coyne, I., Farley, S., Axtell, C., Sprigg, C., Best, L., & Kwok, O. (2017). Understanding the relationship between experiencing workplace cyberbullying, employee mental strain and job satisfaction: A dysempowerment approach. *The International Journal of Human Resource Management, 28*, 945–972. doi:10.1080/09585192.2015.1116454

DePaolis, K., & Williford, A. (2014). The nature and prevalence of cyber victimization among elementary school children. *Child & Youth Care Forum, 44*(3), 377–393. doi:10.1007/s10566-014-9292-8

Didden, R., Scholte, R. H. J., Korzilius, H., de Moor, J. M. H., Vermeulen, A., O'Reilly, M., … Lancioni, G. E. (2009). Cyberbullying among students with intellectual and developmental disability in special education settings. *Developmental Neurorehabilitation, 12*, 146–151. doi:10.1080/17518420902971356

Dooley, J. J., Pyzalski, J., & Cross, D. (2009). Cyberbullying versus face-to-face bullying: A theoretical and conceptual review. *Zeitschrift für Psychologie/Journal of Psychology, 217*, 182–188. doi:10.1027/0044–3409.217.4.182

Einarsen, S. (2000). Harassment and bullying at work: A review of the Scandinavian approach. *Aggression and Violent Behavior, 4*, 371–401.

Englander, E. (2012, November 12). Cyberbullying among 11,700 elementary school students. Paper presented at the annual meeting of the International Bullying Prevention Association, Kansas City, MO.

Farley, S., Coyne, I., Axtell, C. & Sprigg, C. (2016): Design, development and validation of a workplace cyberbullying measure, the WCM. *Work & Stress, 30*, 293–317. doi:10.1080/02678373.2016.1255998

Ford, D. P. (2013). Virtual harassment: Media characteristics' role in psychological health. *Journal of Managerial Psychology, 28*(4), 408–428. doi:10.1108/JMP-12-2012-0398

Francisco, S. M., Simao, A. M. V., Ferreira, P. C., & Martins, M. J. (2015). Cyberbullying: The hidden side of college students. *Computers in Human Behavior, 43*, 167–182. http://dx.doi.org/10.1016/j.chb.2014.10.045

Gardella, J. H., Fisher, B. W., & Teurbe-Tolon, A. R. (2017). A systematic review and meta-analysis of cyber-victimization and educational outcomes for adolescents. *Review of Educational Research, 87*, 283–308. doi:10.3102/0034654316689136

Gardner, D., O'Driscoll, M., Cooper-Thomas, H. D., Roche, M., Bentley, T., Catley, B., … Trenberth, L. (2016). Predictors of workplace bullying and cyberbullying in New Zealand. *International Journal of Environmental Research and Public Health, 13*. doi:10.3390/ijerph13050448

Giumetti, G. W., McKibben, E. S., Hatfield, A. L., Schroeder, A. N., & Kowalski, R. M. (2012). Cyber incivility @ work: The new age of interpersonal deviance. *Cyberpsychology, Behavior, and Social Networking, 15*, 148–154. doi:10.1089/cyber.2011.0336

Görzig, A., Milosevic, T., & Staksrud, E. (2017). Cyberbullying victimization in context: The role of social inequalities in countries and regions. *Journal of Cross-Cultural Psychology, 48*, 1198–1215. doi:10.1177/0022022116686186

Hershcovis, M. S. (2011). Incivility, social undermining, bullying … Oh my! A call to reconcile constructs within workplace aggression research. *Journal of Organizational Behavior, 32*, 499–519. doi:10.1002/job.689

Hinduja, S., & Patchin, J. W. (2010). Bullying, cyberbullying, and suicide. *Archives of Suicide Research, 14*(3), 206–221. doi:10.1080/13811118.2010.494133

Jenaro, C., Flores, N., & Frias, C. P. (2018). Systematic review of empirical studies on cyberbullying in adults: What we know and what we should investigate. *Aggression and Violent Behavior, 38*, 113–122. doi:10.1016/j.avb.2017.12.003

Kowalski, R. M., Giumetti, G. W., Schroeder, A. N., & Lattanner, M. R. (2014). Bullying in the digital age: A critical review and meta-analysis of cyberbullying research among youth. *Psychological Bulletin, 140*(4), 1073–1137. doi:10.1037/a0035618

Kowalski, R. M., & Limber, S. P. (2007). Electronic bullying among middle school students. *Journal of Adolescent Health, 41*(6, Suppl), S22–S30. doi:10.1016/j.jadohealth.2007.08. 017

Kowalski, R. M., & Limber, S. P. (2013). Psychological, physical, and academic correlates of cyberbullying and traditional bullying. *Journal of Adolescent Health, 53*, S13–S20. doi:10.1016/j.jadohealth.2012.09doi:018

Kowalski, R. M., Limber, S. E., & Agatston, P. W. (2012). *Cyberbullying: Bullying in the digital age* (2nd ed.). Malden, MA: Wiley-Blackwell.

Kowalski, R. M., Morgan, C. A., Drake-Lavelle, K., & Allison, B. (2016). Cyberbullying among college students with disabilities. *Computers in Human Behavior, 57*, 416–427. doi:10.1016/j.chb.2015.12.044

Kowalski, R. M., Toth, A., & Morgan, M. (2018). Bullying and cyberbullying in adulthood and the workplace. *The Journal of Social Psychology, 158*, 64–81. doi:10.1080/00224545.2017.1302402

Leisring, P. A., & Giumetti, G. W. (2014). Sticks and stones may break my bones, but abusive text messages also hurt: Development and validation of the Cyber Psychological Abuse scale. *Partner Abuse, 5*(3), 323–341. doi:10.1891/1946-6560.5. 3. 323

Lim, V. K. G., & Teo, T. S. H. (2009). Mind your E-manners: Impact of cyber incivility on employees' work attitude and behavior. *Information & Management, 46*, 419–425. doi:10.1016/j.im.2009. 06. 006

Livingstone, S., & Haddad, L. (2009). EU Kids Online. *Zeitschrift Für Psychologie/Journal of Psychology, 217*(4), 236.

Lund, E. M., & Ross, S. W. (2017). Bullying perpetration, victimization, and demographic differences in college students: A review of the literature. *Trauma, Violence, and Abuse, 18*, 348–360. doi:10.1177/1524838015620818

Menesini, E., Nocentini, A., Palladino, B. E., Frisén, A., Berne, S., Ortega-Ruiz, R., …. Smith, P. K. (2012). Cyberbullying definition among adolescents: A comparison across six European countries. *Cyberpsychololgy, Behavior, and Social Networking, 15*, 455–463. doi:10.1089/cyber.2012.0040

Mishna, F., Cook, C., Gadalla, T., Daciuk, J., & Solomon, S. (2010). Cyber bullying behaviors among middle and high school students. *American Journal of Orthopsychiatry, 80* (3), 362–374. doi:10.1111/j.1939-0025.2010.01040.x

Modecki, K. L., Minchin, J., Harbaugh, A. G., Guerra, N. G., & Runions, K. C. (2014). Bullying prevalence across contexts: A meta-analysis measuring cyber and traditional bullying. *Journal of Adolescent Health, 55*(5), 602–611. doi:10.1016/j.jadohealth.2014.06.007

Monks, C., Robinson, S., & Worlidge, P. (2012). The emergence of cyberbullying: A survey of primary school pupils' perceptions and experiences. *School Psychology International, 33*(5), 477–491. doi:10.1177/0143034312445242

Monks, C., Worlidge, P., Robinson, S., & Ortega, R. (2009). Cyberbullying among primary school-aged pupils. *Kwartalnik Pedagogiczny, 4*(214), 167–182.

Nocentini, A., Calmaestra, J., Schultze-Krumbholz, A., Scheithauer, H., Ortega, R., & Menesini, E. (2010). Cyberbullying: Labels, behaviours and definition in three European countries. *Australian Journal of Guidance and Counseling, 20*, 129–142. doi:10.1375/ajgc.20. 2. 129

Olweus, D. (1993). *Bullying at school: What we know and what we can do*. New York: Blackwell.

Olweus, D. (2013). School bullying: Development and some important challenges. *Annual Review of Clinical Psychology, 9*, 1–14. doi:10.1146/annurev-clinpsy-050212-185516

Palladino, B. E., Menesini, E., Nocentini, A., Luik, P., Naruskov, K., Ucanok, Z., … Scheithauer, H. (2017). Perceived severity of cyberbullying: Differences and similarities across four countries. *Frontiers in Psychology, 8*, 1–12, doi:10.3389/fpsyg.2017.01524

Privitera, C., & Campbell, M. A. (2009). Cyberbullying: The new face of workplace bullying? *Cyberpsychology & Behavior, 12*(4), 395–400. doi:10.1089/cpb.2009.0025-

Sawyer, A. L., Bradshaw, C. P., & O'Brennan, L. M. (2008). Examining ethnic, gender, and developmental differences in the way children report a victim of "bullying" on self-report measures. *Journal of Adolescent Health, 43*, 106–114. doi:10.1016/j.jadohealth.2007.12.011

Selkie, E. M., Kota, R., Chan, Y.-F., & Moreno, M. (2015). Cyberbullying, depression, and problem alcohol use in female college students: A multisite study. *Cyberpsychology, Behavior, and Social Networking, 18*(2), 79–86. doi:10.1089/cyber.2014.0371

Selkie, E. M., Kota, R., & Moreno, M. (2016). Cyberbullying behaviors among female college students: Witnessing, perpetration, and victimization. *College Student Journal, 50*, 278–287.

Slonje, R., & Smith, P. K. (2008). Cyberbullying: Another main type of bullying? *Scandinavian Journal of Psychology, 49*, 147–154. doi:10.1111/j.1467–9450.2007.00611.x

Slonje, R., Smith, P. K., & Frisén, A. (2013). The nature of cyberbullying, and strategies for prevention. *Computers in Human Behavior, 29*, 26–32.

Smith, P. K., Mahdavi, J., Carvalho, M., Fisher, S., Russell, S., & Tippett, N. (2008). Cyberbullying: Its nature and impact in secondary school pupils. *Journal of Child Psychology and Psychiatry, 49*(4), 376–385. doi:10.1111/j.1469-7610.2007.01846.x

Snyman, R., & Loh, J. M. (2015). Cyberbullying at work: The mediating role of optimism between cyberbullying and job outcomes. *Computers in Human Behavior, 53*, 161–168. doi:10.1016/j.chb.2015.06.050

Staude-Müller, F., Hansen, B., & Voss, M. (2012). How stressful is online victimization? Effects of victim's personality and properties of the incident. *European Journal of Developmental Psychology, 9*(2), 260–274. doi:10.1080/17405629.2011.643170

Tsitsika, A., Janikian, M., Wójcik, S., Makaruk, K., Tzavela, E., Tzavara, C., & … Richardson, C. (2015). Cyberbullying victimization prevalence and associations with internalizing and externalizing problems among adolescents in six European countries. *Computers in Human Behavior, 51*(Pt A), 1–7. doi:10.1016/j.chb.2015. 04. 048

Vranjes, I., Baillien, E., Vandebosch, H., Erreygers, S., & DeWitte, H. (2017). The dark side of working online: Towards a definition and an emotion-reaction model of workplace cyberbullying. *Computers in Human Behavior, 69*, 324–334. doi:10.1016/j.chb.2016.12.055

Watts, L. K., Wagner, J., Velasquez, B., & Behrens, P. I. (2017). Cyberbullying in higher education: A literature review. *Computers in Human Behavior, 69*, 268–274. doi:10.1016/j.chb.2016.12.038

Weatherbee, T., & Kelloway, E. (2006). A case of cyberdeviancy: Cyberaggression in the workplace. In E. K. Kelloway, J. Barling, & J. Hurrell (Eds.), *Handbook of workplace violence* (pp. 445–488). Thousand Oaks, CA: Sage.

Zweig, J. M., Lachman, P., Yahner, J., & Dank, M. (2014). Correlates of cyber dating abuse among teens. *Journal of Youth and Adolescence, 43*(8), 1306–1321. doi:10.1007/s10964-013-0047-x

2

DIFFERENCES IN TECHNOLOGY USE AMONG DEMOGRAPHIC GROUPS

Implications for Cyberbullying Research

Robin M. Kowalski, Gary W. Giumetti, and Hayden Cox

In June, 2017, Michelle Carter was convicted of involuntary manslaughter in the 2016 suicide of her boyfriend, Conrad Roy III. While readers unfamiliar with the case may think involuntary manslaughter and suicide seem paradoxical, the case hinged on hundreds of text messages that Michelle Carter sent her boyfriend, who suffered from depression, encouraging him to bring to fruition his claims that he was ready to take his own life. While the case is troubling on many levels, it highlights several things that would not have been at issue just a few decades ago. First, the medium upon which the case hinged involved the use of Information and Communication Technologies (or ICTs). Second, Michelle Carter was 17 at the time, highlighting not only the use of texting by individuals within this age bracket but also raising the issue of whether younger or older individuals would have engaged in similar behavior using the same electronic means. Third, the case raises the question of whether Carter's behavior constitutes cyberbullying.

In the current chapter, we take a look at the prevalence rates of ICT use among different demographic groups. In particular, we explore age, gender, and racial/ethnic differences in technology use. After examining these differences, we look at the literature on cyberbullying and summarize evidence related to demographic differences in cyberbullying. We end the chapter by proposing a few possible directions for future research.

Introduction to ICTs

The use of technology has become a central element in our culture in the last few decades. In particular, mobile phones, tablets, computers, and other forms of electronic communication have become increasingly common throughout society. In the 2017 report published by the Center for the Digital Future at the USC Annenberg School, 92% of Americans reported that they were Internet users, with an average 23.6 hours a week spent online (Center for the Digital Future at USC Annenberg, 2017). While ICTs seem commonplace today, it was not too long ago that these items and their capabilities were little more than dreams within the mind of great innovators. Now, these devices and their ability to share information and communication have paved the way for a variety of new facets in both industry and social life. ICTs are commonly operated by nearly every age group, from small children playing tablet games in their mother's laps to older adults in retirement homes using Facebook and email to connect with their grandchildren.

Depending on their age, people use ICTs for a variety of reasons. Children use tablets to watch videos and play online games (Englander, 2012). Teens often use smartphones to access social media so they can establish and maintain friendships and relationships (Lenhart, 2015). Among adults, common uses of ICTs include "getting directions, recommendations, or other information related to one's location" (71%), "listening to an online radio or music service, such as Pandora or Spotify" (54%), and "buying a product online, such as books, music, toys, or clothing" (48%) (Pew Research Center, 2015a). The use of the Internet at work by employed adults is also becoming more ubiquitous (Purcell & Rainie, 2014). In addition, adults are increasingly using ICTs to establish relationships via online dating sites. Not surprisingly, younger adults are more likely to use ICTs for dating purposes than older adults.

Clearly, there are many beneficial reasons why people use ICTs. However, ICTs are also the vehicle by which cyberbullying occurs (Kowalski, Limber, & Agatston, 2012). As noted by Kowalski, Giumetti, Schroeder, and Lattanner (2014, p. 2), "certain features of online communications, including reproducibility, lack of emotional reactivity, perceived uncontrollability, relative permanence, and 24/7 accessibility, make it more likely for online misbehavior to occur." Which form of electronic communication is used to perpetrate cyberbullying depends on the most common form of technology in vogue at a particular time and among a particular demographic group (Juvonen & Gross, 2008; Katzer, Fetchenhauer, & Belschak, 2009; Kowalski et al., 2014; Kowalski & Limber, 2007). Whereas online gaming is the most popular activity among elementary school children (Englander, 2012), social media assumes an increasingly important role among middle and high school students as well as college students (Kowalski et al., 2012). In the workplace, email and social media predominate as vehicles for electronic communication (Purcell & Rainie, 2014). Whereas the majority of the research on cyberbullying has focused on middle school aged youth, more recent research has demonstrated that cyberbullying is not limited to individuals in this age group. Thus, it is important to understand the use of ICTs across different demographic groups to provide a context for understanding when and how cyberbullying is likely to occur. In the next section, we examine the use of ICTs across different demographic groups, with a particular focus on age. A portion of the data included in this chapter are drawn from the Pew Institute.

Elementary School Aged Youth and Technology

A recent campaign called "Wait Until 8th" encourages parents to hold off getting children a smartphone until they are in at least the 8th grade ("Wait Until 8th", 2017). In keeping with this, many parents say that they limit their young children's access to technology and that they would not allow their children to have access to a smartphone until they are a teenager. However, they readily provide them with an iPad and access to "kid-friendly" social media sites, such as Disney's Club Penguin Island. Indeed, technology use among elementary school aged youth is widespread. In a study by Pearson (2015), 66% of elementary school students said that they *used* a laptop, 53% a smartphone, and 78% a tablet. Thirty-five percent said they *owned* a laptop, 36% a smartphone, and 69% a tablet (Pearson, 2015). Importantly, use was not dictated by provision of said technology by the school attended as only 19% of students in elementary, middle, and high school indicated that their school provided a laptop or tablet to each student to use. A survey of parents with children under the age of 6 found that 53% allow their child to use a tablet, 42% a smartphone, and 32% a computer (Erikson Institute, 2016). Notably, however, 84% of these parents indicated that either they or another adult in the home used the technology with the child, with 35% indicating that they spend 30 to 60 minutes a day in this endeavor. Only 6% of parents stated that they did not spend time jointly involved in technological endeavors with their young child. In the report by the Center for the Digital Future (Center for the Digital Future at USC Annenberg, 2017), 65% of parents reported that they monitor the activities of their children on social networking sites. Among those who indicated that they did not monitor their child's activity, the reasons included trusting their child (35%), not wanting to show lack of trust (12%), and lack of time (10%). This collaboration between parent and child will be important in examining statistics, particularly those related to cyberbullying, across age demographics in the coming years. As parents become more digitally savvy and more in-tune with both the costs and benefits associated with online activity, will young children develop more online civility than has been characteristic of many youth in recent years?

Table 2.1 includes, among other statistics, data obtained in the United Kingdom looking at the use of technology among elementary and middle school aged youth. Two things are noteworthy. First, whereas the remainder of the data discussed in this chapter are based on American samples, the data about these children, as noted, are from another country. Second, the fact that we are using data from the United Kingdom highlights the paucity of data within the United States on technology use among young children. The data in Table 2.1 support research showing a preponderance of technology use among teenagers and young adults. However, the data in the table also indicate that the use of ICTs is not age specific. Although the specific type of technology most often used may vary by age, the use of technology is clearly a womb to tomb phenomenon.

TABLE 2.1 Technology Use Across Age Groups

	Age Groupings								
	3–4	*5–7*	*8–11*	*13–14*	*15–17*	*18–29*	*30–49*	*50–64*	*65+*
Smartphone	0	2	32	68	76	92	88	74	42
Tablet	55	67	80	61	56	50	57	37	32
Online gaming	25	52	74	80	81	67	58	40	25
Facebook	___	___	55	57	80	88	84	72	62
Instagram	___	___	43	44	58	59	33	18	8
Twitter	___	___	8	21	42	36	23	21	10

Note: Numbers reflect percentages. Data included in the table were obtained from the following sources: Anderson (2015); Anderson and Perrin (2017); Erikson Institute (2016); Lenhart (2015); Ofcom (2016); Pearson (2015). In order to reflect the most comprehensive age coverage based on survey data collected across studies, age 12 was omitted.

Teens and Technology

Referred to as the "always on" generation, teens appear to be forever tethered to their technology (Belsey, 2017). Given the pervasive use of technology among elementary school aged youth, the continued and increased use of technology among teens is hardly surprising. Whereas a generation ago, teenagers, like most other age groups, would mostly engage with their peers in face-to-face conversations (Gray, 2013), now it seems as if these face-to-face conversations have largely been replaced by ICTs. In the section that follows, we explore not only the use of various ICTs by teens, but, more specifically, how the use of these ICTs among teens varies by age, gender, and race/ethnicity. Among teens, these demographic variables will be discussed in terms of the type of technology used.

Mobile Phones/Smartphones

Key among the ICTs used by teens are mobile phones. Among teenagers 13 to 17, 88% own a mobile phone of some sort (e.g., smart phone, flip phone). This is particularly surprising given that, according to the National Center for Children in Poverty, 44% of children under 18 live in low-income households, 21% of these are in poor households (Jiang, Ekono, & Skinner, 2016). Considering the high percentage of teens that either own or have access to a mobile phone of some type, it is not surprising to see so many teens communicating with their peers through call, text, and other mobile phone applications (Lenhart, 2015).

Smartphone use among teens, however, varies with age and race. Unsurprisingly, smartphone prevalence increases with age, as 90% of 17-year-old teens own or have access to a smartphone compared to only 69% of 13-year-old teens

(Lenhart, 2015). This makes sense, as it is likely that, the older a child becomes, the more likely parents are to trust their child with greater responsibilities.

Regarding racial differences, Black/African American teens (85%) are more likely to own or have access to a smartphone than white (71%) or Hispanic (71%) youth (Lenhart, 2015). This is particularly interesting when you consider the income distribution of all three races. According to the 2016 census data, considering the three racial groups, "Black," "Hispanic," and "White," those who identified as black had the lowest income. Respondents who identified as black reported a median income of $37,211 compared to a Hispanic median income of $45,148 and a White median income of $62,950 (Proctor, Semega, & Kollar, 2016). Considering the expense of purchasing and owning mobile phones (e.g., call, text, and data plans), the importance of mobile phones to teens (even those from lower income brackets) becomes clear.

There are many possible explanations for the racial differences observed in mobile phone ownership among teens. One could be that the ownership of cell phones among teenagers is seen as more acceptable in the Black/African American community. Another could be the makeup of said households. Of the three racial groups described, Blacks/African Americans are less likely to grow up in a home owned by two married parents (34%), compared to Hispanics (60%) and Whites (74%) (US Census, 2015). Because phones are a common form of communication, they may serve as a tool for single parents to stay in closer contact with their children. Uses of technology, such as maintaining communication with parents, will be important to keep in mind later in the chapter when we discuss race and cyberbullying involvement.

Desktops/Laptops/Gaming Consoles/Tablets

However, the use of technology by teens is not limited to smartphones. Eighty-seven percent of teens report access to a desktop or laptop computer, 81% a gaming console, and 58% a tablet. As with mobile phones, variations in use of these forms of technology by teens exist by race, age, and gender. Whereas Black/African American teens are more likely to own smartphones than White or Hispanic teens, they are less likely to own other forms of technology. White teens report having more access to desktops or laptops (91%) than Hispanic teens (82%) or Black/African American teens (79%). Similar percentages had access to gaming consoles, with White teens (85%) reporting similar access to Black/African American teens (84%), but greater access than Hispanic teens (71%) (Lenhart, 2015).

As for age, not surprisingly, older teens (90%) report having greater access to laptops than younger teens (84%). However, there were few age differences in access to game consoles, as younger teens (80%) reported similar levels of access to older teens (81%) (Lenhart, 2015). This is not surprising given the high prevalence of online gaming among elementary school aged youth. Regarding gender, there was little difference between teen boys (87%) and girls (88%) with availability to desktops/laptops; however, more males (91%) than females (70%) owned or had access to a gaming console (Lenhart, 2015).

Social Media

Whether via mobile phones, laptops, or another form of technology, 92% of teenagers between the ages of 13 to 17 report going online almost daily, with a significant portion (24%) reporting that they are online "almost constantly" (Lenhart, 2015). With this information, the widespread presence of teens on social media is not surprising. Seventy-one percent of teenagers indicated having profiles on multiple social media platforms, with the most popular being Facebook (71%), Instagram (52%), and Snapchat (41%) (Lenhart, 2015). Approximately equal numbers of males (72%) and females (70%) use Facebook. However, girls are significantly more likely to use Instagram (61% vs. 44%) and Snapchat (51% vs. 31%) than boys (Lenhart, 2015). The average teen reports having 145 friends on Facebook, 150 followers on Instagram, and 95 followers on Twitter (Lenhart, 2015).

Older teens (aged 15–17) seem to have a larger presence on social media than younger teens (aged 13–14). This is true of Facebook (80% vs. 57%), Instagram (58% vs. 44%), Snapchat (47% vs. 31%), Twitter (42% vs. 21%), and Tumblr (16% vs. 10%) (Lenhart, 2015). This is not all that surprising as older teens (81%) are significantly more likely to use social media on their cellphones than younger teens (68%) (Lenhart, 2015). Importantly, particularly for possible cyberbullying victimization, 10% of 13- to 14-year-old youth and 12% of 15- to 17-year-olds report subscribing to anonymous messaging apps, such as Whisper and Ask.FM (Lenhart, 2015).

Many teens acquire technology, such as smartphones, as a means for their parents to track or keep in touch with them, particularly once the teens reach driving age. Many parents report using cell phones if they need to contact their children quickly (Lenhart, 2015). Texting, calling, emailing, and messaging on social media make up 92% of responses for how parents get in touch with their child quickly, with texting being the most common (48%) followed by calling (41%) (Lenhart, 2015). Teens aged 15–17 (52%) are significantly more likely to receive a text message from parents who want to reach them quickly than teens aged 13–14 (43%) (Lenhart, 2015); however, younger teens are slightly although not significantly more likely to receive a phone call (43%) from parents than older teens (40%). There are slight gender differences here as well. Girls (51%) are more likely to receive texts in this situation than boys (46%). However, parents are more likely to call boys (43%) than girls (39%) (Lenhart, 2015).

Adults and Technology

Unlike the previous age groups discussed, adulthood represents a wide expanse of time that encompasses a great deal of life change and experience. Whereas individuals who are 18 years old are considered adults, the experiences and comfort level of an 18-year-old with technology are likely to be different from those of an 80-year-old. Survey reports not only support this contention but also highlight that an examination of technology use in adulthood must take into account particular phases of adulthood.

Ninety-five percent of all adults in the US report that they own a mobile phone of some sort, with 77% indicating that the phone is a smartphone (Pew Research Center, 2017). Researchers at the Pew Center note, however, that "reliance on smartphones for online access is especially common among younger adults, non-whites, and lower-income Americans" (Pew Research Center, 2017; see also Center for the Digital Future at USC Annenberg, 2017). As would be expected, younger adults are more likely to report having both a mobile phone and a mobile phone that is a smartphone than older adults. Among young adults age 18 to 29, 100% own a mobile phone, with 92% owning a smartphone. Percentages of mobile/smart phone ownership among older age groups are as follows: 30–49-year-olds (99%/88%), 50–64-year-olds (97%/74%), 65+ (80%/42%) (Pew Research Center, 2017). Similar data are observed with other forms of technology. In 2016, 51% of all adults used tablets, compared to only 32% of senior adults 65 and older (Anderson & Perrin, 2017). During that same year, 69% of all adults accessed social media, compared to only 34% of senior adults. While this relative difference is important, perhaps even more notable is the rapid increase in technology use and access among adults in recent years. In 2008, for example, only 21% of adults and 2% of senior adults accessed social media. In 2011, only 35% of adults and 11% of senior adults used smartphones (Anderson & Perrin, 2017). Furthermore, among older adults, younger older adults are more likely to both use and be comfortable with technology (see Table 2.2). In their survey of over 3000 senior adults, Anderson and Perrin (2017) found that, whereas 59% of adults 66 to 69 owned a smartphone, only 17% of those 80 and over did so. Part of this difference is a comfort level with technology. In response to the statement "When I get a new electronic device, I usually need someone else to set it up or show me how to use it," 6% of individuals 18 to 29 stated that the statement described them very well compared to 48% of senior adults 65 and older.

As shown in Table 2.1, use of social media also varies among adults with, not surprisingly, younger adults using social media more often than older adults. Importantly, however, the relative patterns of use across social media platforms are similar across age demographics. Specifically, for all adult groups, Facebook is the most common social media platform used, followed by Instagram and Twitter (Greenwood, Perrin, & Duggan, 2016). Additionally, and with potential implications for cyberbullying involvement, younger adults (10%) are more likely than older adults age 50 and over (<1%) to use messaging apps on which they can chat or post anonymously. Examples would include the now defunct Yik Yak and Whisper (Greenwood et al., 2016). Later in the chapter, we will discuss the link between anonymity and online harassment and cyberbullying.

TABLE 2.2 Technology Use Among Senior Adults

	Age Groupings			
	65–69	*70–74*	*75–79*	*80+*
Smartphone	59	49	31	17
Tablet	41	32	28	20
Internet use	82	75	60	44
Social media use	47	41	24	17

Note: Numbers reflect percentages. Data included in the table were obtained from Anderson and Perrin (2017).

Among adults, race/ethnicity and income also influence access. According to the Pew Center (Pew Research Center, 2017), differences in technology usage by race/ethnicity are relatively small, as adult Hispanic Americans report similar levels of owning a mobile phone (98%) and a smartphone (75%) as compared to White (94%/77%) or Black/African American (94%/72%) adult respondents. Reliance on solely a smartphone for online access is higher among individuals earning less than $30,000 annually (21%) compared to those earning more than $75,000 (5%).

The Workplace

Not surprisingly given the amount of time that most adults spend at work, technology plays a key role in the workplace. In the Digital Future Project report (2017), workers reported spending an average of 14.3 hours a week using the Internet at work. In a survey of 1,066 Internet users conducted by Purcell and Rainie (2014) at the Pew Center, 53% reported being employed full- or part-time in occupations that were classified as either office-based ("white-collar") or non office-based ("blue-collar"). Among these workers, 61% indicated that email was very important to their job activities and 54% reported that the Internet was very important to performance of their job activities. Few, however, reported the utility of social networking sites such as Facebook for job-related activities. Females (55%) were about as likely to consider the internet as very important to their job than males (54%) and non-White participants (60%) were more likely to say the same thing than White participants (52%) (Purcell & Rainie, 2014).

Purcell and Rainie (2014) found both positive and negative outcomes associated with technology use in the workplace. On the negative side, 35% of workers found that technology, including the Internet, email, and cellular phones, had increased the amount of time they spent working. Importantly, however, this was more true for workers in office-based as opposed to non office-based occupations. On the positive side, 46% of workers stated that the Internet had made them more productive at work. In fact, for only 7% had the Internet made them less productive at work (Purcell & Rainie, 2014; see also Center for the Digital Future at USC Annenberg, 2017).

With possible implications for cyberbullying and cyber incivility at work, 46% of workers indicated that their employer blocked employee access to certain websites, with an identical percentage reporting that their employer regulated what employees were allowed to post or communicate online. Eighteen percent were unsure whether their employer blocked access to particular sites, and 27% were unsure whether their company had rules regarding what employees were allowed to communicate online. These percentages of uncertainty were higher among non office-based workers (Purcell & Rainie, 2014).

ICTs and Cyberbullying

Research has consistently shown that time spent online is correlated with cyberbullying involvement (Kowalski et al., 2014). Thus, based on the pattern of usage reported thus far in this chapter, one should be able to predict cyberbullying involvement across varying age, race, and gender demographics. Whereas that is true to a degree, the predictions are not as clean as one might think. One reason for this is that, even within a given demographic, wide variability exists in reported prevalence rates due to, among other things, varying definitions of cyberbullying, the sample used, the time parameter used to determine when the cyberbullying occurred (1 month, 2 months, 6 months, lifetime), and the conservative (2 to 3 times a month or more) versus liberal (at least once) criterion used to determine whether cyberbullying occurred (Olweus, 2013). Nevertheless, there do appear to be some general trends in cyberbullying involvement related to the use of ICTs. Across age groups, as reported in the 2017 Digital Future Project report, 14% of respondents said they had been bullied or harassed online (14% of men; 13% of women). Not surprisingly, younger as opposed to older individuals were more likely to report online harassment and bullying with 27% of respondents under 18 stating they had been bullied or harassed online compared to only 6% of those 55 and older. Over 30% indicated that they knew someone who had been bullied or harassed online (31% men; 36% women). Once again, more younger individuals reported knowing someone who had been cyberbullied (58% of those younger than 18 compared to 16% of those 55 and over) (Center for the Digital Future at USC Annenberg 2017).

Few studies have been conducted examining cyberbullying as it occurs among elementary school aged children (for reviews, see Chapter 5, this volume; and, Kowalski & Giumetti, 2016). Englander (2012) found that very young children were more likely to be cyberbullied via online gaming because that was the online activity in which they most often engaged. In terms of prevalence, Arslan, Savaser, Hallet, and Balci (2012) examined a sample of Turkish children ages 8–11 and found that 27.4% reported experiencing cyberbullying victimization, whereas 17.5% reported engaging in cyberbullying perpetration. DePaolis and Williford (2018) reported a much lower prevalence rate. Specifically, they found that 9 to 15% of a sample of 660 elementary school students in the Midwestern US experienced cyberbullying victimization. With regard to possible correlates of cyberbullying involvement among elementary school aged children, DePaolis and Williford (2018) reported that children who experienced initial levels of cyberbullying victimization were more likely to have lower self-esteem and school connection a year later. Additionally, Arslan et al. (2012) reported that cyberbullying involvement (as either a bully or a victim) was linked with lower school satisfaction and achievement.

More data are available regarding cyberbullying victimization and perpetration among teens. However, as noted above, these statistics are highly variable. Kowalski and Limber (2007) found, for example, that 18% of over 3000 middle school youth had been cyberbully victims and 11% had been cyberbully perpetrators at least once within the previous two months. A large-scale study of Canadian youth found that 9.1% experienced cyberbullying victimization (Kim, Colwell, Kata, Boyle, & Georgiades, 2018). A study of more than 10,000 adolescents across six European countries found that 21.4% of the adolescents experienced cyber victimization during the previous 12 months (Tsitsika et al., 2015). Another study of over 1,000 adolescents in Belgium found that 32% of LGBQ youth experienced cyber victimization as compared to 26% of non-LGBQ youth (DeSmet et al., 2018). Across studies, prevalence estimates typically range between 10 and 40% (e.g., Kowalski et al., 2014; Lenhart, 2015; O'Brennan, Bradshaw, & Sawyer, 2009). For example, a meta-analysis of studies focusing on adolescent samples reported that, on average across studies, the prevalence rate for cyberbullying victimization was 15.5% and the prevalence rate for cyberbullying perpetration was 15.2% (Modecki, Minchin, Harbaugh, Guerra, & Runions, 2014).

Among youth, sex differences in cyberbullying victimization have been widely debated in the literature. Some researchers have suggested that females are more likely to be both victims and perpetrators of cyberbullying than males (Connell, Schell-Busey, Pearce, & Negro, 2014; Kowalski & Limber, 2007). Others have found no sex differences in either cyberbullying victimization or perpetration (e.g., Robson & Witenberg, 2013). Still others have observed that females are more likely to be cyberbullying victims (e.g., Beckman, Hagquist, & Hellström, 2013; Kim et al., 2018; Kowalski, Morgan, & Limber, 2012) whereas males are more likely to perpetrate cyberbullying (e.g., Coelho, Sousa, Marchante, Brás, & Romão, 2016; Shapka, Onditi, Collie, & Lapidot-Lefler, 2018; Topcu & Erdur-Baker, 2012). Yet others have suggested that observed differences are a function of the type of technology being investigated with males perpetrating cyberbullying more via multi-player online games (Ballard & Welch, 2017) and females more via chat messaging (Lee & Shin, 2017). Again, looking at patterns of technology use by sex, such as highlighted in the Pew report, helps to elucidate the different patterns of victimization and perpetration by sex that are observed. Even for a given age, the fact that males and females are differentially active on various social media platforms, all of which may make them more vulnerable to cyberbullying victimization, may negate any sex differences that might actually exist.

Patterns of usage of ICTs by age and race also help to elucidate cyberbullying patterns among these same demographics. While the prevalence of cyberbullying among middle school students has been noted, even within this age demographic, age variations are observed, with rates of cyberbullying increasing across middle school grades (Williams & Guerra, 2007). With the understanding that objective prevalence rates ignore differences by age in the venue by which cyberbullying occurs (Smith et al., 2008), research has also indicated that over 30% of college students reported that their initial experience with cyberbullying was during college (Kowalski, Giumetti, Schroeder, & Reese, 2012). In the same study, 43% of college students stated that the majority of the cyberbullying that they experienced occurred in college.

Few studies have examined race as it relates to cyberbullying victimization and perpetration. In addition, in some of these studies the contributions of race to cyberbullying involvement have been difficult to extricate from those of culture and geographical setting (i.e., rural/urban) (Price, Chin, Higa-McMillan, Kim, & Frueh, 2013). One study found that White students were more likely than African American middle school students to report being victims of cyberbullying (Rice et al., 2015). Hinduja and Patchin (2008), on the other hand, found no significant differences by race in cyberbullying victimization or perpetration. Again, the patterns of cyberbullying involvement by race are interesting when examined in the context of technology use. For example, African American teens are more likely to own or have access to smartphones than White or Hispanic teens (Lenhart, 2015). However, they are less likely to be involved in cyberbullying. While there is not a 1:1 correspondence between technology use and cyberbullying involvement, this relationship highlights the need to look further and examine the specific uses of ICTs across different demographic groups.

While the term cyberbullying is often not used with adult samples, other terms reflective of similar types of behavior are used instead, including online harassment and cyber incivility. Regardless of the terminology used, adults are not immune from negative experiences online. In a survey of over 3,600 adults, Kowalski and colleagues found that a fifth (20%) reported having experienced the majority of their cyberbullying victimization during adulthood; 30% of these respondents had been bullied in the workplace at least once (Kowalski, Toth, & Morgan, 2018). A 2017 survey by the Pew Center on online harassment found that 41% of 4,248 American adults surveyed reported having experienced harassment online (Duggan, 2017). Another 66% said they witnessed such behavior online. The online behavior reported took a variety of forms, some more severe than others including offensive name-calling (27%), purposeful embarrassment (22%), physical threats (10%), ongoing harassment (7%), stalking (7%), and sexual harassment (6%).

Reports of the experience of online harassment varied with age, race/ethnicity, and sex (Duggan, 2017). Not surprisingly, the largest percentage of individuals reporting having experienced online harassment were younger adults, ranging in age from 18 to 29. Sixty-seven percent of respondents in this age range indicated that they had experienced harassment online, with 41% saying that the harassment was severe. Forty-nine percent of respondents aged 30 to 49 had experienced online harassment followed by 22% of respondents age 50 and older. Importantly, all of these statistics represent increases from a similar survey conducted by the Pew Center in 2014.

With regard to race/ethnicity differences in online harassment among adults, 59% of Black/African Americans, 41% of White Americans, and 48% of Hispanics reported that they had been harassed online. Eighty-two percent of Black/African Americans, 71% of White Americans, and 71% of Hispanics reported having witnessed online harassment. Among Black/African Americans, a quarter reported that they had been harassed online because of their race/ethnicity, compared to 3% of Whites and 10% of Hispanics. The Pew report highlighted that online harassment for physical or personal characteristics other than race/ethnicity was common, including politics (14%), physical appearance (9%), gender (8%), and sexual orientation (3%) (Duggan, 2017).

Contrary to some studies on cyberbullying among youth (e.g., Kowalski & Limber, 2007), the Pew findings from an adult sample indicate that women (37%) reported experiencing online harassment less frequently than men (44%). Importantly, the form that the harassment took varied between men and women. Whereas men were more likely than women to be called offensive names or to be physically threatened online, women, particularly in the 18 to 29 year age range, were more likely to report having been sexually harassed including receiving uninvited sexts (that is, text messages that are sexual in nature; Duggan, 2017).

Additionally, similar to youth, many adults reported being harassed online by a stranger or not knowing the identity of the perpetrator (54%) (Duggan, 2017). Perhaps in part because of the anonymous nature of the online harassment and the disconcerting feelings stemming from that, it is not surprising that adults would experience negative consequences as a result of being harassed online. These consequences are similar to those experienced by youth victims of cyberbullying. Many experience mental health issues, such as depression and anxiety, some, particularly those who have been threatened online, fear for their personal safety, and others suffer damage to their reputations on- and off-line (Duggan, 2017).

Conclusion

This chapter has reported on the usage of technology across different demographic groups, with a special focus on gender, age, and race/ethnicity. With regard to age, the most common use of technology among children is for online game playing (Englander, 2012), whereas students in middle school through college most often use technology to access social networking sites or communicate with each other via text messaging (Kowalski et al., 2012; Lenhart, 2015). Among adults, the most common uses for technology include texting and emailing (Newport, 2014), and, in the workplace, the most common use of technology is for email and peer-to-peer communication (Purcell & Rainie, 2014). Regarding gender, few studies have examined elementary aged children, but research on teens indicates that females use the social media sites Instagram and Snapchat more than males (Lenhart, 2015). Among adults, gender differences are generally small (Smith, 2016), although evidence from a 2015 Pew Research Center study found that females were slightly more likely to use social media than males (Perrin, 2015). Lastly, findings related to race/ethnicity differences in technology usage indicate that among teens, a slightly higher percentage of Black/African Americans own or have access to a smartphone (85%) as compared to White or Hispanic individuals (71%; Lenhart, 2015). However, these race/ethnic differences appear to diminish by adulthood (Pew Research Center, 2017).

Based on these patterns of technology use, we have described recent studies that have examined differences in cyberbullying prevalence across demographic groups. Evidence suggests that time spent online is correlated with cyberbullying involvement (Kowalski et al., 2014); however, there do appear to be age differences in the prevalence of cyberbullying. Particularly, researchers have suggested that cyberbullying appears to peak in adolescence (like traditional bullying; Due et al., 2005), and slowly declines as individuals grow older (e.g., see Kann et al., 2015). Regarding gender differences, evidence is mixed, with some studies reporting that females are more likely to experience cyberbullying victimization than males (e.g., see Kim et al., 2018) and other studies reporting that males are more likely to perpetrate cyberbullying (e.g., see Coelho et al., 2016). However, other studies have reported opposite findings or no gender differences. Similarly, findings related to race/ethnicity differences in cyberbullying prevalence are also mixed, with some studies reporting that White students are more likely to be victims of cyberbullying than Black/African American students (Rice et al., 2015), whereas other studies found no race/ethnicity differences (Hinduja & Patchin, 2008).

Considering these demographic differences in cyberbullying, we propose a few directions for future research. Firstly, additional research is needed that examines other demographic and individual difference variables as they relate to cyberbullying prevalence and outcomes. For example, how might rates of cyberbullying perpetration and victimization differ depending on culture or socioeconomic status? Other chapters in this volume explore differences in cyberbullying depending on culture (see Chapters 4, 7, and 10, this volume). Regarding socioeconomic status, data from the Pew Research Center suggest that the percentage of middle-income households is shrinking, while the percentage of the US population in upper and lower income households is increasing (Pew Research Center, 2015b). Hong et al. (2016) reported that SES was negatively associated with cyberbullying and traditional bullying victimization among a national US sample of children in grades 6–10. That is, individuals from higher income families are less likely to experience cyber or traditional bullying victimization, and children from lower income families are more likely to experience cyber or traditional bullying victimization. Given the increasing size of the lower-income group in the US (Pew Research Center, 2015b), further research is needed into how SES might impact the venues or modalities of cyberbullying, and whether there may be differential outcomes as a result of exposure to cyberbullying depending on SES.

Future research is also needed that examines changes in cyberbullying perpetration and victimization across time. Whereas much more longitudinal research examining cyberbullying is needed in general, we know little about how cyberbullying experiences change as individuals move through the lifespan as well as how these experiences shape individual and social outcomes. That is, do children who experience cyberbullying victimization in elementary school continue to experience cyberbullying victimization in high school, college, and the workplace? Additionally, are individuals who engage in cyberbullying perpetration in elementary school more likely to engage in cyberbullying perpetration in middle school, high school, college, and the workplace? Further, how does experiencing cyberbullying victimization at a young age relate to adult functioning?

Longitudinal research may also shed light on changing patterns of technology and cyberbullying behavior. New forms of technology appear regularly, with many presenting both new avenues for cyberbullying to occur (particularly anonymous messaging apps) and new challenges for both parents and researchers as they navigate the cyberbullying terrain. With time and better prevention/intervention strategies along with increased awareness of cyberbullying behavior, perhaps observed prevalence rates of the behavior will begin to wane.

References

Anderson, M. (2015, October 29). *Technology device ownership: 2015*. Retrieved from http://assets.pewresearch.org/wp-content/uploads/sites/14/2015/10/PI_2015-10-29_device-ownership_FINAL.pdf

Anderson, M., & Perrin, A. (2017, May 17). *Tech adoption climbs among older adults*. Retrieved from www.pewinternet.org/2017/05/17/tech-adoption-climbs-among-older-adults/

Arslan, S., Savaser, S., Hallett, V., & Balci, S. (2012). Cyberbullying among primary school students in Turkey: Self-reported prevalence and associations with home and school life. *Cyberpsychology, Behavior, and Social Networking, 15*(10), 527–533. doi:10.1089/cyber.2012.0207

Ballard, M. E., & Welch, K. M. (2017). Virtual warfare: Cyberbullying and cyber-victimization in MMOG play. *Games and Culture: A Journal of Interactive Media, 12*(5), 466–491. doi:10.1177/1555412015592473

Beckman, L., Hagquist, C., & Hellström, L. (2013). Discrepant gender patterns for cyberbullying and traditional bullying: An analysis of Swedish adolescent data. *Computers in Human Behavior, 29*(5), 1896–1903. doi:10.1016/j.chb.2013.03.0doi:10

Belsey, B. (2017). *Cyberbullying: An emerging threat to the "always on" generation*. Retrieved from https://pdfs.semanticscholar.org/d4b9/5d4ad8599e86cd726290f4e4a5d8309f6bda.pdf

Center for the Digital Future at USC Annenberg. (2017). *2017 Digital Future Project Survey.* Retrieved from www.digitalcenter.org/wp-content/uploads/2013/10/2017-Digital-Future-Report.pdf

Coelho, V. A., Sousa, V., Marchante, M., Brás, P., & Romão, A. M. (2016). Bullying and cyberbullying in Portugal: Validation of a questionnaire and analysis of prevalence. *School Psychology International, 37*(3), 223–239. doi:10.1177/0143034315626609

Connell, N. M., Schell-Busey, N. M., Pearce, A. N., & Negro, P. (2014). Badgrlz? Exploring sex differences in cyberbullying behaviors. *Youth Violence and Juvenile Justice, 12*(3), 209–228. doi:10.1177/1541204013503889

DePaolis, K. J., & Williford, A. (2018). Pathways from cyberbullying victimization to negative health outcomes among elementary school students: A longitudinal investigation. *Journal of Child and Family Studies.* Advance Online Publication. doi:10.1007/s10826-018-1104-6

DeSmet, A., Rodelli, M., Walrave, M., Soenens, B., Cardon, G., & De Bourdeaudhuij, I. (2018). Cyberbullying and traditional bullying involvement among heterosexual and non-heterosexual adolescents, and their associations with age and gender. *Computers in Human Behavior, 83*, 254–261. doi:10.1016/j.chb.2018. 02. 010

Due, P., Holstein, B. E., Lynch, J., Diderichsen, F., Gabhain, S. N., Scheidt, P., & Currie, C. (2005). Bullying and symptoms among school-aged children: International comparative cross sectional study in 28 countries. *European Journal of Public Health, 15*(2), 128–132. doi:10.1093/eurpub/cki105

Duggan, M. (2017, July 11). *Online harassment 2017.* Retrieved from www.pewinternet.org/2017/07/11/online-harassment-2017/

Englander, E. (2012, November). *Cyberbullying among 11,700 elementary school students.* Paper presented at the annual meeting of the International Bullying Prevention Association, Kansas City, MO.

Erikson Institute. (2016). *New research from the TEC Center at Erikson Institute.* Retrieved from http://teccenter.erikson.edu/publications/tec-parent-survey/

Gray, P. (2013). *Free to learn: Why unleashing the instinct to play will make our children happier, more self-reliant, and better students for life.* New York: Perseus.

Greenwood, S., Perrin, A., & Duggan, M. (2016November 11). *Social media update 2016.* Retrieved from www.pewinternet.org/2016/11/11/social-media-update-2016/

Hinduja, S., & Patchin, J. W. (2008). Cyberbullying: An exploratory analysis of factors related to offending and victimization. *Deviant Behavior, 29*, 129–156. doi:10.1080/01639620701457816

Hong, J. S., Lee, J., Espelage, D. L., Hunter, S. C., Patton, D. U., & Rivers, T. J. (2016). Understanding the correlates of face-to-face and cyberbullying victimization among U.S. adolescents: A social-ecological analysis. *Violence and Victims, 31*(4), 638–663. doi:10.1891/0886-6708.VV-D-15-00014

Jiang, Y., Ekono, M., & Skinner, C. (2016). *Basic facts about low-income children: Children under 18 years, 2014.* Retrieved from www.nccp.org/publications/pdf/text_1145.pdf

Juvonen, J., & Gross, E. F. (2008). Extending the school grounds? Bullying experiences in cyberspace. *Journal of School Health, 78*, 496–505. doi:10.1111/j.1746-1561.2008.00335.x

Kann, L., McManus, T., Harris, W. A., Shanklin, S. L., Flint, K. H., Hawkins, J., … Zaza, S. (2015). Youth risk behavior surveillance – United States, 2015. Centers for Disease Control. *Morbidity and Mortality Weekly Report, 65*, 1–180. Retrieved from www.cdc.gov/healthyyouth/data/yrbs/pdf/2015/ss6506_updated.pdf

Katzer, C., Fetchenhauer, D., & Belschak, F. (2009). Cyberbullying: Who are the victims? A comparison of victimization in Internet chatrooms and victimization in school. *Journal of Media Psychology, 21*, 25–36. doi:10.1027/1864-1105.21.doi:1.25

Kim, S., Colwell, S. R., Kata, A., Boyle, M. H., & Georgiades, K. (2018). Cyberbullying victimization and adolescent mental health: Evidence of differential effects by sex and mental health problem type. *Journal of Youth and Adolescence*. doi:10.1007/s10964-017-0678-4

Kowalski, R. M., Giumetti, G. W., Schroeder, A. W., & Reese, H. H. (2012). Cyber bullying among college students: Evidence domains of college life. In C. Wankel & L. Wankel (Eds.), *Misbehavior online in higher education* (pp. 293–321). Bingley, UK: Emerald Publishing Group.

Kowalski, R. M., & Giumetti, G. W. (2016). Cyberbullying among children 0 to 8 years. In O. N. Saracho (Ed.), *Contemporary perspectives on research on bullying and victimization in early childhood education* (pp. 157–175). Charlotte, NC: US IAP Information Age Publishing.

Kowalski, R. M., Giumetti, G. W., Schroeder, A. N., & Lattanner, M. R. (2014). Bullying in the digital age: A critical review and meta-analysis of cyberbullying research among youth. *Psychological Bulletin, 140*(4), 1073–1137. doi:10.1037/a0035618

Kowalski, R. M., & Limber, S. E. (2007). Electronic bullying among middle school students. *Journal of Adolescent Health, 41*, S22–S30.

Kowalski, R. M., Limber, S. E., & Agatston, P. W. (2012). *Cyberbullying: Bullying in the digital age* (2nd ed.). Malden, MA: Wiley-Blackwell.

Kowalski, R. M., Morgan, C. A., & Limber, S. P. (2012). Traditional bullying as a potential warning sign of cyberbullying. *School Psychology International, 33*(5), 505–519. doi:10.1177/0143034312445244

Kowalski, R. M., Toth, A., & Morgan, M. (2018). Bullying and cyberbullying in adulthood and the workplace. *Journal of Social Psychology, 158*(1), 64–81. doi:10.1080/00224545.2017.1302402

Lee, C., & Shin, N. (2017). Prevalence of cyberbullying and predictors of cyberbullying perpetration among Korean adolescents. *Computers in Human Behavior, 68*, 352–358. doi:10.1016/j.chb.2016. 11. 047

Lenhart, A. (2015, April 9). *Teens, social media, and technology overview 2015*. Retrieved from www.pewinternet.org/2015/04/09/teens-social-media-technology-2015/

Modecki, K. L., Minchin, J., Harbaugh, A. G., Guerra, N. G., & Runions, K. C. (2014). Bullying prevalence across contexts: A meta-analysis measuring cyber and traditional bullying. *Journal of Adolescent Health, 55*(5), 602–611. doi:10.1016/j.jadohealth.2014. 06. 007

Newport, F. (2014, November). *The new era of communication among Americans*. Retrieved from https://news.gallup.com/poll/179288/new-era-communication-americans.aspx

O'Brennan, L. M., Bradshaw, C. P., & Sawyer, A. L. (2009). Examining developmental differences in the social-emotional problems among frequent bullies, victims, and bully/victims. *Psychology in Schools, 46*, 100–115. doi:10.1002/pits.20357

Ofcom. (2016, November). *Children and parents: Media use and attitudes report*. Retrieved from www.ofcom.org.uk/__data/assets/pdf_file/0034/93976/Children-Parents-Media-Use-Attitudes-Report-2016.pdf

Olweus, D. (2013). School bullying: Development and some important challenges. *Annual Review of Clinical Psychology, 9*, 751–780. doi:10.1146/annurev-clinpsy-050212-185516

Pearson. (2015). *Pearson student mobile device survey 2015.* Retrieved from www.pearsoned.com/wp-content/uploads/2015-Pearson-Student-Mobile-Device-Survey-Grades-4-12.pdf

Perrin, A. (2015, October). *Social media usage: 2005–2015.* Retrieved from www.pewinternet.org/2015/10/08/social-networking-usage-2005-2015/

Pew Research Center. (2015a, July). *Gaming, jobs, and broadband: June 10 – July 12, 2015.* Retrieved from www.pewinternet.org/dataset/june-2015-gaming-jobs-broadband/

Pew Research Center. (2015b, December). *The American middle class is losing ground.* Retrieved from www.pewsocialtrends.org/2015/12/09/the-american-middle-class-is-losing-ground/

Pew Research Center (2017, January). *Mobile fact sheet.* Retrieved from www.pewinternet.org/fact-sheet/mobile/

Price, M., Chin, M. A., Higa-McMillan, C., Kim, S., & Frueh, C. B. (2013). Prevalence and internalizing problems of ethnoracially diverse victims of traditional and cyber bullying. *School Mental Health, 5*(4), 183–191. doi:10.1007/s12310-013-9104-6

Proctor, B. D., Semega, J. L., & Kollar, M. A. (2016). *U.S. Census Bureau, Current population reports, P60–256(RV), Income and poverty in the United States: 2015.* Washington, DC: U.S. Government Printing Office.

Purcell, K., & Rainie, L. (2014, December). *Technology's impact on workers.* Retrieved from www.pewInternet.org/2014/12/30/technologys-impact-on-workers/

Rice, E., Petering, R., Rhoades, H., Winetrobe, H., Goldbach, J., Plant, A., Montoya, J., & Kordic, T. (2015). Cyberbullying perpetration and victimization among middle school students. *American Journal of Public Health, 105,* e66–e72. doi:10.2105/AJPH.2014.302393

Robson, C., & Witenberg, R. T. (2013). The influence of moral disengagement, morally based self-esteem, age, and gender on traditional bullying and cyberbullying. *Journal of School Violence, 12*(2), 211–231. doi:10.1080/15388220.2012.762921

Shapka, J. D., Onditi, H. Z., Collie, R. J., & Lapidot-Lefler, N. (2018). Cyberbullying and cybervictimization within a cross-cultural context: A study of Canadian and Tanzanian adolescents. *Child Development, 89,* 89–99. doi:10.1111/cdev.12829

Smith, A. (2016, February 11). *15% of Americans have used online dating sites or mobile dating apps.* Retrieved from www.pewinternet.org/2016/02/11/15-percent-of-american-adults-have-used-online-dating-sites-or-mobile-dating-apps/

Smith, P. K., Mahdavi, J., Carvalho, M., Fisher, S., Russell, S., & Tippett, N. (2008). Cyberbullying: Its nature and impact in secondary school pupils. *Journal of Child Psychology and Psychiatry, 49*(4), 376–385. doi:10.1111/j.1469-7610.2007.01846.x

Topcu, Ç., & Erdur-Baker, Ö. (2012). Affective and cognitive empathy as mediators of gender differences in cyber and traditional bullying. *School Psychology International, 33*(5), 550–561. doi:10.1177/0143034312446882

Tsitsika, A., Janikian, M., Wojcik, S., Makaruk, K., Tzavela, E., Tzavara, C., … Richardson, C. (2015). Cyberbullying victimization prevalence and associations with internalizing and externalizing problems among adolescents in six European countries. *Computers in Human Behavior, 51,* 1–7. doi:10.1016/j.chb.2015. 04. 048

US Census. (2015). *America's families and living arrangements: 2015 Table C-2.* Retrieved from www.census.gov/data/tables/2015/demo/families/cps-2015.html

Wait until 8th. (2017). Retrieved from www.waituntil8th.org.

Williams, K. R., & Guerra, N. G. (2007). Prevalence and predictors of internet bullying. *Journal of Adolescent Health, 41,* 14–21. doi:10.1016/j.jadohealth.2007. 08. 018

3

CYBERBULLYING IN SCHOOLS

A Review of Research in the United States

Sheri Bauman and Diana Meter

Research on cyberbullying is a 21st century development. Although there were uses of the word *cyberbullying* in the popular press in the 1990s (Bauman, 2011), empirical research on the phenomenon began a bit later, with the first empirical studies appearing in 2004 (Ybarra, 2004; Ybarra & Mitchell, 2004a; Ybarra & Mitchell, 2004b). Unlike research on bullying, which was dominated by European scholars, these publications on cyberbullying included a US presence from the beginning. These early papers focused on the association of cyberbullying involvement with depression and psychosocial problems. They also explored the relations between bullying and cyberbullying (called Internet harassment by Ybarra) (Zych, Ortega-Ruiz, & Del Rey, 2015). In the period between 2006 and 2010, the quantity of publications on cyberbullying increased, with US scholars contributing 49% of articles to the scholarly literature (Zych et al., 2015). Since 2011, the volume of publications has continued to grow, with US scholars having the largest proportion of articles (32.4%). The level of interest in the problem suggests that US researchers will continue to be important in building a knowledge base on this topic.

Platforms

One of the challenges in cyberbullying research is the speed at which new innovations in technology change the parameters for social interaction. For example, Internet access once meant having an available desktop or laptop computer. The advent of tablets and especially smartphones means that most young people have Internet access in their pockets. Anderson and Jiang (2018) report that 95% of US teens have a smartphone or have access to one at home. Furthermore, 45% reported being online "almost constantly" (p. 2).

As device creators add features, and devices perform at increased speed, the number of platforms available for interpersonal communication (including various messaging apps) and social media sites (e.g., Snapchat) proliferate and innovate, and new sites offer new features and easy accessibility on smartphones. Thus, researchers must scramble to keep up with changes in cyberspace, which is no easy task.

Trends change with time; Facebook, once the most popular social media platform among teens, has now been eclipsed by YouTube, Instagram, and Snapchat, with the largest proportion of youth saying the one they use most often is Snapchat, with Instagram a close second (Anderson & Jiang, 2018). Some demographic differences were detected: Facebook is used more often by youth from low-income households, girls report Snapchat as their favored platform more than boys, while the reverse is true for YouTube. In addition, teens who identify as White are more likely to select Snapchat as their preferred site than Hispanic or Black teens, while Black teens are more likely than Whites to prefer Facebook (Anderson & Jiang, 2018).

Internet and social media use is almost ubiquitous among young people, leading to concern about threats to internet safety, including cyberbullying. According to Cox, an internet service provider that conducts annual surveys of internet safety, among the participants interviewed (1,307 youth aged 13–17, 16% African American, 10% Hispanic, from 13 US states), 54% had seen cyberbullying on social media and 24% were victimized (Rossi, 2014). Of those, 39% observed it on Facebook, 29% on YouTube, 22% on Twitter, and 22% on Instagram. Sixty-one percent indicated they were cyberbullied about their appearance, 25% regarding their academic achievement or intelligence, 17% about race, and 15% about sexuality.

A study published in 2012 described the ways in which eighth graders reported having been cyberbullied: cell phones (77%), instant messaging (75%), social networking sites (46%), email (28%), and chatrooms (12%) (Holfield & Grabe, 2012a). These researchers also inquired about the relationship of the target with the perpetrator of cyberbullying, and found that classmates were most often named (56%), followed by former (52%) and current (44%) friends, ex-romantic partners (36%), strangers (27%), many people (11%), and don't know (8%). It is likely that new studies with similar samples would produce different findings given the changes described above.

A series of studies with college student samples investigated cyberbullying occurring via social media. Surprisingly, the proportion of participants experiencing their first incident of cyberbullying was the same in college as in middle school (Whittaker & Kowalski, 2015). Whittaker and Kowalski (2015) found that 18.2% of their college sample had been victimized online in the previous year, and 12% acknowledged having cyberbullied others in that time frame. The most commonly endorsed platforms for being victimized were (in order of frequency): texting, Twitter, Facebook, Instagram, and YouTube. Cyberbullying and cybervictimization were significantly correlated. Half the perpetrators were friends of the victim, 54.3% were other students at the school, almost 8% were siblings, and almost 3% were teachers. Those who were targeted responded in a variety of ways, including by doing nothing, reporting the incident, requesting that the cyberbully cease the behavior, retaliating by cyberbullying the bully, saving the evidence, and blocking the perpetrator (Whittaker & Kowalski, 2015).

In another study, Whittaker and Kowalski (2015) used sophisticated software to extract social media content that were potential instances of cyberbullying. Of the 180,215 total posts that were extracted, a random sample of 3,000 were coded. The analysis revealed that a large majority of aggression was detected in the comments sections of websites, that the targets were most often persons known online only, except for on Facebook, where peers were the most common victims.

This section demonstrated that, in the changing universe of cyberspace, researchers have been able to monitor the ways in which the population accesses and uses devices and platforms, but these data are mostly descriptive and sometimes overlook recently emerging applications. More theoretically based and nuanced research that focuses on the distinguishing features of platforms and examines whether those features are uniquely prone to misuse by cyberbullies would better inform efforts to prevent and reduce cyberbullying.

Risk Factors

One area of inquiry for researchers has been to identify risk factors or characteristics of young people involved in cyberbullying. In that way, prevention programs can target vulnerable groups. Many US studies of risk factors associated with cyberbullying involvement are cross-sectional, limiting our ability to make causal inferences. Nevertheless, some of the findings are intriguing and merit further exploration in longitudinal studies. Gender differences have been explored as a predictor of cyberbullying and cybervictimization, but results vary and there is no firm conclusion that can be made. Researchers reporting no gender differences in rates of cyberbullying include Patchin and Hinduja (2006), Tokunaga (2010), and Varjas, Henrich, and Meyers (2009). On the other hand, Holfield and Grabe (2012a) found girls in their sample were more involved in cyberbullying than boys as bullies, victims, and observers. Kowalski and Limber (2007) also found that girls were more likely to be involved in cyberbullying than boys. However, Wang, Iannotti, and Nansel (2009) found that boys were more likely to cyberbully others, and that girls were more likely to be victimized. It appears that the jury is still out on the association of gender and cyberbullying vulnerability.

Age as a risk factor, like gender, has yielded varied findings. A meta-analysis by Bartlett and Coyne (2014) examined sex and age together. The overall analysis found that boys were more likely to report cyberbullying others than girls. However, this was not the case for the younger samples, in which girls engaged in more cyberbullying than boys, while boys were more likely to cyberbully in late adolescence and during college. Tokunaga (2010), in his meta-synthesis concluded that the highest rates of cybervictimization were found in 7th and 8th grades. Kowalski, Giumetti, Schroeder, and Reese (2012) found that college students were cyberbullied at high rates, with 30% having their first experience in college and 43% saying that the most cyberbullying occurred when they were in college. However, it may be that different methods of cyberbullying are more common at different ages (Kowalski, Giumetti, Schroeder, & Lattanner, 2014).

Racial and ethnic differences in cyberbullying have been reported in only a few studies. For example, Wang et al. (2009) found that African American adolescents cyberbullied others more and were victimized less than other groups, whereas Tynes, Giana, Williams, and Thompson (2008) found that African Americans and students who selected "other/multiracial" on the survey were more likely to be victimized online in racially based incidents. Among middle school students in the Los Angeles area, White participants were more likely to be in the cyberbully-cybervictim group compared to uninvolved students than Latinos compared to uninvolved students (Rice et al., 2015). In a short-term longitudinal study with early adolescents in the mid-western US, Low and Espelage (2013) included race, gender, family conflict, non-physical traditional bullying, and alcohol and drug use as potential predictors of cyberbullying at the third time point, and found that parental monitoring measured at Time 1 was negatively associated with cyberbullying "via alcohol and drug use, but only for White females" (p. 39).

One demographic group that has consistently been found to be at higher risk for cyberbullying is LGBT youth and those with atypical gender expression (Cooper & Blumenfeld, 2012; Hinduja & Patchin, 2008; Rice et al., 2015; Schneider, O'Donnell, Stueve, & Coulter, 2012; Varjas, Meyers, Kiperman, & Howard, 2013; Wensley & Campbell, 2012). Widerhold (2014) noted that a previous study found that LGBT youth reported cyberbullying at a rate twice that of their heterosexual peers. She expressed concern that cyberbullying has been linked not only to depression, but also suicidal thoughts and attempts, and self-harm at higher rates than among non-LGBT youth. She reminds us that it is imperative to find effective ways to reduce this problem.

Other potential risk factors include individual differences among youth. Lonigro et al. (2015) concluded that trait anger was associated with cyberbullying involvement, as was state anger but to a lesser degree. Many studies have found that adolescents are more likely to experience cyberbullying if they spend more time online (Kowalski et al., 2014: Twyman, Saylor, Taylor, & Comeaux, 2010). Using the Internet for more hours per day, sending more texts per day, and engaging in risky online behaviors have been found to be more common among those involved in cyberbullying (e.g., Rice et al., 2015). Further, individuals' risk for cyberbullying increases if they engage in risky online behaviors (e.g., sharing passwords, revealing personal information) (Walrave & Heirman, 2011). Nixon (2014) pointed out that the link between cybervictimization and depression extends to college students. Furthermore, it has been noted that being a cyberbully increases the risk for cybervictimization, and vice versa (Bauman, 2010; Bauman & Pero, 2010; Kowalski et al., 2014).

We have reviewed the research that seeks to understand involvement in cyberbullying by identifying factors that increase the likelihood of such involvement. The one consistent factor that elevates the risk for cyberbullying involvement is identifying as LGBT. Researchers and practitioners must begin to implement and study interventions to mitigate this risk, as the negative outcomes are serious and long term. In the next section, we look at research on the consequences of being involved in cyberbullying, as a perpetrator or victim.

Consequences of Cyberbullying

A question that has guided much of the research on consequences of cyberbullying is whether the consequences of this type of bullying are similar to those of traditional bullying, or whether they might be more severe. The literature points to the unique aspects of the digital context (possible anonymity, speed of dissemination, large audience, 24/7 availability, permanence of content, etc.) as reasons to suspect that consequences will be more severe. No US research has confirmed this empirically.

Tokunaga (2010), in his review, noted that decreased school performance (see also Abreu & Kenny, 2017, and Holfield & Grabe, 2012b), increased truancy, diminished concentration, and increases in carrying weapons have been associated with victimization by cyberbullying. Holfield and Grabe (2012b) provided only descriptive data, but reported that 53% of participants noted that their social relationships had been harmed by cyberbullying, and 45% only felt safe at school "sometimes." Additionally, Cooper and Blumenfeld (2012) surveyed 310 secondary students from 40 US states who identified as LGBT or attracted to same-sex others or as LGBT allies to assess the prevalence and impact of cyberbullying in this group. Participants in this study indicated that as a result of being victimized online, they were afraid to attend school (24% LGBT participants), and that their grades had declined (23%). For perpetrators of cyberbullying, increases in delinquency and other forms of rule violations have been detected (Tokunaga, 2010; Ybarra & Mitchell, 2007).

One of the most consistently reported consequences of cyberbullying is depressive symptoms (Bauman, Toomey, & Walker, 2013; Raskauskas & Stoltz, 2007; Ybarra & Mitchell, 2004a). Wang, Nansel, and Iannotti (2011) reported that the frequency of victimization was related to levels of depression so that more frequent victims were more depressed than those who were only occasionally victimized. Among LGBT students, 56% of cybervictims reported feeling depressed compared to 33% of allies (Wang et al., 2011). Unfortunately, longitudinal studies in the US are lacking, limiting our ability to infer causality.

Suicidal ideation has also been implicated as an outcome of cyberbullying involvement. Kowalski and Limber (2007) found such a relation but cautioned that the effects were quite small. Bauman et al. (2013) found that depression was a mediator of the link between cybervictimization and suicidal thoughts, but among girls only. In another study, suicidal thoughts were reported by 35% of LGBT and 19% of allied cybervictims (Cooper & Blumenfeld, 2012). Furthermore, 15% of LGBT and 5% of allies reported having made a suicide attempt after being cyberbullied.

Finally, it is important to note that involvement in cyberbullying is also associated with psychosomatic problems (sleep difficulties, headaches, and stomach aches), and that externalizing difficulties such as substance abuse and delinquent behavior have been found to be associated with cyberbullying (Nixon, 2014). While it is perhaps not surprising to find such links, it is important that we find a way to prevent these harmful sequelae.

Overlap between Cyberbullying, Cybervictimization, Traditional Bullying, and Traditional Victimization

Some researchers have purported that cyberbullying is an extension of traditional face-to-face bullying (Olweus & Limber, 2018). Evidence for this includes participants' reports that they often know those who victimize them online, and that these perpetrators are often peers from school (Holfield & Grabe, 2012a; Juvonen & Gross, 2008). Statistical models suggest that those who are victims in one context tend to be victimized in the other, and those who perpetrate aggression in one context similarly tend to perpetrate aggression toward peers in the other context. The overlap between cyberbullying and school bullying tends to be substantial. Meta-analytically combined results show an overlap of cyberbullying perpetration and traditional bullying perpetration to be 0.45. The overlap of cybervictimization and traditional victimization was 0.40, but we note that this meta-analysis included studies from throughout the world (Kowalski et al., 2014). When traditional bullying or victimization are broken down into different forms (physical, verbal, relational), there still seems to be overlap in bullying and victimization in the traditional and digital context as evidenced by medium-sized correlations between each form of traditional bullying and victimization and cyberbullying and victimization (Varjas et al., 2009). Being victimized by traditional teasing and via rumor-spreading were correlated with victimization via text messaging and on websites/chat rooms. Traditional bullying perpetration by teasing, rumor-spreading, exclusion, and physical aggression was positively correlated to a medium degree with bullying via text messages and websites/chat rooms (Raskauskas & Stoltz, 2007). In another study, bullying perpetration through physical aggression, verbal aggression, social exclusion, and rumor-spreading correlated to a medium degree with cyberbullying perpetration (Wang, Iannotti, & Luk, 2012). Overall, there is evidence that it is common for traditional bullying involvement and cyberbullying involvement to overlap.

The effects of traditional (Card, Stucky, Sawalani, & Little, 2008) and cyberbullying (Bauman et al., 2013; Wang et al., 2011) perpetration and victimization are known to be harmful, but youth who experience peer victimization in both the traditional and digital context seem to be at even higher risk for adjustment problems (Schneider et al., 2012). Further, cybervictimization may cause harm to children and adolescents above and beyond the effects of traditional victimization. One study found that, controlling for the effect of traditional bullying, cyberbullying perpetration and victimization predicted school truancy, lower grades, and leaving school early from illness, depression and anxiety, and lower self-esteem and physical health (Giumetti & Kowalski, 2015). Beyond the effect of traditional victimization, Dempsey and colleagues found an effect of cybervictimization on social anxiety (Dempsey, Sulkowski, Nichols, & Storch, 2009). In another study, effects of cybervictimization were found on self-esteem, social stress, anxiety and depression, and locus of control after controlling for school victimization. Cybervictimization also predicted lower self-efficacy, but this effect was no longer significant once school victimization was included in the model (Fredstrom, Adams, & Gilman, 2011). A large-scale study found that victimization in either context positively predicted substance use, violent behavior, risky sexual behavior, and suicidal behavior, with cybervictimization accounting for slightly more variance in the outcomes than traditional (physical) victimization (Litwiller & Brausch, 2013). It seems that cyberbullying and cybervictimization may uniquely predict some adjustment problems that traditional bullying involvement does not (Giumetti & Kowalski, 2015). For youth who experience victimization in a single context, it is important to consider that the victimization may eventually spill over into other contexts.

What remains unknown is whether the *same* incidents are occurring in face-to-face and digital spaces. One seldom considered form of cyberbullying is the recording and sharing of traditional bullying incidents, sometimes called "happy slapping." For example, physical aggression can be easily video recorded with hand-held devices and posted for others to view, moving traditional bullying into the digital context. Similarly, acts of traditional bullying may move into digital spaces when the perpetrators continue the torment via digital communication after school hours. A person could be excluded from the lunch table via a group text message, or could see evidence of their exclusion from an activity via social media.

Much of the research on cyberbullying and cybervictimization has been modeled after traditional bullying research, which has consistently found groups of perpetrators, victims, and a smaller group (about 6% of youth; Nansel et al., 2001) who are aggressive toward peers *and* are targeted by other aggressive children, referred to as bully-victims. Although this model was useful in first exploring aggressive behavior in digital contexts, mounting evidence suggests that perpetrators and victims are not as distinct in cyberbullying. In multiple studies including US samples, cyberbullying victimization and cyberbullying perpetration were highly correlated ($r = 0.63$, Bauman & Pero, 2010; $r = 0.42$, Kowalski, Morgan, & Limber, 2012; $r = 0.88$, Varjas et al., 2009; $r = 0.55$, Bauman et al., 2013). Meta-analytically combined results inclusive of US and international samples support these findings. The correlation between cyberbullying perpetration and victimization across 91 studies was 0.51 (Kowalski et al., 2014).

With knowledge of the substantial overlap between a) being a perpetrator in the traditional and digital context, b) being a victim in each context, and c) cyberbullying perpetration and victimization, an important next step will be to further investigate these comorbidities. There is, to our knowledge, no research considering the overlap of specific victimization incidents in different contexts. Youth who are teased or threatened in person and then receive additional abuse in the digital context or vice versa regarding the same theme may experience more adjustment problems. It is important to better establish why youth who are both perpetrators and victims in the cyber context suffer more adjustment problems than youth who are either bullies or victims (Schneider et al., 2012), as is the case with traditional "bully-victims" (Haynie et al., 2001; Kowalski & Limber 2013). Further, it is of interest to know specific predictors and consequences of being a cyber bully-victim. Researchers may also be interested in studying possible developmental trajectories from non-involvement in cyberbullying to involvement as a victim, to involvement as a bully, or vice versa in the digital context. There is also a current need to investigate factors that may decrease involvement in cyberaggression with attention to the prevalence of cyber "bully-victims."

Online Gaming

Although we know that online gaming is a popular activity for young people (and adults), US research on the topic is sparse, and there are methodological limitations that detract from the rigor of the few existing research studies. However, a 2014 report indicated that teens between 13 and 17 years old are online five hours 38 minutes per day, of which half is spent playing online games (Rossi, 2014), suggesting that online gaming is likely an important context in which to investigate cyberbullying.

Ballard and Welch (2017) describe features of the online gaming environment that make it fertile ground for cyberbullying. One potent motivation to engage in any form of bullying is to gain status, dominance, or power. In online games, rank (an indicator of status in the game world, attained by earning points for conquests and completing challenges, etc.) is a feature that lends itself to such behavior. There are other aspects of online gaming that make aggression more likely: aggression is modeled and reinforced within the game, players are desensitized to violence, and there are numerous opportunities to observe violence in the gaming world. In addition, players are aware that the game is not the "real world," because all manner of actions (fighting and killing) are expected and perhaps necessary for survival. Thus, players may consider other negative behaviors to also be acceptable because they take place in the digital and not the "real" world.

Much of the gaming activity takes place in massively multiplayer online games (MMOGs; Warner & Raiter, 2005). These games take their name from the fact that thousands of people (usually known only by screen names) of many ages in various locations engage in the game activities within online worlds. The games have goals, which players achieve either individually or in teams. Players or teams gain and lose points for their actions, and the social structure in these "worlds" can be quite complex. There are typically online forums, and sometimes direct messaging features, that allow for discussions about the game. Cybervictimization behavior in the MMOG context may involve intentionally causing distress to others (known as "griefing").

Ballard and Welch (2017) provided evidence that online games encouraged misogyny and that pejorative racial, sexual, and homophobic terms were widely used in the gaming context. In a sample of 151 US university students who indicated they had recently played MMOGs, 52% indicated they had been victimized in a game world, and 35% admitted to perpetrating cyberbullying, although frequency varied from once or twice to multiple times per week. Half of those who had been victimized reported the behavior occurred in only one gaming session. The most common reason players were victimized and bullied others was rank in the game. Cyberbullying included name-calling, exclusion, threats, and lies. Men in the sample had higher rates of cyberbullying, but cybervictimization did not differ by gender. Women reported more frequent sexual harassment and "excessive sexual pursuit" than men.

Fryling, Cotler, Rivituso, Mathews, and Pratico (2015) received surveys from 1033 members of an online gaming forum. Participants' mean age was 22, with 73% being 18 or older; 62% women, 38% men. In this study, 38% of participants reported they did not play a specific game because they worried about cyberbullying, and 54% had left a game in response to cyberbullying. About 64% of respondents considered cyberbullying in online gaming to be a serious issue. Interestingly, 53% of men and 67% of women indicated that cyberbullying occurs often or always in online games. Self-reported decline in self-esteem was greatest for victimized women. Furthermore, women (aged 12–37) with high levels of gaming experience were most likely to be victims and witnesses to cyberbullying within the game, and men were most likely to be engaged in cyberbullying others. These researchers concluded that there are negative outcomes associated with cyberbullying in gaming environments, and that both victims and witnesses are more likely to cyberbully others in this context.

These few studies about cyberbullying and gaming confirm that the online gaming context, including the widely played MMOGs, are worthy of further study, as cyberbullying is a part of that experience for many users.

Parental Monitoring and Cyberbullying/Victimization

As mentioned previously, many children and most adolescents in the United States have access to internet-connected devices, either owning their own or using friends', and have private social media accounts (Lenhart, Purcell, Smith, & Zickuhr, 2010). Parents and children have reported different techniques for monitoring children's online behavior. Restricting which websites youth are allowed to visit was a successful strategy related to less cybervictimization among one US sample (Mesch, 2009). Monitoring more generally was related to less cybervictimization in another sample (Taiariol, 2010). Importantly, not all research has found an association between parental monitoring and cyberbullying involvement either as a cyberbully, victim, or both (Aoyama, Barnard-Brock, & Talbert, 2011). In one study, parental monitoring of online behavior positively predicted cyberbullying involvement, although this could have been an effect of the concurrent nature of the data, or due to relying on child reports of parents' parental monitoring of their online behavior (Meter & Bauman, 2016).

Because of the difficulty parents have monitoring children and adolescents' online and social media activity, parents might need to request access to their child's accounts through friending so they can keep abreast of positive and negative behavior enacted by peers in the child's network as well as their own child's behavior toward others. On the other hand, youth may create multiple accounts on the same social media site, and friend parents on the one sanitized for parental scrutiny.

Further, parental monitoring might affect cyberbullying involvement indirectly (Low & Espelage, 2013). Additional research might test whether parental monitoring might affect cyberbullying and cybervictimization via known predictors, or could investigate whether parental monitoring buffers the effect of these risk factors. For example, parental monitoring has been found to be negatively associated with cybervictimization directly, and also through reducing youth time on social networking sites (Khurana, Bleakley, Jordan, & Romer, 2015). This study investigated parental restriction of online behavior and more general parental monitoring of child behavior and found that, although parental restriction had indirect effects on online harassment of youth, the more positive parental monitoring had stronger effects.

Policies, Laws, and Legal Ramifications

After several high-profile suicides following cyberbullying there was an impetus to create policies and laws to address the problem. According to Green (2016), all 50 states have passed anti-bullying legislation. In general, these laws make school bullying illegal and describe the duties of schools with respect to dealing with bullying; all of these laws also explicitly cover cyberbullying. Generally, schools have a duty to protect students from harm, including harm from cyberbullying.

There are no federal laws against cyberbullying, but the existence of the First Amendment of the constitution makes legal issues somewhat muddy. While students have the right to free speech guaranteed by the First Amendment, the Supreme Court has upheld some restrictions on free speech in the school setting to protect students from harm caused by disruptive speech (Hofheimer, 2013). Lawsuits have challenged the courts to specify what types of off-campus speech can be restricted and under what conditions. That is, some school rules might be in conflict with the First Amendment rights of students. The legal precedent cited in these cases is that of *Tinker v. Des Moines Independent Community School District* (n.d.), in which the court concluded that, when speech causes a "material and substantial disruption" of the learning environment at school, the school has the authority to impose disciplinary consequences on the creator of the speech. Another standard that has been applied in legal challenges is that there must be a "nexus" between the speech and the school when the speech is created off-campus. That means the speech must be connected to a school and that the potential for disruption of the educational function of the school must be foreseeable (Hofheimer, 2013).

In 2011, the Fourth Circuit Court of Appeals ruled that the Berkeley County Schools were within their authority to discipline Kara Kowalski, a high school student who had created an online group that maligned and disparaged another student (Gerston, 2011). The Tinker case was the rationale for the ruling. In the same year, the Third Circuit Court of Appeals ruled that JS (the student identifier) should not have been suspended for the parody MySpace profile she created for her principal (J.S. v Blue Mtn. Sch. Dist., 2011). There are other examples of conflicting rulings on similar cases.

Until the Supreme Court makes a definitive ruling regarding the limits of free speech as it relates to cyberbullying that is committed off-campus, individual courts are likely to disagree about specific cases. This does not mean, however, that cyberbullying can be perpetrated without consequences. In the absence of federal anti-bullying statutes, there are civil rights prohibitions against discrimination that are based on race, ethnicity, gender, and other protected groups, and cyberbullying incidents may be perpetrated in situations where these laws apply, providing school districts the opportunity to discipline those who commit cyberbullying infractions against peers.

Another concern in regard to legal consequences of cyberbullying involves the sharing of nude pictures of minors. Although sexting typically first occurs between two individuals, explicit photos have been known to be forwarded to peers without consent. In some states, sharing nude pictures of minors is considered sexual exploitation and child pornography. Seven percent of those arrested for producing child pornography were teens whose exchange of nude images was consensual (Wolak, Finkelhor, & Mitchell, 2012). That means that sexting by two minors could result in conviction for a felony and addition to the sex offender database under the laws that prohibit the possession of child pornography; many believe such a penalty is too severe for youth under 18.

Consequences for minors engaging in sharing this material varies across states; in some, penalties can include imprisonment and sex offender registration while in others, counseling or education might be imposed (Botelho & Martinez, 2015). Nineteen states have passed laws that impose lesser penalties for minors (e.g., warnings, fines, probation, or detention (DeHoyos, 2018)). Hasinoff (2016) summarized the conundrum this way:

> Teenagers who sext are in a precarious legal position. Though in most states teenagers who are close in age can legally have consensual sex, if they create and share sexually explicit images of themselves, they are technically producing, distributing or possessing child pornography. The laws that cover this situation, passed decades ago, were meant to apply to adults who exploited children and require those convicted under them to register as sex offenders. *(Paragraph 1)*

Future Directions

The most obvious need in cyberbullying research among US youth is for more longitudinal research and more sophisticated research designs. Longitudinal studies can provide stronger support for causal relationships. Potential moderating and mediating variables (e.g., age, gender, sexual orientation, race/ethnicity, disability status, coping styles) also merit investigation to broaden our understanding of this phenomenon. Furthermore, more representative samples should be used so that results can be generalized. Much existing work is based on convenience samples; including cyberbullying-relevant items in national surveys would be extremely valuable. The Youth Risk Behavior Surveys (YRBS) have added several items related to bullying and cyberbullying (one each for bullying and cyberbullying, and one each for victimization and cybervictimization), but more specific items are needed. We know that time spent online and being involved in traditional bullying are risk factors, and social support is protective. It is likely that other factors play a role as well, and understanding those would enhance models of intervention.

Regarding areas that are in particular need of further investigation are cyberbullying based on race/ethnicity and sexual orientation. It is clear that racial/ethnic and sexual minorities are at high risk for involvement in cyberbullying, but we need more than prevalence studies. Are there additional risk or protective factors that can be identified? Perhaps age, or presence of a disability, or enrollment in special education, personality traits, or achievement status in school (high achievers and low achievers) are worthy of investigation. The Low and Espelage (2013) study attempted to identify predictors beyond demographics, and the study is an excellent example of the kind of research that is needed. That said, the sample was from four schools in one geographic area, included only African American and White students, and did not inquire about sexual orientation. The focus on grades five through seven is useful, although extending the range through middle and late adolescence would be more informative.

Finally, there are very few programs to reduce cyberbullying with any empirical evidence of efficacy or effectiveness (see Campbell & Bauman, 2018, for examples). It is important that we involve youth in the development of strategies that are appealing and relevant to the target population. Programs tend to be developed by adults, and if they are to make a difference in youth behavior, youth need to be consulted and involved in their creation.

Summary

In this chapter, we have reviewed what is known about cyberbullying and victimization in US schools and suggested possible directions for new research. It is clear that cyberbullying involves and affects young people to an important degree and that it will continue to concern researchers, educators, and the public. We reviewed existing research on prevalence, demographic differences in involvement, relations to traditional bullying and victimization, consequences of involvement, parental roles, and risk factors for involvement. In addition, we discussed cyberbullying in online gaming, which has received insufficient attention in the literature. We addressed the thorny issue of legislation and court rulings, which have yet to be clarified by the Supreme Court. It is obvious that social media will continue to proliferate and provide many avenues for cyberbullying; researchers need to focus on identifying the characteristics or features of these venues that are problematic, and devise strategies, prevention and intervention programs that work across platforms. Creativity, and perhaps youth involvement in prevention efforts, is needed to address the problems of cyberbullying and cybervictimization.

References

Abreu, R. L. & Kenny, M. C. (2017). Cyberbullying and LGBT youth: A systematic literature review and recommendations for prevention and intervention. *Journal of Child & Adolescent Trauma, 11*, 81–97. doi:10.1007/s40653–40017–0175–0177

Anderson, M., & Jiang, J. (2018, May). *Teens, social media, and technology 2018.* Report from Pew Research Center. Retrieved from www.pewinternet.org/2018/05/31/teens-social-media-technology-2018/

Aoyama, I., Barnard-Brock, L., & Talbert, T. L. (2011). Cyberbullying among high school students: Cluster analysis of sex and age differences and the level of parental monitoring. *International Journal of Cyber Behavior, Psychology and Learning, 1*, 25–35. doi:10.4018/ijcbpl.2011010103

Ballard, M. E., & Welch, K. M. (2017). Virtual warfare: Cyberbullying and cyber-victimization in MMOG play. *Games and Culture, 12*, 466–491. doi:10.1177/1555412015592473

Bartlett, C., & Coyne, S. M., (2014). A meta-analysis of sex differences in cyber-bullying behavior: The moderating role of age. *Aggressive Behavior, 40*, 474–488. doi:10.1002/ab.21555

Bauman, S. (2010). Cyberbullying in a rural intermediate school: An exploratory study. *The Journal of Early Adolescence, 30*, 803–833. doi:10.1177/0272431609350927

Bauman, S. (2011). *Cyberbullying: What counselors need to know*. Alexandria, VA: American Counseling Association.

Bauman, S., & Pero, H. (2010). Bullying and cyberbullying among deaf students and their hearing peers: An exploratory study. *Journal of Deaf Studies and Deaf Education, 16*, 236–253.

Bauman, S., Toomey, R. B., & Walker, J. L. (2013). Associations among bullying, cyberbullying, and suicide in high school students. *Journal of Adolescence, 36*, 341–350. doi:10.1016/j.adolescence.2012.12.001

Botelho, G., & Martinez, M. (2015, December 9). *DA: No charges against Colorado students in sexting scandal.* Retrieved from www.cnn.com/2015/12/09/us/colorado-sexting-scandal-canon-city/

Campbell, M., & Bauman, S. (Eds.) (2018). *Reducing cyberbullying in schools: International evidence-based best practices.* Sydney, AU: Academic Press.

Card, N. A., Stucky, B. D., Sawalani, G. M., & Little, T. D. (2008). Direct and indirect aggression during childhood and adolescence: A meta-analytic review of gender differences, intercorrelations, and relations to maladjustment. *Child Development, 79,* 1185–1229. doi:10.1111/j.1467-8624.2008.01184.x

Cooper, R. M., & Blumenfeld, W. J. (2012). Responses to cyberbullying: A descriptive analysis of the frequency of and impact on LGBT and allied youth. *Journal of LGBT Youth, 9,* 153–177. doi:10.1080/19361653.2011.649616

DeHoyos, B. (2018, March 13). Sexting laws in the United States. *Lifewire.* Retrieved from www.lifewire.com/sexting-laws-in-united-states-1949957

Dempsey, A. G., Sulkowski, M. L., Nichols, R., & Storch, E. A. (2009). Differences between peer victimization in cyber and physical settings and associated psychosocial adjustment in early adolescence. *Psychology in the Schools, 46,* 962–972. doi:10.1002/pits.20437

Fredstrom, B. K., Adams, R. E., & Gilman, R. (2011). Electronic and school-based victimization: Unique contexts for adjustment difficulties during adolescence. *Journal of Youth and Adolescence, 40,* 405–415. doi:10.1007/s10964-010-9569-7

Fryling, M., Cotler, J., Rivituso, J., Mathews, L., & Pratico, S. (2015). Cyberbullying or normal game play? Impact of age, gender, and experience on cyberbullying in multi-player online gaming environments: Perceptions from one gaming forum. *Journal of Information Systems Applied Research, 8,* 4–15.

Gerston, E. (2011). *Appeals court back school punishment for W. Va. Students' MySpace group.* Retrieved from www.splc.org/article/2011/07/appeals-court-backs-school-punishment-for-w-va-students-myspace-group

Giumetti, G. W., & Kowalski, R. M. (2015). Cyberbullying matters: Exploring the incremental impact of cyberbullying on outcomes over and above traditional bullying in North America. In R. Navarro, S. Yubero, & E. Larrañaga (Eds.), *Cyberbullying across the globe: Gender, family, and mental health* (pp. 117–130). New York: Springer.

Green, L. (2016). *Cyberbullying: Challenging legal issues for schools.* Retrieved from www.nfhs.org/articles/cyberbullying-challenging-legal-issues-for-schools/

Hasinoff, A. A. (2016). Teenage sexting is not child porn. *New York Times.* Retrieved from www.nytimes.com/2016/04/04/opinion/teenage-sexting-is-not-child-porn.html?_r=0

Haynie, D. L., Nansel, T., Eitel, P., Crump, A. D., Saylor, K., Yu, K., & Simons-Morton, B. (2001). Bullies, victims, and bully/victims: Distinct groups of at-risk youth. *The Journal of Early Adolescence, 21,* 29–49. doi:10.1177/0272431601021001002

Hinduja, S., & Patchin, J. W. (2008). Cyberbullying: An exploratory analysis of factors related to offending and victimization. *Deviant Behavior, 29,* 129–156. doi:10.1080/01639620701457816

Hofheimer, A. (2013). Saved by the Bell? Is online, off-campus student speech protected by the First Amendment? *Florida State University Law Review, 40,* 971–993.

Holfield, B., & Grabe, M. (2012a). Middle school students' perceptions of and response to cyberbullying. *Journal of Educational Computing Research, 46,* 395–413.

Holfeld, B., & Grabe, M. (2012b). An examination of the history, prevalence, characteristics, and reporting of cyberbullying in the United States. In Q. Li, D. Cross, & P. K. Smith (Eds.),

Cyberbullying in the global playground: Research from international perspectives (pp. 117–142). West Sussex, UK: Wiley.

J.S. v. Blue Mtn. Sch. Dist., No. 08–4138 (3d Cir. 2011)

Juvonen, J., & Gross, E. F. (2008). Extending the school grounds? Bullying experiences in cyberspace. *Journal of School Health, 78*, 496–505. doi:10.1111/j.1746-1561.2008.00335.x

Khurana, A., Bleakley, A., Jordan, A. B., & Romer, D. (2015). The protective effects of parental monitoring and internet restriction on adolescents' risk of online harassment. *Journal of Youth and Adolescence, 44*, 1039–1047. doi:10.1007/s10964-014-0242-4

Kowalski, R. M., Giumetti, G. W., Schroeder, A. N., & Lattanner, M. R. (2014). Bullying in the digital age: A critical review and meta-analysis of cyberbullying research among youth. *Psychological Bulletin, 140*, 1073–1137. doi:10.1037/a0035618

Kowalski, R. M., Giumetti, G. W., Schroeder, A. N., & Reese, H. H. (2012). Cyber bullying among college students: Evidence domains of college life. In C. Wankel & L. Wankel (Eds.), *Misbehavior online in higher education* (pp. 293–321). Bingley, UK: Emerald Publishing Group.

Kowalski, R. M., & Limber, S. P. (2007). Electronic bullying among middle school students. *Journal of Adolescent Health, 41*, S22–S30. doi:10.1016/j.jadohealth.2007. 08. 017

Kowalski, R. M., & Limber, S. P. (2013). Psychological, physical, and academic correlates of cyberbullying and traditional bullying. *Journal of Adolescent Health, 53*, S13–S20. doi:10.1016/j.jadohealth.2012.09.018

Kowalski, R. M., Morgan, C. A., & Limber, S. P. (2012). Traditional bullying as a potential warning sign of cyberbullying. *School Psychology International, 33*, 505–519. doi:10.1177/0143034312445244

Lenhart, A., Purcell, K., Smith, A., & Zickuhr, K. (2010). Social media & mobile Internet use among teens and young adults. *Pew Internet & American Life Project*. Retrieved from http://files.eric.ed.gov/fulltext/ED525056.pdf

Litwiller, B. J., & Brausch, A. M. (2013). Cyber bullying and physical bullying in adolescent suicide: The role of violent behavior and substance use. *Journal of Youth and Adolescence, 42*, 675–684. doi:10.1007/s10964-013-9925-5

Lonigro, A., Schneider, B. H., Laghi, F., Baiocco, R., Pallini, S., & Brunner, T. (2015). Is cyberbullying related to trait or state anger? *Child Psychiatry & Human Development, 46*, 445–454. doi:10.1007/s10578-014-0484-0

Low, S., & Espelage, D. (2013). Differentiating cyber bullying perpetration from non-physical bullying: Commonalities across race, individual, and family predictors. *Psychology of Violence, 3*, 39–52. doi:10.1037/a0030308

Mesch, G. S. (2009). Parental mediation, online activities, and cyberbullying. *CyberPsychology & Behavior, 12*, 387–393. doi:10.1089/cpb.2009.0068

Meter, D. J., & Bauman, S. (2016). Moral disengagement about cyberbullying and parental monitoring: Effects on traditional bullying and victimization via cyberbullying involvement. *The Journal of Early Adolescence, 38*, 303–326. doi:10.1177/0272431616670752

Nansel, T. R., Overpeck, M., Pilla, R. S., Ruan, W. J., Simons-Morton, B., & Scheidt, P. (2001). Bullying behaviors among US youth: Prevalence and association with psychosocial adjustment. *Journal of the American Medical Association, 285*, 2094–2100. doi:10.1001/jama.285.16.2094

Nixon, C. L. (2014). Current perspectives: The impact of cyberbullying on adolescent health. *Adolescent Health, Medicine and Therapeutics, 5*, 143–158. doi:10.2147/AHMT.S36456

Olweus, D. & Limber, S. P. (2018). Some problems with cyberbullying research. *Current Opinion in Psychology, 19*, 139–143. doi:10.1016/j.copsyc.2017. 01. 012

Patchin, J. W., & Hinduja, S. (2006). Bullies move beyond the schoolyard: A preliminary look at cyberbullying. *Youth Violence and Juvenile Justice, 4*, 148–169. doi:10.1177/1541204006286288

Raskauskas, J., & Stoltz, A. D. (2007). Involvement in traditional and electronic bullying among adolescents. *Developmental Psychology, 43*, 564–575. doi:10.1037/0012-1649.43. 3. 564

Rice, E., Petering, R., Rhoades, H., Winetrobe, H., Goldbach, J., Plant, A., ... & Kordic, T. (2015). Cyberbullying perpetration and victimization among middle-school students. *American Journal of Public Health, 105*, e66–e72. doi:10.2105/AJPH.2014.302393

Rossi, J. (2014). 2014 Teen Internet Safety Survey. Report by Cox Communications. Retrieved from www.cox.com/content/dam/cox/aboutus/documents/tween-internet-safety-survey.pdf

Schneider, S. K., O'Donnell, L., Stueve, A., & Coulter, R. W. (2012). Cyberbullying, school bullying, and psychological distress: A regional census of high school students. *American Journal of Public Health, 102*, 171–177. doi:10.2105/AJPH.2011.300308

Taiariol, J. (2010). *Cyberbullying: The role of family and school.* (Wayne State University Dissertations, Paper No. 118). Retrieved from http://digitalcommons.wayne.edu/oa_dissertations/118

Tinker v. Des Moines Independent Community School District. (n.d.). Oyez. Retrieved from www.oyez.org/cases/1968/21

Tokunaga, R. S. (2010). Following you home from school: A critical review and synthesis of research on cyberbullying victimization. *Computers in Human Behavior, 26*, 277–287. doi:10.1016/j.chb.2009.11.0doi:14

Twyman, K., Saylor, C., Taylor, D. A., & Comeaux, C. (2010). Comparing children and adolescents engaged in cyberbullying to matcher peers. *Cyberpsychology, Behavior, and Social Networking, 13*, 195–199. doi:10.1089.cyber.2009.0137

Tynes, B. M., Giang, M. T., Williams, D. R., & Thompson, G. N. (2008). Online racial discrimination and psychological adjustment among adolescents. *Journal of Adolescent Health, 43*, 565–569. doi:10.1016/j.jadohealth.2008. 08. 021

Varjas, K., Henrich, C. C., & Meyers, J. (2009). Urban middle school students' perceptions of bullying, cyberbullying, and school safety. *Journal of School Violence, 8*, 159–176. doi:10.1080/15388220802074165

Varjas, K., Meyers, J., Kiperman, S., & Howard, A. (2013). Technology hurts? Lesbian, gay, and bisexual youth perspectives of technology and cyberbullying. *Journal of School Violence, 12*, 27–44. doi:10.1080/15388220.2012.731665

Walrave, M., & Heirman, W. (2011). Cyberbullying: Predicting victimization and perpetration. *Children and Society, 25*, 59–72. doi:10.1111/j.1099-0860.2009.00260.x

Wang, J.Iannotti, R. J., & Luk, J. W. (2012). Patterns of adolescent bullying behaviors: Physical, verbal, rumor, and cyber. *Journal of School Psychology, 50*, 521–534. doi:10.1016/j.jsp.2012. 03. 004

Wang, J., Nansel, T. R., & Iannotti, R. (2011). Cyber and traditional bullying: Differential association with depression. *Journal of Adolescent Health, 48*, 415–417. doi:10.1016/j.jadohealth.2010.07.2012

Wang, J., Iannotti, R. J., & Nansel, T. R. (2009). School bullying among adolescents in the United States: Physical, verbal, relational, and cyber. *Journal of Adolescent Health, 45*, 368–375. doi:10.1016/j.jadohealth.2009. 03. 021

Warner, D. E., & Raiter, M. (2005). Social context in massively-multi-player online games (MMOGs): Ethical questions in shared space. *International Review of Information Ethics*, 4, 46–52.

Wensley, K., & Campbell, M. (2012). Heterosexual and nonheterosexual young university students' involvement in traditional and cyber forms of bullying. *Cyberpsychology, Behavior, and Social Networking, 15*, 649–654. doi:10.1089/cyber.2012.0132

Whittaker, E., & Kowalski, R. M. (2015). Cyberbullying via social media. *Journal of School Violence, 14*, 11–29. doi:10.1080/15388220.2014.949377

Widerhold, B. K. (2014). Cyberbullying and LGBT youth: A deadly combination. *Cyberpsychology, Behavior, and Social Networking, 17*, 1–2. doi:10.1089/cyber.2014.1521

Wolak, J., Finkelhor, D. & Mitchell, K. J. (2012, April). *Trends in arrests for child pornography production: The third National Juvenile Online Victimization study (NJOV-3).* Durham, NH: Crimes Against Children Research Center, University of New Hampshire.

Ybarra, M. L. (2004). Linkages between depressive symptomatology and Internet harassment among young regular Internet users. *CyberPsychology & Behavior,* 7, 247–257. doi:10.1089/109493104323024500

Ybarra, M. L., & Mitchell, K. J. (2004a). Online aggressor/targets, aggressors, and targets: A comparison of associated youth characteristics. *Journal of Child Psychology and Psychiatry, 45*, 1308–1316. doi:10.1111/j.1469-7610.2004.00328.x

Ybarra, M. L., & Mitchell, K. J. (2004b). Youth engaging in online harassment: Associations with caregiver–child relationships, Internet use, and personal characteristics. *Journal of Adolescence, 27*, 319–336. doi:10.1016/j.adolescence.2004. 03. 007

Ybarra, M. L., & Mitchell, K. J. (2007). Prevalence and frequency of Internet harassment instigation: Implications for adolescent health. *Journal of Adolescent Health, 41*(2), 189–198.

Zych, I., Ortega-Ruiz, R., & Del Rey, R. (2015). Scientific research on bullying and cyberbullying: Where have we been and where are we going. *Aggression and Violent Behavior, 24*, 188–198. doi:10.1016/j.avb.2015. 05. 015

4

CYBERBULLYING IN SCHOOLS

Cross-Cultural Issues

Peter K. Smith, Anke Görzig, and Susanne Robinson

Over the last two decades, research into cyberbullying has gained momentum as researchers endeavour to consider and understand the nature of the behaviour and its wider reaching impact on all concerned. There is not universal agreement on the definition of bullying, but there does exist some consensus that it is aggressive behaviour, intended to hurt or harm another, with two further criteria: repetition – the hurtful behaviour happens more than once; and power imbalance – it is difficult for the victim to defend himself or herself (Olweus, 1999; Smith, 2014). Cyberbullying is usually defined by extending the above to electronic communication media; however, the latter two criteria, i.e., repetition and power imbalance, are particularly debated when it comes to the definition of cyberbullying (Slonje, Smith, & Frisén, 2013).

Cyberbullying has been recognised as an international issue with much of the research having been conducted within North America, Europe, and Australia (Smith & Berkkun, 2017; Zych, Ortega, & del Rey, 2015). However, there has been a tradition of research in the Asian Pacific Rim countries (Smith, Kwak, & Toda, 2016), and growing research in other areas such as South-East Asia (Sittichai & Smith, 2015) and India (Smith et al., 2018) whilst there is a scarcity of research on the phenomena in the Global South (Livingstone, Stoilova, & Kelly, 2016).

Cyberbullying and victimization tend to be most prevalent among school aged children and young adults (Ševčíková & Šmahel, 2009). They often occur outside of school (Migliaccio & Rauskauskas, 2015; Monks, Ortega, Robinson, & Worlidge, 2009; Smith et al., 2008), perhaps as a result of restrictions schools have in place, such as firewalls and the blocking of certain content or key words (Tomazin & Smith, 2007; UK Safer Internet Centre, 2017).

Country Differences in Cyberbullying Rates

A few studies have compared rates of cyberbullying in a small number of countries. For example, Genta et al. (2012) reported on cyberbullying among 12 to 15 year olds in Italy (*n*=1,964, 39 schools), England (*n*=2,227, 14 schools), and Spain (*n*=1,671, 7 schools). They compared mobile and internet cyberbullying over the previous two months, using a definition consistent with that suggested by Olweus (1999). Percentages for severe (two or three times a month or more) mobile bullying perpetration ranged across the three countries from 0.9 to 2.7%, and internet bullying from 1.0 to 1.6%, for mobile victimization from 0.5 to 2.2%, and internet victimization from 1.3 to 2.6%. Country differences varied by type of involvement, with Italy consistently having the highest rates for both victimization and perpetration.

Aoyama, Utsumi, and Hasegawa (2011) assessed cyberbullying in Japanese and US high school samples and found both cyber perpetration and victimization rates to be higher in the United States. Similarly, Barlett et al. (2014) gathered data from college-aged participants in the United States (*n*=293) and Japan (*n*=722) (number of institutions not specified). Rates were higher in the United States for all measures – cyberbullying perpetration, reinforcement, and positive attitudes to cyberbullying.

Wright et al. (2015) examined differences in cyber aggression perpetration and victimization among 1,637 adolescents living in China (*n*=683, 2 schools), India (*n*=480, 6 schools), and Japan (*n*=474, 2 schools). Adolescents from India had the highest levels of cyber aggression involvement when compared to adolescents from China or Japan. Chinese adolescents engaged in more cyber aggression perpetration and were victimized more by cyber aggression when compared to Japanese adolescents.

However, there are two large-scale surveys which provide self-reported rates of cyberbullying across a large number of countries. These are the EU Kids online survey (EUKO) across 25 European countries, and the Health Behaviour of School-aged Children survey (HBSC), carried out every four years from 42 countries mainly from Europe and North America. EUKO provided data from 2010 on cyberbullying perpetration and cyber victimization (Livingstone, Haddon, Görzig, & Ólafsson, 2011a). Although HBSC surveys have been going since 1993, only the most recent survey of 2013/2014 included two questions on cyber victimization (Inchley et al., 2016). Other cross-national surveys that include questions on bullying, namely the Global School Health Survey (GSHS), Trends in International Mathematics and Science Study (TIMSS), and Programme for International Student Assessment (PISA), do not include questions on cyberbullying or refer to it in any definition given.

Smith, Robinson, and Marchi (2016) examined concordance across country differences for bullying generally, amongst EUKO, HBSC, GSHS, and TIMSS; although within survey correlations (across ages, genders, survey periods) were high (around 0.8, 0.9), across survey correlations were much more modest; the highest was 0.57, and most were around 0.2–0.4. Smith and López-Castro (2017) calculated how PISA compared with the other surveys. Correlations obtained were generally more acceptable than in the previous comparisons, and especially satisfactory for comparing PISA with TIMSS (correlations around 0.8, comparable to within survey correlations). This may be because both are behaviour-based rather than definition-based surveys.

In this chapter, we report on comparisons between EUKO and HBSC, specifically as regards rates of cyber victimization. We first give an account of each survey, and the range of country rates reported. We then discuss some of the challenges in comparing country rates, both within a survey, and between surveys. This is followed by some discussion of how country differences in cyberbullying rates might be explained. Finally, we make suggestions for future research in this area.

The EU Kids Online Survey and What It Found

Livingstone et al. (2011a) reported findings on traditional bullying and cyberbullying from 25 European countries, from the EU Kids Online survey carried out in spring/summer 2010. The samples were based on random stratified sampling of some 1,000 children, aged 9 to 16 years old, in each country. Self-report survey questionnaires were given face-to-face in children's homes. The survey was on internet use, risks, and safety. A section on bullying did not use the term 'bullying', but started with a statement:

> Sometimes children or teenagers say or do hurtful or nasty things to someone and this can often be quite a few times on different days over a period of time. For example, this can include: teasing someone in a way this person does not like; hitting, kicking or pushing someone around; leaving someone out of things.

The interviewer explained that these activities could be face-to-face, or via mobile phone calls or texts, or on the internet. With regards to the Olweus-type definition, a range of activities was, therefore, covered, as well as the repetition criterion, although the imbalance of power criterion was not explicitly mentioned (Slonje et al., 2013). The child or young person was then asked whether someone had acted in this hurtful or nasty way to them in the past 12 months (response options: 'yes', 'no'). Following on from this, they were asked if they themselves had acted in a hurtful or nasty way to others in the last year. If so, they were asked how this had happened.

The majority of bullying reported was face-to-face, but taking any time over the past 12 months, 6% said they had acted in that kind of way on the internet, and 3% by mobile phone calls or messages. Both these percentages showed a steady rise with age, from 9 to 16 years. Taking part in bullying others by the internet averaged 3% and by mobile phones 2%. Across the entire sample of European countries, being a victim of cyberbullying via the internet, although averaging 6%, varied by country. The range was from 2% in Italy up to 14% in Estonia.

The Net Children Go Mobile project in 2013 used a follow up version of the EUKO questionnaire in 7 of the 25 countries (i.e., Denmark, Italy, Romania, the UK, Belgium, Ireland, and Portugal) which involved a random stratified sample of approximately 500 internet using 9–16 year old children per country. A similar definition of bullying was used as in the EUKO questionnaire; however, response options were changed to include levels of being upset: 'Yes, and I was very upset', 'Yes, and I was a little upset', 'Yes, but I was not at all upset', 'No, I haven't experienced this'. Victim rates of cyberbullying via the internet ranged from 5% in Portugal to 21% in Denmark. In all countries, victimization rates were somewhat higher than for the EUKO survey conducted in 2010 within the same country, the average increasing from 9% to 12% (Mascheroni & Cuman, 2014).

Using a similar survey, the Latin Kids Online project in Brazil found that 9%, 12%, and 15% reported being victims of online bullying in 2012 (n=1,580, 9–16 year olds), 2013 (n=2,261, 9–17 year olds) and 2014 (n=2,105, 9–17 year olds), respectively (Brazilian Internet Steering Committee, 2015).

The HBSC 2013/2014 Survey and What It Found

The HBSC surveys collect data from 11, 13, and 15 year olds from nationally representative samples every four years, starting in 1993/1994: there is a minimum of 1,500 respondents per age group annually in each participating country. These are classroom-based, anonymous, self-report questionnaire surveys. The reports on bullying have been based on a single victim item and a single bully item, adapted from the Olweus questionnaire, which asks about experiences over the past couple of months, with five standard response options. Victim or bully rates are usually calculated from 'at least two or three times in the past couple of months' or more (thus ignoring 'it only happened once or twice'). A standard definition of bullying is given (mentioning repetition and imbalance of power).

In the most recent survey from 2013/14, HBSC included two additional questions on being a victim of cyberbullying. These were whether someone sent mean instant messages, wall-postings, emails, and text messages or created a website that made fun of them; and whether someone took unflattering or inappropriate pictures of them without permission and posted them online. Responses to the first question were analysed and presented in Inchley et al. (2016), on the basis of being a victim at least two to three times a month. For 11 year olds, the mean value was 3.5%; for 13 year olds, 3.5%; and 15 year olds, 3%. However, there were large country differences. Several countries, such as Greece and Armenia, have low rates of 1% or 2% at each age. Others, notably Russian Federation, Greenland, and Lithuania (the top three at each age group) report rates of around 9%, 8%, and 6% at the three age levels, respectively. In the Annex to the report, data are also provided for rates using the more lenient criterion of being bullied at least once in the past couple of months. This then yields higher prevalence rates. Countries such as Greece and Iceland reported rates of around 3% to 7% (at different ages), whereas countries such as Greenland and Lithuania reported rates of around 20% to 32% (at different ages).

The Annex to Inchley et al. (2016) also provides some data on the second question. For being a victim at least two to three times a month, the average rates were 2%, 3%, and 2% at each age (11, 13, and 15 years). This varied from lows of 0% and 1% in countries such as Greece, to highs of around 5% to 8% in countries such as Bulgaria and Russian Federation. For the criterion of at least once in the past couple of months, the average rates were 7%, 9%, and 9% at each age range. This varied from lows of 2% in countries such as Greece, to highs of around 18% to 20% in countries such as Russian Federation and Lithuania.

Gender Differences

The area of gender differences in cyberbullying has been accurately described as 'fraught with inconsistent findings' (Tokunaga, 2010, p. 280). In their meta-analysis, Kowalski, Giumetti, Schroeder, and Lattanner (2014, p. 54) did not enter gender as a main predictor of cyber perpetrator or victim rates, but did conclude that 'further research is needed in this area to understand the role that gender plays'. In a review of 109 research articles, Barlett and Coyne (2014) found that, for cyberbullying perpetration, overall males did more than females, but this varied by age: up to early adolescence, females did more than males, then, in later adolescence, males did more than females. Besides age, another factor may be type of technological resource by which the cyberbullying takes place (Kowalski et al., 2014). As regards being a victim of cyberbullying, Bauman, Toomey, and Walker (2013) suggest no difference in the proportion of males to females reporting involvement. Examples can be found of boys being more involved than girls (e.g., Calvete, Orue, Estévez, Villardón, & Padilla, 2010), few or no significant differences (e.g., Smith et al., 2008), and girls being more involved than boys (e.g., Rivers & Noret, 2010). The usual finding is that boys are more often involved as victims of traditional bullying (Cook, Williams, Guerra, Kim, & Sadek, 2010), so there may be relatively greater involvement of girls in cyberbullying, just as there is in relational bullying, when compared to traditional physical (mainly boys) or verbal bullying, which is consistent with seeing cyberbullying as more similar to relational bullying.

Gender ratios for cyberbullying do vary by country. Smith, López-Castro, Robinson, and Görzig (2018) analysed the data from EUKO and HBSC to provide ratios for male and female rates for reported cyber victimization (here a ratio of 1 signals equality, more than 1 a male preponderance, and less than 1 a female preponderance). The EUKO data show that girls report more often being a victim of cyberbullying than boys (the boy/girl ratio is 0.78, $t = -4.78$, $p < .001$ over 25 countries (Smith et al., 2018); by contrast the ratio for being an offline victim is 1.07, $t = 1.80$, n.s.). The HBSC data from 2013/14, however, show that boys are more often cyber victims at 11 years (ratio is 1.22, t=2.41, p<.05). This reverses at 13 years (ratio is 0.88, t= -1.44, n.s.) and then reverts to boys more often at 15 years (ratio 1.06, t=0.68, n.s.), but both of the latter were non-significant over the 42 countries involved.

Country Differences

We noted earlier that Genta et al. (2012) found rates of cyber victimization higher in Italy than in England or Spain; yet, Italy came out lowest of all the EU countries sampled (including England and Spain) in the EUKO survey. This signals up the issue of possible discrepancies between surveys as regards country differences in this area.

Previous research findings for both EUKO and HBSC reported country/regional differences in response rates for cyber victimization. It would not be unreasonable to expect that countries would be ranked similarly across these two surveys, given that both are based on self-report data from children of broadly similar ages. However, which countries appear as high or low on cyber victimization are rather different when comparing the two surveys. Data were obtained from the websites of the surveys; plus, for EUKO, from Livingstone et al. (2011a, 2011b), supplemented by additional data from the EuKidsOnline team. Table 4.1 shows the correlations obtained across countries (for the 21 countries they have in common), of the EUKO prevalence measure in each country, with the HBSC prevalence measures for the three ages, and for males and females separately. For example, the top left figure of 0.19 indicates a quite small but positive correlation, across countries, between the EUKO figures and the HBSC figures for 11 year old males – the two surveys tended to agree, but only slightly, on which countries scored high on cyber victimization for this group, and which countries scored low.

The pattern of correlations across countries between EUKO and HBSC is broadly similar for males and females, but varies more by age. For 11 year olds, the correlations are small but positive. However, for 13 year olds and 15 year olds, they are even smaller, but negative. None of the correlations approach significance. These correlations are surprising and disappointing bearing in mind that EUKO and HBSC have 21 countries in common. However, a lack of consensus

TABLE 4.1 Comparing Cyber Victim Prevalence Across Countries for 3 Age Groups, and for Males and Females

	11 years	*13 years*	*15 years*
Males	0.19	-0.06	-0.04
Females	0.13	-0.03	-0.15
Total	0.17	-0.05	-0.09

Note: n=21. Data are from EU Kids Online and HBSC. Correlations are over countries, between the two surveys.

between EUKO and HBSC for victimization rates in bullying generally had been previously noted by Smith, Robinson, and Marchi (2016). Possible reasons are considered below.

As regards gender differences, a comparison between EUKO and HBSC across 21 countries for gender ratios yields correlations of 0.16 for 11 year olds, 0.03 for 13 year olds, and 0.21 for 15 year olds. None of these approach significance. There is essentially very little agreement on gender differences across countries in these two surveys.

The strength of these two surveys is their similarities, in that they have large data sets (1000 participants minimum per country/region), and that there is sufficient overlap of those countries to facilitate, examine, and make comparisons for each country/region. Both surveys collected data on victim rates through the completion of self-report questionnaires. So what might explain the differences/discrepancies in their findings? In fact, a number of challenges face researchers examining cross-national differences. There are challenges even comparing within a survey, and these are augmented when comparing different surveys. We discuss both these sets of issues in turn.

Challenges in Examining Country Differences Within a Survey

Sampling Issues and Non-response Rates

Procedural differences between countries in survey methodology can cause non-random or systematic variations in the data, which can be problematic for the interpretation of cross-national differences. Sampling methods between countries can differ due to appropriate cultural practices. For the EUKO survey, for example, address selection methods differed between countries. A random walk technique was used for most countries, which is the random selection of a seed address from which the interviewer proceeds in a pre-defined route to select the next addresses. For some countries, where the population density was very low, the random walk technique was impractical, so it was complemented by preselecting households from national registers and/or using telephone rather than face-to-face recruitment. Different address selection methods may then imply different degrees of sample representativeness as well as differing causes for non-response.

Response rates can be a source of unaccounted for cross-national differences. There are several sources for non-response and each of them may be susceptible to cultural differences impacting on cross-national differences in survey estimates such as for cyberbullying. Non-response can occur upon making first contact with the potential respondents (contact rates) and when obtaining consent to complete the survey (cooperation rates). In the example of EUKO, contact rates ranged from 31% in Germany to 89% in Romania and cooperation rates from 36% in the Netherlands to 100% in Poland and Greece. Overall response rates ranged from 17% in the Netherlands to 83% in Romania. Some of this variation was related to differences in fieldwork procedures between countries, such as using preselected address registers versus a random walk technique and the number of interviewers employed in each country (Görzig, 2012).

A further related issue is missing responses to the particular survey question addressing cyberbullying. Again, there can be variation in those missing responses between countries that may be associated with methodological issues (e.g., was the parent/guardian present during the interview) or cross-cultural differences in social desirability or other factors not necessarily related to the issue of cyberbullying. To complicate matters, those children whose address could not be contacted, who did not cooperate in the survey, and /or chose not to indicate whether or not they have been a victim of cyberbullying may be more likely to be a victim in some countries and more likely to not be a victim in other countries, making it impossible to appraise the impact of those missing responses on the cross-national differences in cyberbullying reported by the survey.

In the example for EU Kids Online above, measures for sampling methods and response rates showed only a few statistically significant and mostly unproblematic relations between fieldwork indicators and sampling procedures – although the associations with country estimates for cyberbullying were not specifically addressed (Görzig, 2012). Other surveys, such as HBSC, show similar issues of cross-national variations in sampling methods, response rates, and missing responses (Currie et al., 2014). Hence, as unavoidable for most cross-national surveys, country comparisons for both surveys suffer from a certain degree of inaccuracy. Moreover, there will be differences between surveys in the way that those issues affect them, contributing further to cross-survey variations in country differences (Harkness et al., 2010).

Linguistic Issues

Questionnaires are normally given in the native language of the country concerned. A particular issue will be how a word such as *bullying* is translated, since it is a word with a rather precise definition which often has no close equivalent in many other languages (Smith et al., 2002). The HBSC questionnaires use the term *bullying* and give an Olweus-type definition, but no information is provided about how *bullying* is translated in each country. This can make a difference. In Italy, for example, in early research on bullying, terms such as *prepotenza* were often used. This yielded quite high rates of 'bullying', but *prepotenza* has a broader meaning spectrum than *bullying* and picked up more behavioural episodes. Researchers and also the general public in Italy now use the term *il bullismo*, which is defined in the same way as *bullying* (Menesini, 2000). EUKO does not use the term *bullying*, but even words or phrases such as *teasing* or *hurtful or nasty things* may have different shades of meaning when translated into different languages.

Setting and Social Desirability

Survey responses may be affected by differences in perception/response rather than in the phenomenon itself. Guillaume and Funder (2016) review a number of such challenges. Administration bias refers to how aspects of the setting and administration of the survey may impact differently depending on culture – for example, what the physical setting is like, whether testing is on- or off-line, and how the presence and attitude of the researcher may affect responses. Response styles refer to how participants may tend to give socially desirable responses, or how they use scales or engage in extreme responding; these may vary by culture. Responses may also be influenced by reference group effects, whereby one compares oneself to the norms of the culture one is in. Administration procedures (see below) may also interact with country comparisons if they are not consistent across different countries in the survey.

Challenges in Examining Country Differences Between Surveys

There is a set of further issues involved in comparing different surveys, which may account for the discrepancies in findings between EUKO and HBSC. These include age range, sampling issues, dates of surveys, administration of survey, definition of cyberbullying, time reference period, types of cyber victimization assessed, and frequency scale.

Age

EUKO gathered data from young people ranging from the ages of 9 to 16, while HBSC collected data from more specific age groups (i.e., 11, 13, and 15 year olds, with boys and girls separately). Thus, both surveys collected data from young people primarily at secondary school level; however, EUKO also collected data which includes students at primary school level (aged 9–10 years old). If countries differed in terms of how age related to risk of cyber victimization, this would lead to discrepancies.

Sampling Issues

Both surveys collected data from relatively large samples. EUKO had about 1000 participants per country. HBSC had a minimum of 1500 participants per country; a nationally representative sample was drawn and, where it was not possible, a regional one was drawn (Roberts et al., 2009). Notably, EUKO only sampled young people with access to the internet; this was not a participation criterion for HBSC. Although internet penetration is now very high in most countries, it does vary; for example, during the EUKO survey period, it was estimated to vary from 55% in Italy, 87% in France, to 98% in the UK (Livingstone et al., 2011b).

Countries low in internet penetration might yield lower cyber victimization rates in HBSC (where those without internet would be included) than in EUKO (where they would be excluded).

Dates of the Survey

EUKO data collection was in 2009/2010 and the latest HBSC survey in 2013/2014. While only four years apart, it could be that increasing awareness of intervention and prevention programmes impact on the prevalence of victimization over time (see for example Waasdorp, Pas, Zablotsky, & Bradshaw, 2017, for an example of longitudinal change in Maryland, USA). Especially as regards cyberbullying, technological advances with young people having much easier access to the internet via smart phones and tablets and freer access to all sorts of cyber platforms may also affect countries differentially over even a four year period.

Even when dates of surveys are similar, regional or national events in a country may impact on survey responses (cf. Stoop, 2007); these might be new legal requirements, or new national anti-bullying interventions, for example.

Administration Procedures

If procedural issues vary by country, they may impact on cross-national differences in cyberbullying. These include the type of interview administration (e.g., paper and pencil or computer-administered), and the timing and length of the fieldwork period (e.g., school term or holiday periods). For example, computer based questionnaires mostly contain automatic routing while, in paper and pencil version, the respondent needs to filter out irrelevant content themselves. This means that, in some countries, children, who previously responded they had not been bullied at all, may not have been exposed to the follow up question on cyber victimization while in other countries all children will have received that question. As another example, if children were interviewed during the school holidays, responses may have been lower due to a reduced interaction with their peers in general. If the fieldwork took place during school holidays for some countries but not others, responses might not be equally comparable.

Both EUKO and HBSC surveys were completed using pupil self-report; however, there were differences in how these self-report surveys were administered. HBSC conducted whole school administrations with questionnaires that were long and contained questions covering many health and educational related topics. Respondent fatigue could be a factor, which might vary by country. Also, HBSC surveys were completed by the young person in class. Being in the presence of peers that may have been involved in cyberbullying episodes with the respondent might have an impact on responses, despite whatever precautions regarding confidentiality are taken. In contrast, EUKO conducted face-to-face interviews with the young person followed by a self-report questionnaire. These interviews were usually conducted in the young person's home with a parent present in the vicinity as part of the survey, and it is possible that this parental presence had an impact on responses from the young person.

Definition of Cyberbullying

EUKO and HBSC differed in how they asked about bullying and cyberbullying. In particular, the imbalance of power aspect in the Olweus definition used by HBSC was absent from the preamble provided by EUKO. Repetition and power imbalance are widely considered as defining criteria for bullying, but are debated when it comes to the definition of cyberbullying (Slonje et al., 2013).

Time Reference Period

For EUKO, the time reference period was the past 12 months. For HBSC 2013/14, the time reference period was the last couple of months. Time reference period obviously impacts on prevalence rates, but may also impact on the kinds of incidents reported; a pupil may preferentially report serious impact events if asked about a long time period, but regard less serious incidents as more relevant if the time reference period is short (Schwarz & Oyserman, 2001). Time reference periods may also interact with age, with younger children usually taking shorter time spans into account than older children. What is particularly at issue here is whether the effect of these variables may differ by country – for example, drawing on Hofstede categories, is time reference period going to have more of an influence in long-term orientation societies?

Types of Bullying Assessed

EUKO participants were asked if 'someone acted in this kind of hurtful or nasty way to you in the past 12 months?' by mobile phone (text, calls, image/video texts) or on the internet (social networking sites, instant messaging, email, gaming websites, chat room, some other way on the internet). HBSC asked if they had been a victim through someone sending mean instant messages, wall-postings, emails, and text message or had created a website that made fun of them; or if someone took unflattering or inappropriate pictures of them without permission and posted them online. While for the EUKO survey, it was made explicit that 'this kind of hurtful or nasty way' included 'leaving someone out of things', social exclusion is not explicitly pronounced in the HBSC items. In contrast, the HBSC includes 'inappropriate pictures', while the EUKO survey dedicated other sections of the questionnaire to sexual images and sexual messages that are separate from the bullying section.

We know that the relative frequency of different types of bullying does vary between countries – for example, between England (more physical) and Japan (more relational) (Kanetsuna, 2016). Clearly, if surveys weight different types of bullying to different extents, and countries vary in this too, some survey discrepancies will result.

Frequency Scale

Both surveys used frequency scales to report victim experiences, but they differed slightly. EUKO participants are asked to choose one of six options: every day or almost every day, once or twice a week, once or twice a month, less often, never, or don't know. HBSC participants are asked to choose one of five options: I have not been bullied in this way in the past couple of months; only once or twice; 2 or 3 times a month; about once a week; several times a week. While probably a minor factor, this could cause survey discrepancies if countries vary in the way cyber victim responses are distributed along the frequency spectrum.

Explanations for Country Differences

Even though agreement on country differences between EUKO and HBSC is very low, it appears that there are large country differences. How might they be explained? We suggest that the model proposed by EUKO, and shown in Figure 4.1, can be a useful way forward. Put forward as a framework for looking at internet risks, it is suitable for looking at causes of cyberbullying at various levels. Adopting an ecological

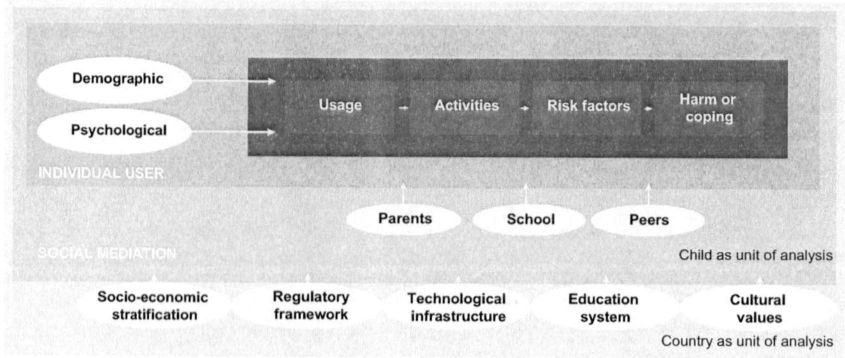

FIGURE 4.1 EU Kids Online model
Source: Livingstone, Haddon, Görzig, & Ólafsson (2011a)

perspective, it includes factors about the individual user, their social network (parents, peers, school), and broader country factors.

The country level comprises five aspects: Cultural values (e.g., power distance, tradition, benevolence, individualism vs. collectivism); Education system (e.g., levels by age, grade retention, class groupings, school and class size, structure of school day, break times, and supervision); Technological infrastructure (e.g., penetration of mobile phones, smart phones, and internet); Regulatory framework (e.g., school policies, legal aspects, anti-bullying initiatives); and, Socio-economic stratification (e.g., income, internet access, health, crime). We consider these in turn. There is rather little evidence directly related to cyberbullying, so we also mention evidence related to traditional bullying, given the large overlap between the two (Kowalski et al., 2014).

Cultural Values (e.g., Power Distance, Tradition, Benevolence, Individualism vs. Collectivism)

Hofstede, Hofstede, and Minkov (2010) proposed six main dimensions of cultural values: power distance, individualism-collectivism, masculinity-femininity, uncertainty avoidance, long-term orientation, and indulgence vs. restraint. Predictions can be made about how these affect bully and victim rates (Campbell, Kettle, & Sundaram, 2018; Smith, Kwak, & Toda, 2016). For example, victim and bully rates are predicted to be higher in more individualist (IDV) societies (less social cohesion: Ji, Zhang, & Jones, 2016). In contrast, Migliaccio and Rauskauskas (2015) informally compared countries on HBSC data, finding bullying *lower* in high IDV countries. In work in progress, we have confirmed this counter-predicted finding systematically, for HBSC, EUKO, GSHS, and TIMSS data; we hypothesized this was due to greater regulatory framework in higher individualist societies, but this is, as yet, untested.

Considering other Hofstede dimensions, predictions could be made regarding Power distance (this might affect the proportions of same-age or cross-age bullying), Masculinity-Femininity (this might affect the extent of male-female differences in bullying), and Uncertainty avoidance (bias, prejudice or identity-based (cyber)bullying can be predicted to be higher in high Uncertainty Avoidance (UAI) societies) (Smith, Kwak, & Toda, 2016). Besides Hofstede categories, categories from Schwartz (2006) and Gelfand (Gelfand et al., 2011) might be considered.

Education System (e.g., Levels by Age, Grade Retention, Class Groupings, School and Class Size, Structure of School Day, Break Times, and Supervision)

These have been reviewed systematically by Jessel (2016). Some effects on victim and bully rates have been documented; for example, Kanetsuna (2016) invoked use of home room classes, and supervision of break times, in explaining differences between *ijime* in Japan and *bullying* in England. Grade retention, whereby pupils performing less well are held back in a grade, has been linked to bullying rates in Portugal (Pereira, Mendonça, Neto, Valente, & Smith, 2004).

Technological Infrastructure (e.g., Penetration of Mobile Phones, Smart Phones, and Internet; Violent Media Exposure)

This is clearly very relevant for cyberbullying. From EUKO data, Helsper, Kalmus, Hasebrink, Sagvari, and de Haan (2013) derived a four-fold classification: supported risky explorers; semi-supported risky gamers; unprotected networkers; and 'protected by restrictions'. Use of other media beyond the internet may be important: Calvete et al. (2010), in Spain, and Fanti, Demetriou, and Hawa (2012), in Cyprus, found links from violent media exposure (on television, internet, movies, video games), to both cyberbullying and cyber victimization, and Hamer, Konijn, and Keijer (2014) suggested a 'Cyclic Process' model of this.

Regulatory Framework (e.g., School Policies, Legal Aspects, Anti-bullying Initiatives)

There is limited evidence on the quality of school anti-bullying policies affecting general victim rates (Smith et al., 2012). In the USA, Hatzenbuehler, Schwab-Reese, Ranapurwala, Hertz, and Ramirez (2015) found that having some anti-bullying laws was associated with reduced rates of being both bullied and cyberbullied across 25 states. Ramirez, Ten Eyck, Peek-Asa, Onwuachi-Willig, and Cavanaugh (2016) found an increase in victim rates in Iowa after an anti-bullying law was introduced, possibly due to increased reporting, but then a decrease for offline but not online victim rates.

Socio-economic Stratification (e.g., Income, Internet Access, Health, Crime)

These have been examined primarily with HBSC data. In relation to bullying generally (using earlier surveys), prevalence rates have been linked to lower country wealth (Chaux, Molano, & Podlesky, 2009; Elgar et al., 2009; Viner et al., 2012) and greater income inequality (Elgar et al., 2009; Elgar, Craig, Boyce, Morgan, & Vella-Zarb, 2015; Viner et al., 2012). For being a cyber victim specifically, Inchley et al. (2016) examined family affluence as a factor in cyber victimization rates; they reported a relationship in a few countries and regions, but, of those that did show a relationship, more cyberbullying was generally reported by those with lower affluence. Using a sample of 18 countries from EUKO, Görzig, Milosevic, and Staksrud (2017) found that regional level cyber victimization rates were positively linked with GDP and crime rates, while they showed a negative relationship with life expectancy and population density.

Social Dominance Theory

Social Dominance Theory (SDT; Pratto, Sidanius, & Levin, 2006) is a complex theoretical framework of intergroup relations derived from the observation that societies are organised in group-based hierarchies. More than a decade of research has supported arguments that social power imbalances originate from multiple levels (e.g., cultural policies and practices as well as individual relations). Power imbalances on the individual level (e.g., bullying) have been linked with power imbalances on cultural contextual levels. Developmental researchers have used SDT to explain general forms of bullying that include both physical and social aggression (Walcott, Upton, Bolen, & Brown, 2008). Addressing multiple levels of the socio-ecological system while explicitly proposing mechanisms that maintain social power imbalances, SDT lends itself well to make predictions about the directions of the effects for the factors proposed within the EUKO model.

It is proposed that culturally shared ideologies (i.e., legitimising myths) exist to maintain or enhance societal hierarchies. For example, it is argued that the predominantly Western value of individual achievement would enhance social comparison processes leading to individual discrimination (ingroup favouritism) (Pratto, Sidanius, Stallworth, & Malle, 1994) (cf. Hofstede's individualism). On the contextual level, legitimising myths can be linked with cultural values and attitudes towards social equality. For example, attitudes towards equality have been found to be inversely linked with cyberbullying rates on the country-level within EUKO (Görzig & Machackova, 2016). SDT links social hierarchies with institutional discrimination (discrimination by governmental and business institutions); this relates to fewer resources for low hierarchy group members (e.g., health provision, income, education) as well as differential treatment by the authorities (e.g., longer prison sentences, higher police violence). Some of those variables have already established links with bullying prevalence rates (e.g., GDP, life expectancy; see above), but further indicators may need to be explored more systematically. Predictions can be derived for contextual level factors relating to socio-economic stratification (e.g., income inequality), technological infrastructure (e.g., digital divide), education system (e.g., educational disparity), as well as regulatory framework (e.g., human rights and welfare).

Summary and Suggestions for Future Research

While there have been several small-scale studies of country differences in cyberbullying, large-scale surveys across many countries are currently limited to two – EUKO and HBSC. Unfortunately, although both are based on pupil self-report, agreement between them on country differences in cyberbullying is slight. This parallels the situation regarding bullying generally, including other large-scale surveys as well (Smith, Robinson, & Marchi, 2016).

Many factors can affect cross-national comparisons, both within a survey and between surveys, and we have outlined what we consider to be the most relevant. What is important in considering these is whether any particular factor interacts with country. For example, consider types of cyberbullying, which are mentioned somewhat differently in the EUKO and HBSC surveys. This would matter if the pattern of different types of cyberbullying varies between countries. For example, consider two countries X and Y with similar rates of overall cyberbullying. If, in country X, social exclusion types of cyberbullying were relatively more frequent, compared to country Y where posting inappropriate pictures was more common, then country X will tend to score higher in the EUKO survey but country Y in the HBSC survey. However, we know rather little about how the various factors identified vary in importance across countries, and more research is needed here.

Even if EUKO and HBSC disagree on country differences, we can be rather confident that they exist. The range of prevalence rates across countries is very large, typically varying by a factor of 7 or more, depending on survey and criteria. This huge range requires explanation, and we propose the EUKO model as an entry point to investigating this. The five factors in the EUKO model at the country level can be studied in relation to EUKO data for both cyber victim and cyberbully rates and HBSC data for online victim rates only. But to do so effectively, a better understanding of discrepancies between surveys is needed. Building such comprehensive models at the country level has not yet been attempted. This should be a target for future research.

References

Aoyama, I., Utsumi, S., & Hasegawa, M. (2011). Cyberbullying in Japan. In Q. Li, D. Cross, & P. K. Smith (Eds.), *Cyberbullying in the global playground: Research from international perspectives* (pp. 183–201). Chichester, England: Wiley-Blackwell.

Barlett, C. & Coyne, S. M. (2014). A meta-analysis of sex differences in cyber-bullying behavior: The moderating role of age. *Aggressive Behavior, 40*, 474–488. doi:10.1002/ab.21555

Barlett, C.P., Gentile, D.A., Anderson, C.A., Suzuki, K., Sakamoto, A., Yamaoka, A., & Katsura, R. (2014). Cross-cultural differences in cyberbullying behavior: A short-term longitudinal study. *Journal of Cross-Cultural Psychology, 45*, 300–313. doi:10.1177/0022022113504622.

Bauman, S., Toomey, R.B., & Walker, J. (2013). Associations among bullying, cyberbullying, and suicide in high school students. *Journal of Adolescence, 36*, 341–350.

Brazilian Internet Steering Committee – CGI.br (2015). *Survey on Internet Use by Children in Brazil – ICT Kids Online Brazil 2014.* São Paulo: CGI.br. Retrieved from www.lse.ac.uk/media@lse/research/EUKidsOnline/EUKidsIV/PDF/TIC-K
ids-2014-livro-eletronico.pdf

Calvete, E., Orue, I., Estévez, A., Villardón, L., & Padilla, P. (2010). Cyberbullying in adolescents: Modalities and aggressors' profile. *Computers in Human Behavior, 26*, 1128–1135.

Campbell, M., Kettle, M., & Sunduram, S. (2018). Societal and cultural considerations in understanding peer bullying in India. In P. K. Smith, S. Sundaram, B. Spears, B. Blaya, M. Schafer, & D. Sandhu (Eds.), *Bullying, cyberbullying and pupil well-being in schools:*

Comparing European, Australian and Indian perspectives. Cambridge: Cambridge University Press.

Chaux, E., Molano, A., & Podlesky, P. (2009). Socio-economic, socio-political and socio-emotional variables explaining school bullying: A country-wide multilevel analysis. *Aggressive Behavior, 35*, 520–529.

Cook, C. R., Williams, K. R., Guerra, N. G., Kim, T. E., & Sadek, S. (2010). Predictors of bullying and victimization in childhood and adolescence: A meta-analytic investigation. *School Psychology Quarterly, 25*(2), 65–83. doi:10.1037/a0020149

Currie, C., Inchley, J., Molcho, M., Lenzi, M., Veselska, Z., & Wild, F. (Eds.). (2014). *Health Behaviour in School-aged Children (HBSC) Study Protocol: Background, Methodology and Mandatory items for the 2013/14 Survey*. St Andrews: CAHRU.

Elgar, F. J., Craig, W., Boyce, W., Morgan, A., & Vella-Zarb, R. (2009). Income inequality and school bullying: Multilevel study of adolescents in 37 countries. *Journal of Adolescent Health, 45*, 351–359.

Elgar, F.J., McKinnon, B., Walsh, S.D., Freeman, J., Donnelly, P.D., de Matos, M.G. ... Currie, C. (2015). Structural determinants of youth bullying and fighting in 79 countries. *Journal of Adolescent Health, 57*, 643–650.

Fanti, K.A., Demetriou, A.G., & Hawa, V.V. (2012). A longitudinal study of cyberbullying: Examining risk and protective factors. *European Journal of Developmental Psychology, 9*, 168–181.

Gelfand, M. J., Raver, J. L., Nishii, L., Leslie, L. M., Lun, J., Lim, B. C., ... Yamaguchi, S. (2011). Differences between tight and loose cultures: A 33-nation study. *Science, 332*, 1100–1104.

Genta, M. L., Smith, P. K.Ortega, R., Brighi, A., Guarini, A., Thompson, F., ... Calmaestra, J. (2012). Comparative aspects of cyberbullying in Italy, England and Spain: findings from a DAPHNE Project. In Q. Li, D. Cross, & P. K. Smith (Eds), *Cyberbullying in the global playground: Research from international perspectives* (pp. 15–31). Chichester: Wiley-Blackwell.

Görzig, A. & Machackova, H. (2016). Cyberbullying in Europe: A review of evidence from cross-national data. In M. Wright (Ed.), *A social-ecological approach to cyberbullying* (Chapter 17). Hauppauge, NY: Nova Science.

Görzig, A. (2012). Methodological framework: The EU Kids Online project. In S. Livingstone, L. Haddon, & A. Görzig (Eds.), *Children, risk and safety online: Research and policy challenges in comparative perspective* (pp. 15–32). Bristol: The Policy Press.

Görzig, A., Milosevic, T., & Staksrud, E. (2017). Cyberbullying victimisation in context: The role of social inequalities in countries and regions. *Journal of Cross-Cultural Psychology, 48*(8), 1198–1215.

Guillaume, E., & Funder, D. (2016). Theoretical and methodological issues in making cross-national and cross-cultural comparisons. In P.K. Smith, K. Kwak, & Y. Toda (Eds.), *School bullying in different cultures: Eastern and western perspectives* (pp. 211–228). Cambridge: Cambridge University Press.

Hamer, A. den, Konijn, E. A., & Keijer, M. G. (2014). Cyberbullying behavior and adolescents' use of medias with antisocial content: A cyclic process model. *Cyberpsychology, Behavior, and Social Networking, 17*, 74–81.

Harkness, J. A., Braun, M., Edwards, B., Johnson, T. P., Lyberg, L., Mohler, P. P. ... Smith, T. W. (2010). *Survey methods in multinational, multiregional, and multicultural contexts*. Hoboken, NJ: Wiley.

Hatzenbuehler, M. L., Schwab-Reese, L., Ranapurwala, S. I., Hertz, M. F., & Ramirez, M. R. (2015). Associations between antibullying policies and bullying in 25 states. *JAMA Pediatrics, 169*(10), e152411.

Helsper, E. J., Kalmus, V., Hasebrink, U., Sagvari, B. & de Haan, J. (2013). *Country classification: Opportunities, risks, harm and parental mediation*. London: EU Kids Online, LSE.

Hofstede, G., Hofstede, G. J., & Minkov, M. (2010). *Cultures and organizations: Software of the mind*. New York: McGraw-Hill.

Inchley, J., Currie, D., Young, T., Samdal, O., Torsheim, T., Augustson, L., … Barnekow, V. (Eds.) (2016). *Growing up unequal: Gender and socioeconomic differences in young people's health and well-being: Health Behaviour in School-aged Children (HBSC) study: International report from the 2013/2014 survey*. Copenhagen: WHO Regional Office for Europe.

Jessel, J. (2016). Educational systems: A basis for some comparative perspective. In P.K. Smith, K. Kwak, & Y. Toda (Eds.), *School bullying in different cultures: Eastern and western perspectives* (pp. 229–258). Cambridge: Cambridge University Press.

Ji, L., Zhang, W. & Jones, K. (2016). Children's experience of and attitudes towards bullying and victimization: A cross-cultural comparison between China and England. In P. K. Smith, K. Kwak, & Y. Toda (Eds.), *School bullying in different cultures: Eastern and western perspectives* (pp. 170–188). Cambridge: Cambridge University Press.

Kanetsuna, T. (2016). Comparisons between English bullying and Japanese ijime. In P.K. Smith, K. Kwak, & Y. Toda (Eds.), *School bullying in different cultures: Eastern and western perspective* (pp. 153–169). Cambridge: Cambridge University Press.

Kowalski, R. M., Giumetti, G. W., Schroeder, A. N., & Lattanner, M. R. (2014). Bullying in the digital age: A critical review and meta-analysis of cyberbullying research among youth. *Psychological Bulletin, 140*, 1073–1137. doi:10.1037/a0035618

Livingstone, S., Haddon, L., Görzig, A., & Ólafsson, K. (2011a). *Risks and safety on the internet: The perspective of European children: Full findings*. London, UK: EU Kids Online, London School of Economics and Political Science: EU Kids Online.

Livingstone, S., Haddon, L. G., Görzig, A., & Olafsson, K. (2011b). *Technical Report and User Guide: The 2010 EU Kids Online Survey*. London, UK: London School of Economics and Political Science.

Livingstone, S., Stoilova, M., & Kelly, A. (2016). Cyberbullying: Incidence, trends and consequences. In *Ending the torment: Tackling bullying from the schoolyard to cyberspace* (pp. 115–120). New York: United Nations Office of the Special Representative of the Secretary-General on Violence against Children.

Mascheroni, G., & Cuman, A. (2014). *Net Children Go Mobile: Final Report* (with country fact sheets). Deliverables D6.4 and D5.2. Milano: Educatt. Retrieved from netchildrengomobile.eu/ncgm/wp-content/uploads/2013/07/NCGM_FinalReport_Country_DEF.pdf

Menesini, E. (Ed.). (2000). *Bullismo: Che fare?*Florence: Giunti.

Migliaccio, T., & Rauskauskas, J. (2015). *Bullying as a social experience: Social factors, prevention and intervention*. London: Routledge.

Monks, C. P., Ortega, R., Robinson, S., & Worlidge, P. (2009). Cyberbullying among primary school-aged pupils. *Kwartalnik Pedagogiczny*, 214, 167–181.

Olweus, D. (1999). Norway. In P. K. Smith, Y. Morita, J. Junger-Tas, D. Olweus, R. Catalano, & P. Slee (Eds.), *The nature of school bullying. A cross-national perspective* (pp. 28–48). London: Routledge.

Pereira, B., Mendonça, D., Neto, C., Valente, L., & Smith, P. K. (2004). Bullying in Portuguese schools. *School Psychology International, 25*, 241–254.

Pratto, F., Sidanius, J., & Levin, S. (2006). Social dominance theory and the dynamics of intergroup relations: Taking stock and looking forward. *European Review of Social Psychology, 17*(1), 271–320.

Pratto, F., Sidanius, J., Stallworth, L. M., & Malle, B. F. (1994). Social dominance orientation: A personality variable predicting social and political attitudes. *Journal of Personality and Social Psychology, 67*(4), 741–763.

Ramirez, M., Ten Eyck, P., Peek-Asa, C., Onwuachi-Willig, A. & Cavanaugh, J. E. (2016). Evaluation of Iowa's anti-bullying law. *Injury Epidemiology, 3*(1), 15.

Rivers, I. & Noret, N. (2010). 'I h8 u': Findings from a five year study of text and email bullying. *British Educational Research Journal, 36*, 643–671.

Roberts, C., Freeman, J., Samdal, O., Schnohr, C., Looze, M., Nic Gabhainn, S., & Iannotti, R. (2009). The Health Behaviour in School-aged Children (HBSC) study: Methodological developments and current tensions. *International Journal of Public Health, 54*(Suppl 2), 140–150. doi:10.1007/s00038-009-5405-9

Schwarz, N., & Oyserman, D. (2001). Asking questions about behavior: Cognition, communication, and questionnaire construction. *American Journal of Evaluation, 22*(2), 127–160. doi:10.1016/S1098-2140(01)00133-3

Schwartz, S. H. (2006). Value orientations: Measurement, antecedents and consequences across nations. In R. Jowell, C. Roberts, R. Fitzgerald, & G. Eva (Eds.), *Measuring attitudes cross-nationally - lessons from the European Social Survey* (pp. 161–193). London: Sage.

Ševčíková, A., & Šmahel, D. (2009). Online harassment and cyberbullying in the Czech Republic: Comparison across age groups. *Zeitschrift Für Psychologie/Journal of Psychology, 217*(4), 227–229. doi:10.1027/0044-3409.217.4.227

Sittichai, R., & Smith, P.K. (2015). Bullying in South-East Asian countries: A review. *Aggression and Violent Behavior, 23*, 22–35.

Slonje, R., Smith, P. K., & Frisén, A. (2013). The nature of cyberbullying, and strategies for prevention. *Computers in Human Behavior, 29*(1), 26–32.

Smith, P. K. (2014). *Understanding school bullying: Its nature & prevention strategies*. London: Sage.

Smith, P. K., & Berkkun, F. (2017). How research on cyberbullying has developed. In C. Mc Guckin & L. Corcoran (Eds.). *Bullying and cyberbullying: Prevalence, psychological impacts and intervention strategies* (pp. 11–27). Hauppauge, NY: Nova Science.

Smith, P. K., Cowie, H., Olafsson, R., & Liefooghe, A. (2002). Definitions of bullying: a comparison of terms used, and age and sex differences, in a 14-country international comparison. *Child Development, 73*, 1119–1133.

Smith, P.K., Kupferberg, A., Mora-Merchan, J.A., Samara, M., Bosley, S., & Osborn, R. (2012). A content analysis of school anti-bullying policies: A follow-up after six years. *Educational Psychology in Practice, 28*, 61–84.

Smith, P.K., Kwak, K. & Toda, Y. (2016). Reflections on bullying in eastern and western perspectives. In P.K. Smith, K. Kwak, & Y. Toda (Eds.), *School bullying in different cultures: Eastern and western perspectives* (pp. 399–419). Cambridge: Cambridge University Press.

Smith, P.K., & López-Castro, L. (2017). Cross-national data on victims of bullying: How does PISA measure up with other surveys? *International Journal of Developmental Science, 11*, 87–92.

Smith, P.K., López-Castro, L., Robinson, S., & Görzig, A. (2018). Consistency of gender differences in bullying in different cross-cultural surveys. *Aggression and Violent Behavior*. Advance online publication. doi:10.1016/j.avb.2018. 04. 006

Smith, P. K., Mahdavi, J. M., Carvahlo, M., Fisher, S., Russell, S., & Tippett, N. (2008). Cyberbullying: Its nature and impact in secondary school pupils. *Journal of Child Psychology and Psychiatry, 49*(4), 376–385. doi:10.1111/j.1469-7610.2007.01846.x

Smith, P. K., Robinson, S., & Marchi, B. (2016). Cross-national data on victims of bullying: What is really being measured? *International Journal of Developmental Science, 10*, 9–19. doi:10.3233/DEV-150174

Smith, P. K., Sundaram, S., Spears, B., Blaya, C., Schafer, M., & Sandhu, D. (Eds.). (2018). *Bullying, cyberbullying and pupil well-being in schools: Comparing European, Australian and Indian Perspectives*. Cambridge: Cambridge University Press.

Stoop, I. (2007). If it bleeds, it leads: The impact of media-reported events. In R. Jowell, C. Roberts, R. Fitzgerald, and G. Eva (Eds.), *Measuring attitudes cross-nationally. Lessons from the European Social Survey* (pp. 95–111). London: SAGE.

Tokunaga, R. (2010). Following you home from school: A critical review and synthesis of research on cyberbullying victimisation. *Computers in Human Behaviour, 26*, 277–287.

Tomazin, F., & Smith, B. (2007). *The bully you can't see*. Retrieved from www.theage.com.au/news/in-depth/the-bully-you-cant-see/2007/03/09/1173166983566.html?page=fullpage

UK Safer Internet Centre (2017) *Appropriate filtering and monitoring*. Retrieved from www.saferinternet.org.uk/advice-centre/teachers-and-school-staff/appropriate-filtering-a nd-monitoring (accessed 4 January 2018).

Viner, R. M., Ozer, E. M., Denny, S., Marmot, M., Resnick, M., Fatusi, A., & Currie, C. (2012). Adolescence and the social determinants of health. *The Lancet, 379*(9826), 1641–1652.

Waasdorp, T. E., Pas, E. T., Zablotsky, B., & Bradshaw, C. P. (2017). Ten-year trends in bullying and related attitudes among 4th- to 12th-graders. *Pediatrics, 139*, e20162615. doi:10.1542/peds.2016–2615

Walcott, C. M., Upton, A., Bolen, L., & Brown, M. B. (2008). Associations between peer-perceived status and aggression in young adolescents. *Psychology in the Schools, 45*, 550–561.

Wright, M.F., Aoyama, I., Shanmukh V. Kamble, S.V., Li, Z., Soudi, S. … Shu, C. (2015). Peer attachment and cyber aggression involvement among Chinese, Indian, and Japanese adolescents. *Societies, 5*, 339–353.

Zych, I., Ortega-Ruiz, R., & del Rey, R. (2015). Scientific research on bullying and cyberbullying: Where have we been and where are we going. *Aggression and Violent Behavior, 23*, 1–21.

5

CYBERBULLYING IN SCHOOLS

Developmental Perspectives

Elizabeth Englander

Cyberbullying – a form of intentional, repeated aggression, using electronic forms of contact, such as text messaging and social media (Hinduja & Patchin, 2010; Smith et al., 2008) – is a developmentally mediated problem. This chapter will review the differences in cyberbullying prevalence between children of different ages, and will explore some plausible reasons for those differences.

Aggression in general varies between children of different ages, and becomes significantly more common as youth begin to enter adolescence (Liu, Lewis, & Evans, 2013). Unlike research on other types of aggression, however, comparing the prevalence of cyberbullying across studies examining children of different ages is exceptionally challenging because there is no consensus definition of cyberbullying used by researchers (Englander, Donnerstein, Kowalski, Lin, & Parti, 2017). One key question is the similarity and overlap between traditional bullying and cyberbullying. Factors such as intention, repetition, and power imbalance are much more easily identified in traditional bullying, relative to digital behaviors. Still, most researchers who have examined bullying and cyberbullying find that the two behaviors are clearly correlated, suggesting that there is at minimum a substantial amount of co-morbidity (Kowalski, 2015; Ybarra, Espelage, & Mitchell, 2014). Yet the nature and degree of that co-morbidity is still very unclear. Some researchers regard cyberbullying as simply bullying that occurs using digital technology. Others focus their definition on the more observable digital elements and omit others, such as power imbalance, that are central characteristics of traditional bullying but that can be difficult to assess in a digital environment (Patchin & Hinduja, 2006; Ybarra & Chen, 2015).

Further, unlike other types of aggressive behaviors, cyberbullying prevalence is probably mediated by factors such as education regarding the appropriate use of digital technology, and the type of hardware used (Anderson, 2015; Pelfrey &

Weber, 2015). Cyberbullying is a unique form of aggression in these ways. Its obvious reliance on digital technology renders it a form of communication that may, at times, lend itself to aggression or at least miscommunication. As an example, the repetitive nature of communication "threads" (i.e., typed out conversations that are sent in their entirety repeatedly) may increase the intensity of negative emotions (Englander, 2015a; Varjas, Talley, Meyers, Parris, & Cutts, 2010). The availability of digital technology outside of school means that bullies can continue to torment their victims 24/7 (Kowalski, 2015). Victims may not be able to escape the bullying for a mental health respite (Slonje, Smith, & Frisén, 2012). Still, as noted above, digital behaviors are clearly not completely separate from traditional bullying. Most children who are cyberbullied are also bullied in school (Cross, Lester, & Barnes, 2015).

Prevalence Among Children of Different Ages

It must be noted, first and foremost, that even after excluding extreme outliers, prevalence estimates of cyberbullying are significantly varied. Resolving the differences in the definition of cyberbullying utilized between different studies is beyond the scope of this chapter. In addition, the date of the research in question matters, since the rapid and dramatic changes in technology probably render pre-2010 and post-2010 prevalence studies incomparable. For example, teenage owners of clamshell style phones use their devices differently, compared to owners of smartphones (Anderson, 2015). While this may seem like hardware minutiae, how people behave in digital environments changes as hardware changes (Lenhart, 2015). Consider, for example, the effort involved in texting on a flip phone (where each key represents three different letters) versus a smartphone (where a text can even be dictated if desired). As behaviors like texting become simpler, they are engaged in more frequently. Focusing, therefore, on studies done after 2010, most estimates of the prevalence of cyberbullying among adolescents range between roughly 15% and 50% reporting victimization. One meta-analysis of 80 studies from several countries found that the average adolescent victimization prevalence rate was approximately 15% (Modecki, Minchin, Harbaugh, Guerra, & Runions, 2014). Another study that examined more than 20,000 high school students found similar rates of almost 16% (Kessel Schneider, O'Donnell, Stueve, & Coulter, 2012).

Other studies have found higher rates. In 2016, Patchin and Hinduja reviewed prevalence estimates across a variety of studies. Almost all studies reviewed examined children aged 11 or older, although a few included 10-year-olds in their samples. Lifetime prevalence rates varied between 24.1% and 34.6%, with three studies reporting numbers in the 30s and two reporting numbers in the mid- and high-20s. A 2011 retrospective study of several hundred college students found that 41% reported being victims of cyberbullying at some point during the four years of high school (Englander, 2012). Another survey of middle and high school students (n = 2,186) found that slightly fewer than half (49.5%)

indicated they had been bullied online and 33.7% indicated they had bullied others online (Mishna, Cook, Gadalla, Daciuk, & Solomon, 2010).

The above studies focused on prevalence among adolescents. Studies of younger students in North America have generally found possibly even more varied prevalence estimates of victimization. A study of 665 subjects examined middle school students, and found that approximately 20% reported being cyberbullied, with more than half of these victims reporting repeated cyberbullied within the last 30 days (Holfeld & Grabe, 2012). Another study of 660 Midwestern American children in grades 3, 4, and 5 found that almost 18% reported cyberbullying victimization, and further, that such victimization was related to victimization in school through traditional bullying (DePaolis & Williford, 2014). A study of Canadian 10- to 12-year-olds (4, 5, and 6 grades) found that 27% reported, at the end of the school year, that they had experienced cyberbullying victimization during the preceding school year (Holfeld & Leadbeater, 2015).

A handful of other studies on younger children have been completed in the United Kingdom and Europe. In one sample of 7- to 11-year-olds in the U.K., 23% reported being a victim of cyberbullying (Monks, Robinson, & Worlidge, 2012). The Anti-Bullying Alliance found in their research that about 20% of 10- to 11-year-olds were cyberbullied (ABA, 2009). Another study of British children (116 boys and 104 girls) aged 7 to 11 years found that 21% self-identified as cyber victims and 5% reported perpetrating cyberbullying (Monks et al., 2012). A study of 372 Turkish children aged 8 to 11 years old found that 27% of the children studied were victims of cyberbullying; 18% reported being cyberbullying perpetrators; and an additional 15% reported being both cyber bully/victims (Arslan, Savaser, Hallett, & Balci, 2012). Finally, a study of 1,141 students aged 6–11 years old found that 25% reported being cyberbullied at least monthly (Ybarra, Boyd, Korchmaros, & Oppenheim, 2012).

Yet other studies of elementary school-aged samples have found much lower rates of victimization. A 10-year cross-sectional study in the US (with several hundred subjects in 2000, 2005, and 2010) found that digital harassment was reported by 6% of 10–12-year-olds in 2010 (Jones, Mitchell, & Finkelhor, 2012). A 2017 study of more than 4,500 children in third, fourth and fifth grade in the United States found a cyberbullying victimization rate of 9.5%, which was similar to the rate found by the National Crime Victimization Survey (9%) (Englander, 2017; Lessne & Cidade, 2015).

Clearly, the evidence that cyberbullying differs significantly between children of different ages is mixed. However, we cannot yet reject the hypothesis that children of younger ages are victimized less frequently in digital environments, relative to their adolescent peers.

Significance of Variations in Prevalence Estimates

In the struggle to determine the prevalence of cyberbullying in children of different ages, the significance of such data may sometimes be lost. Cyberbullying is part of the dynamic relationships that occur between children. As children increasingly use digital technology, digital forms of communications will naturally increase. Thus, we would expect incidence of cyberbullying to increase as digital communications increase. Still, the prevalence of cyberbullying is important for several reasons. First, higher or lower prevalence may help researchers determine if cyberbullying is a rare and thus more deviant behavior, or one that occurs more commonly, perhaps for a variety of reasons. Second, prevalence, along with motivation, can help researchers understand the dynamics that occur between children of different ages in digital contexts. For example, does cyberbullying typically occur as part of a pattern of ongoing abuse that occurs in school as well as outside of school, between a particular set of children? In such cases, the relationship dynamics may be the most important drivers. Such contexts seem to be more common among younger school age children, relative to their adolescent counterparts (Englander, 2015b). Among teenagers, prevalence clearly increases, and more cases emerge that occur only online, without an ongoing dynamic that is also reflected in person and in school. That raises the possibility that at least some of the cyberbullying that occurs between adolescents is not the result of ongoing relationship dynamics but, rather, can be the result of misinterpretations and misperceptions that occur more easily online (Englander, 2015a).

Developmental Factors, Prevalence, and Cyberbullying

If cyberbullying is less frequent among younger (school age) children, that difference may be attributable to developmental reasons: differential access to digital technology, varied education about how to use social media, and psychological development.

Access to Technology

Mobile technology ownership rates are of interest as a rough measure of Internet exposure and use. Simply owning a cell phone seems to translate into increased time spent online. A Common Sense Media study found that children's average daily Internet use increased along with mobile phone ownership, tripling between 2011 and 2013 (Common Sense Media, 2013). Further, using a smartphone frequently may increase the use of social media. Mascheroni and Olafsson's (2016) study of European children found that daily cell phone users had a 30% to 60% chance of visiting a social networking site, while those who did not use phones daily had a reduced chance of 10% to 35%.

Several studies have noted that increased access and usage of digital technology heightens the probability of involvement in cyberbullying (Hinduja & Patchin, 2008; Holfeld & Leadbeater, 2015; Mishna et al., 2010; Smith et al., 2008). Theoretically, greater access and use increases digital exposure to a potential perpetrator of cyberbullying, in much the same way that greater exposure to a traditional aggressor can increase the odds of in-person victimization (Fisher, Cullen, & Turner, 2002; Wilcox, Jordan, & Pritchard, 2007). A potential target's visibility and accessibility in online spaces can be directly impacted by their frequent use of digital devices (Yar, 2005). One study of adolescents in Singapore found that access to technology, online routine behaviors, and target suitability were all significant predictors of cyberbullying victimization (Holt, Fitzgerald, Bossler, Chee, & Ng, 2016). Among 8- to 11-year-old children, cell phone owners showed an increased tendency to be both a bully and a cyberbully (Englander, 2017). Specifically, cell phone ownership, being a victim of cyberbullying, and being either a traditional bully or a victim of bullying in school all predicted cyberbullying perpetration.

Access to technology clearly increases with age as children progress through childhood. Continuous access to technology in the form of mobile digital technology (cell phones) and wireless access points is widespread among adults and adolescents in the US and Europe, and is increasing rapidly. In 2013, a Pew Center study found that 37% of adolescents owned smartphones; by 2016, that percentage had essentially doubled to 73% (Madden, Lenhart, Duggan, Cortesi, & Gasser, 2013; Pew Research Center, 2017). In contrast, younger children seem to have access to mobile technology at lower rates (although this is changing rapidly). A 2017 study of approximately 4,500 8-, 9-, 10- and 11-year-olds in five states in the US found that 40% of third graders, 50% of fourth graders, and 60% of fifth graders reported that they owned cell phones (Englander, 2017). Other recent studies in Europe have found that between 10% and 40% of 9- to 11-year-olds owned smartphones (with one notable outlier: Denmark, where an astonishing 70% of 9-year-olds own smartphones) (Mascheroni & Olafsson, 2016). Two studies of British children aged 11 and younger found mobile phone ownership rates of approximately 45% (Davie, Panting, & Charlton, 2004; Ofcom, 2016).

Despite lower rates of cell phone ownership among younger children, the trend is clearly towards more ownership of mobile devices. Between 2011 and 2016, the percent of British children using mobile tablets increased dramatically from 6% to 80% (Ofcom, 2016). In the United States, a nationally representative sample of families with children 8 years old or younger revealed that the use of mobile devices nearly doubled between 2011 and 2013 (from 38% to 72%), and families who provided young children with access to a tablet or smartphone increased from 52% to 75% (Common Sense Media, 2013).

Varied Education about Digital Technology Among Children of Different Ages

Training in the use of digital technology, and in how communication changes in digital environments, may reduce cyberbullying. There are several studies that point to a lack of education as one cause of bullying online. One study of 17,000 Canadian teens found that many teens attributed cyberbullying to frequent errors and mistakes made online, such as jokes that go awry (Shapka & Amos, 2012). A dearth of digital skills predicted cyberbullying victimization among younger school-age children as well (Livingstone & Smith, 2014). Adolescent students seem to be aware that education can be helpful in preventing cyberbullying among middle and high school students (Pelfrey & Weber, 2015). Overall, it seems likely that younger children are less educated about cyberbullying. A 2017 study of 4,500 children in five states in the US found that third and fourth grade children were much less able to define the term "cyberbullying," compared to their older peers (Englander, 2017). Cyberbullying education in schools is less common among younger elementary school children, and teachers in the earlier elementary school grades may feel less prepared to teach their students about it (Eden, Heiman, & Olenik-Shemesh, 2013). Teachers of younger students are less likely to be aware of cyberbullying and its implications, and less likely to discuss it with students (Huang & Chou, 2013). They were also more likely than teachers of older students to feel that they needed more education about cyberbullying in order to intervene effectively (Eden et al., 2013).

Education about cyberbullying can take place outside of school, as well. Parents often cite the benefits of giving their child a cell phone, but Englander's (2017) study suggests that giving young children mobile digital devices may incur some risks as well. Pediatricians, counselors, and other stakeholders should educate parents about the risks as well as the benefits when deciding whether or not to provide their elementary school-aged child with a cell phone. A number of experts have called for pediatricians to ask during well-child visits about cell phone ownership and use, and experiences with bullying and cyberbullying (Englander & Raffalli, 2011; Shulman, 2010; Strasburger, Jordan, & Donnerstein, 2012). The American Academy of Pediatrics has recommended that pediatricians should ask patients about all forms of bullying (Committee on Injury, Violence, and Poison Prevention, 2009). However, there is no empirical data on how frequently primary care providers for children (i.e., pediatricians, family physicians) actually query patients about these topics. Boston Children's Hospital has partnered with the Massachusetts Aggression Reduction Center and provides a free checklist with prompts for pediatricians to use during well-child visits (Englander & Raffalli, 2013).

Child Development and Cyberbullying

Studying younger children in a research setting is always somewhat more challenging. One possible interpretation of the studies that found lower prevalence of cyberbullying among school age children is the possibility that younger children were simply more likely to misinterpret questions about bullying, cyberbullying, or cell phone ownership. Because children in Piaget's concrete-operational stage of development may not have mastered abstract phrases and descriptions, surveying young children always raises questions about the accuracy of their comprehension.

Other developmental limitations may explain motivation rather than prevalence. Regardless of whether or not younger children are less likely or equally likely to be victims or perpetrators of cyberbullying, their communication skills may be relevant in determining perpetration or victimization. For example, young children may be more inclined to misinterpret ambiguous online communications, and ambiguity is common in digital environments (Kota, Schoohs, Benson, & Moreno, 2014). Perhaps younger children are more apt to make social errors when using technology (e.g., underestimating the emotional impact of a comment) that could easily lead to social problems both online and in school (Englander, 2015b).

Developmental Differences in Correlates and Outcomes of Cyberbullying

In 2017, a sample of 1,193 college freshman in Massachusetts, Colorado, and Texas were surveyed by the Massachusetts Aggression Reduction Center about their bullying experiences and mental health status in elementary and middle school. Subjects were asked about alcohol and drug use, aggression, family violence, depression, anxiety, problems with self-control, social skills, and academic functioning. They were also asked details about the nature of bullying or cyberbullying they experienced at the hands of their peers. An important developmental difference, which has been noted in many other studies, was the proliferation of digital forms of bullying in middle school (as compared to elementary school) (Donnerstein, 2015). In elementary school, 4% of subjects reported being cyberbullied only online, in comparison to 11.4% who reported online-only bullying while in middle school. The most dramatic change occurred in bullying cases that happened both online and in school: while in elementary school, 9.5% reported this type of bullying, but that number rose to 30% for the middle school years.

Other interesting patterns emerged. When in-school-only and online-only bullying were compared, bullying in school almost always produced more reports of each of the negative psychological and academic factors listed above. However, importantly, for both elementary and middle school years, subjects who reported being bullied *both* online and in school simultaneously reported the highest levels of psychological and academic problems. Not all the negative factors followed the same pattern, moreover. Of the problems studied, depression and anxiety were most frequently endorsed as the result of cyberbullying and combined bullying/cyberbullying. However, depression and anxiety were different from the other factors in one important way. For most variables, combined bullying/cyberbullying produced the most reports of distress, and bullying in school produced the second-highest levels of distress, with online-only cyberbullying producing the least distress. But in the case of depression and anxiety, online-only cyberbullying produced more reports, relative to in-school-only bullying.

This study, in combination with other research, suggests several important developmental conclusions. First, the influence of digital technology clearly grows as children develop. This may be due to increased use of digital devices, and increases in misunderstandings and misperceptions. Second, young children's developmentally mediated cognitive limitations may contribute to some of the problems, like cyberbullying, that are associated with device ownership in younger but not older children (Englander, 2017). Third, unlike other poor outcomes frequently associated with cyberbullying, depression and anxiety may be more commonly associated with online forms of bullying in children of all ages. The variation between depression and anxiety and other noxious outcomes (like aggression) may help explain previous research that has varied in its conclusion about the impact of cyberbullying, relative to traditional bullying (Beckman, 2013).

Conclusions

The prevalence of cyberbullying is not clear. It is fair to estimate that, among adolescents, most estimates are between 20 and 40% of teenagers being victimized online by bullies. Having said that, what is most notable about the literature on prevalence is its variability. Factors such as a lack of a consensual definition of cyberbullying, and the rapid change in technology that limits our ability to generalize across studies of more than a few years, make prevalence estimates even more challenging. What is clear is that, among adolescents, cyberbullying is neither extremely rare nor extremely common. It is a social problem and a type of aggression that occurs between one quarter and one third of youth, roughly. That makes it frequent enough to be a legitimate source of concern.

Among younger children, estimates of prevalence differ even more dramatically than among their older peers. Many studies find that approximately 20 to 25% of school age children are victims of cyberbullying, but a good handful also find that prevalence rates are under 10%, substantially lower. At present, it seems likely that younger children are victimized at lower rates, but we cannot yet say whether their rates of victimization are dramatically or only slightly lower. Having said that, there are theoretical explanations for why older children might be involved in cyberbullying at higher rates. First, older children clearly have more access to technology, particularly mobile technology, which has been reliably associated with increased involvement in cyberbullying. Second, adolescent children may be more educated about cyberbullying; they can define the concept better, their teachers may be more knowledgeable about it, and more willing to discuss it in school. Third, there is a dearth of research examining younger children and cyberbullying. The fact that pre-adolescent children have been neglected in the research literature is probably largely due to the more visible and salient problems experienced by adolescent children online. Adult biases may have also resulted in the minimization or dismissal of the risk and involvement in cyberbullying among children in elementary or primary schools (Englander, 2017).

References

ABA. (2009). *New research on cyberbullying highlights the role of parents in prevention*. United Kingdom: Anti Bullying Alliance. Retrieved from www.anti-bullyingalliance.org.uk/press_centre/news_archive/new_research_on_cyberbullying.aspx

Anderson, M. (2015, August 20). *How having smartphones (or not) shapes the way teens communicate*. Retrieved from www.pewresearch.org/fact-tank/2015/08/20/how-having-smartphones-or-not-shapes-the-way-teens-communicate/

Arslan, S., Savaser, S., Hallett, V., & Balci, S. (2012). Cyberbullying among primary school students in Turkey: Self-reported prevalence and associations with home and school life. *Cyberpsychology, Behavior, and Social Networking*, 15(10), 527–533. doi:10.1089/cyber.2012.0207

Beckman, L. (2013). Traditional bullying and cyberbullying among Swedish adolescents: Gender differences and associations with mental health. Karlstad University, Faculty of Health, Science and Technology, Sweden. Retrieved from www.diva-portal.org/smash/record.jsf?pid=diva2:639930

Committee on Injury, Violence, and Poison Prevention. (2009). Role of the pediatrician in youth violence prevention. *Pediatrics*, *124*(1), 393–402. doi:10.1542/peds.2009-0943

Common Sense Media. (2013). Zero to eight: Children's media use in American 2013. Common Sense Media. Retrieved from www.commonsensemedia.org/file/zero-to-eight-2013pdf-0/download

Cross, D., Lester, L., & Barnes, A. (2015). A longitudinal study of the social and emotional predictors and consequences of cyber and traditional bullying victimisation. *International Journal of Public Health*, *60*(2), 207–217. doi:10.1007/s00038-015-0655-1

Davie, R., Panting, C., & Charlton, T. (2004). Mobile phone ownership and usage among pre-adolescents. *Telematics and Informatics*, *21*(4), 359–373. doi:10.1016/j.tele.2004.04.001

DePaolis, K., & Williford, A. (2014). The nature and prevalence of cyber victimization among elementary school children. *Child & Youth Care Forum*, *44*(3), 377–393. doi:10.1007/s10566-014-9292-8

Donnerstein, E. (2015). Section V: Need for longitudinal research. In *Cyberbullying: Current & Future Research & Directions: A White Paper Submitted to the Institute of Child Development and Digital Media*. New York: Institute of Child Development and Digital Media.

Eden, S., Heiman, T., & Olenik-Shemesh, D. (2013). Teachers' perceptions, beliefs and concerns about cyberbullying: Teachers' perceptions about cyberbullying. *British Journal of Educational Technology*, *44*(6), 1036–1052. doi:10.1111/j.1467-8535.2012.01363.x

Englander, E. (2012). *Research Findings: MARC 2011 Survey Grades 3-12*. Bridgewater, Massachusetts: Massachusetts Aggression Reduction Center, Bridgewater State University. Retrieved from http://webhost.bridgew.edu/marc/MARC%20REPORT-Bullying%20In%20Grades%203-12%20in%20MA.pdf

Englander, E. (2015a). *Cognitive and perceptual factors in digital communications*. Presented at the Science of Character: Teaching Self-Regulation, Resilience, Empathy and Anti-bullying Skills in Children and Teens, Massachusetts Institute of Technology, Cambridge, MA.

Englander, E. (2015b). Section IV: It's not all cyberbullying: Different problem behaviors and perceptual factors online. In *Cyberbullying: Current & Future Research & Directions: A White Paper Submitted to the Institute of Child Development and Digital Media*. New York: Institute of Child Development and Digital Media.

Englander, E. (2017). Risky business: Talking with your patients about cyberbullying and sexting. *Child & Adolescent Psychiatric Clinics of North America, 27*, 287–305. doi:10.1016/j.chc.2017.11.010

Englander, E., Donnerstein, E., Kowalski, R., Lin, C. A., & Parti, K. (2017). Defining cyberbullying. *Pediatrics, 140*(Supplement 2), S148–S151. doi:10.1542/peds.2016-1758U

Englander, E., & Raffalli, P. (2011). Tips for pediatricians: Addressing bullying and cyberbullying in your practice. *Pediatric News.* Retrieved from https://marccenter.webs.com/Tips%20for%20Pediatricians-%20Addressing%20Bullying%20&%20Cyberbullying%20In%20Your%20Practice[2].pdf

Englander, E., & Raffalli, P. (2013). *MARC/BACPAC Pediatric Questionnaire: Bullying and cyberbullying.* Retrieved from www.childrenshospital.org/~/media/centers-and-services/programs/a_e/bacpac/neu_12731_bacpac_tool.ashx?la=en

Fisher, B. S., Cullen, F. T., & Turner, M. G. (2002). Being pursued: Stalking victimization in a national study of college women. *Criminology, 1*(2), 257–308. doi: 10.1111/j.1745-9133.2002.tb00091.x

Hinduja, S., & Patchin, J. W. (2008). Cyberbullying: An exploratory analysis of factors related to offending and victimization. *Deviant Behavior, 29*(2), 129–156. doi:10.1080/01639620701457816

Hinduja, S., & Patchin, J. W. (2010). Bullying, cyberbullying, and suicide. *Archives of Suicide Research*, 14(3), 206–221. doi:10.1080/13811118.2010.494133

Holfeld, B., & Grabe, M. (2012). Middle school students' perceptions of and responses to cyber bullying. *Journal of Educational Computing Research, 46*(4), 395–413. doi:10.2190/EC.46.4.e

Holfeld, B., & Leadbeater, B. J. (2015). The nature and frequency of cyber bullying behaviors and victimization experiences in young Canadian children. *Canadian Journal of School Psychology, 30*(2), 116–135. doi:10.1177/0829573514556853

Holt, T. J., Fitzgerald, S., Bossler, A. M., Chee, G., & Ng, E. (2016). Assessing the risk factors of cyber and mobile phone bullying victimization in a nationally representative sample of Singapore youth. *International Journal of Offender Therapy and Comparative Criminology, 60*(5), 598–615. doi:10.1177/0306624X14554852

Huang, Y., & Chou, C. (2013). Revisiting cyberbullying: Perspectives from Taiwanese teachers. *Computers & Education, 63*, 227–239. doi:10.1016/j.compedu.2012.11.023

Jones, L. M., Mitchell, K. J., & Finkelhor, D. (2012). Trends in youth internet victimization: Findings from three youth internet safety surveys 2000–2010. *Journal of Adolescent Health, 50*(2), 179–186. doi:10.1016/j.jadohealth.2011.09.015

Kessel Schneider, S., O'Donnell, L., Stueve, A., & Coulter, R. W. S. (2012). Cyberbullying, school bullying, and psychological distress: A regional census of high school students. *American Journal of Public Health, 102*(1), 171–177. doi:10.2105/AJPH.2011.300308

Kota, R., Schoohs, S., Benson, M., & Moreno, M. (2014). Characterizing cyberbullying among college students: Hacking, dirty laundry, and mocking. *Societies, 4*(4), 549–560. doi:10.3390/soc4040549

Kowalski, R. (2015). Section II: Overlap between cyberbullying and traditional bullying: Fact or fiction. In *Cyberbullying: Current & Future Research & Directions: A White Paper Submitted to the Institute of Child Development and Digital Media.* New York: Institute of Child Development and Digital Media.

Lenhart, A. (2015). *Teens, social media & technology overview 2015* (Internet American Life Project). Pew Research Center. Retrieved from www.pewinternet.org/2015/04/09/teens-social-media-technology-2015/

Lessne, D., & Cidade, D. (2015). *Student reports of bullying and cyber-bullying: Results from the 2011 school crime supplement to the national crime victimization survey*. National Center for Education Statistics. Retrieved from https://nces.ed.gov/pubsearch/pubsinfo.asp?pubid=2015056

Liu, J., Lewis, G., & Evans, L. (2013). Understanding aggressive behaviour across the lifespan. *Journal of Psychiatric and Mental Health Nursing, 20*(2), 156–168. doi:10.1111/j.1365-2850.2012.01902.x

Livingstone, S., & Smith, P. K. (2014). Harms experienced by child users of online and mobile technologies: The nature, prevalence and management of sexual and aggressive risks in the digital age. *Journal of Child Psychology and Psychiatry, 55*(6), 635–654. https://doi.org/10.1111/jcpp.12197

Madden, M., Lenhart, A., Duggan, M., Cortesi, S., & Gasser, U. (2013). *Teens and technology 2013*. Pew Internet & American Life Project. Retrieved from www.pewinternet.org/2013/03/13/teens-and-technology-2013/

Mascheroni, G., & Olafsson, K. (2016). The mobile Internet: Access, use, opportunities and divides among European children. *New Media & Society, 18*(8), 1657–1679. doi:10.1177/1461444814567986

Mishna, F., Cook, C., Gadalla, T., Daciuk, J., & Solomon, S. (2010). Cyber bullying behaviors among middle and high school students. *American Journal of Orthopsychiatry, 80*(3), 362–374. doi:10.1111/j.1939-0025.2010.01040.x

Modecki, K. L., Minchin, J., Harbaugh, A. G., Guerra, N. G., & Runions, K. C. (2014). Bullying prevalence across contexts: A meta-analysis measuring cyber and traditional bullying. *Journal of Adolescent Health, 55*(5), 602–611. doi:10.1016/j.jadohealth.2014.06.007

Monks, C., Robinson, S., & Worlidge, P. (2012). The emergence of cyberbullying: A survey of primary school pupils' perceptions and experiences. *School Psychology International, 33*(5), 477–491. doi:10.1177/0143034312445242

Ofcom. (2016). *Children and parents: Media use and attitudes report 2016*. Retrieved from www.ofcom.org.uk/research-and-data/media-literacy-research/children/children-parents-nov16

Patchin, J. W., & Hinduja, S. (2006). Bullies move beyond the schoolyard: A preliminary look at cyberbullying. *Youth Violence and Juvenile Justice, 4*(2), 148–169. doi:10.1177/1541204006286288

Patchin, J. W., & Hinduja, S. (2016). *Cyberbullying research in review*. Retrieved from https://cyberbullying.org/Cyberbullying-Research-In-Review.pdf

Pelfrey, W. V., & Weber, N. L. (2015). Student and school staff strategies to combat cyberbullying in an urban student population. *Preventing School Failure: Alternative Education for Children and Youth, 59*(4), 227–236. doi:10.1080/1045988X.2014.924087

Pew Research Center. (2017, April 8). 73% of teens have access to a smartphone; 15% have only a basic phone. Retrieved from www.pewinternet.org/2015/04/09/teens-social-media-technology-2015/pi_2015-04-09_teensandtech_06/

Shapka, J., & Amos, H. (2012, April 13). *Cyberbullying and bullying are not the same: UBC research*. University of British Columbia. Retrieved from www.publicaffairs.ubc.ca/2012/04/13/cyberbullying-and-bullying-are-not-the-same-ubc-research/

Shulman, S. T. (2010). Reducing screen time for children. *Pediatric Annals, 39*(9), 536–537. doi:10.3928/00904481-20100825-01

Slonje, R., Smith, P. K., & Frisén, A. (2012). Processes of cyberbullying, and feelings of remorse by bullies: A pilot study. *European Journal of Developmental Psychology, 9*(2), 244–259. doi:10.1080/17405629.2011.643670

Smith, P. K., Mahdavi, J., Carvalho, M., Fisher, S., Russell, S., & Tippett, N. (2008). Cyberbullying: Its nature and impact in secondary school pupils. *Journal of Child Psychology and Psychiatry, 49*(4), 376–385. doi:10.1111/j.1469-7610.2007.01846.x

Strasburger, V. C., Jordan, A. B., & Donnerstein, E. (2012). Children, adolescents, and the media: *Pediatric Clinics of North America, 59*(3), 533–587. doi:10.1016/j.pcl.2012.03.025

Varjas, K., Talley, J., Meyers, J., Parris, L., & Cutts, H. (2010). High school students' perceptions of motivations for cyberbullying: an exploratory study. *The Western Journal of Emergency Medicine, 11*(3), 269–273.

Wilcox, P., Jordan, C. E., & Pritchard, A. J. (2007). A multidimensional examination of campus safety: Victimization, perceptions of danger, worry about crime, and precautionary behavior among college women in the post-Clery era. *Crime & Delinquency, 53* (2), 219–254. doi:10.1177/0097700405283664

Yar, M. (2005). The novelty of "cybercrime": An assessment in light of Routine Activity Theory. *European Journal of Criminology, 2*(4), 407–427. doi:10.1177/147737080556056

Ybarra, M. L., Boyd, D., Korchmaros, J. D., & Oppenheim, J. K. (2012). Defining and measuring cyberbullying within the larger context of bullying victimization. *The Journal of Adolescent Health: Official Publication of the Society for Adolescent Medicine*, 51(1), 53–58. doi:10.1016/j.jadohealth.2011.12.031

Ybarra, M. L., & Chen, E. (2015). Section III: The importance of differential power and repetition as defining features of cyberbullying. In *Cyberbullying: Current & Future Research & Directions: A White Paper Submitted to the Institute of Child Development and Digital Media*. New York: Institute of Child Development and Digital Media.

Ybarra, M. L., Espelage, D. L., & Mitchell, K. J. (2014). Differentiating youth who are bullied from other victims of peer-aggression: the importance of differential power and repetition. *The Journal of Adolescent Health: Official Publication of the Society for Adolescent Medicine, 55*(2), 293–300. doi:10.1016/j.jadohealth.2014.02.009

6

CYBERBULLYING IN THE WORKPLACE

A Review of the Research

Jenna L. Scisco

Technology is an essential part of communication at work, with e-mail, the Internet, smartphones, and social networking sites being used by both office-based and non-office-based workers (Purcell & Rainie, 2014). This integration of technology into the workplace comes with many perceived benefits for employees, including an expanded communication network, job flexibility, and increased productivity (Purcell & Rainie, 2014). However, these technologies also enable aggressive workplace behaviors to spill over into the cyber realm. For example, employees might have their work publicly criticized on the Internet, be excluded from important work-related information, or receive threatening work-related electronic messages (Farley, Coyne, Axtell, & Sprigg, 2016; Vranjes, Baillien, Vandebosch, Erreygers, & De Witte, 2018). These negative, technology-mediated acts are examples of workplace cyberbullying, a behavior associated with adverse outcomes for individuals and organizations, such as poorer physical and mental health and decreased job performance (Baruch, 2005; Gardner et al., 2016; Vranjes et al., 2018).

The purpose of this chapter is to provide a comprehensive review of the workplace cyberbullying literature. First, the chapter explores the nuances of the conceptual definition and some related constructs within workplace cyberaggression. Then, the chapter summarizes the prevalence, correlates, mediators, and moderators of workplace cyberbullying. Next, the chapter describes recently developed measures of workplace cyberbullying. To conclude, this chapter provides future research directions for the workplace cyberbullying literature and practical implications for organizations and human resources departments.

Workplace Cyberbullying: Conceptual Definition and Related Constructs

Research on cyberbullying in the workplace is an emerging field, and preliminary work has begun to establish a conceptual definition of this phenomenon. Initially, the definition of cyberbullying, regardless of context, varied widely in earlier literature. Tokunaga (2010), identifying the need for a clear definition of cyberbullying, and, synthesizing past definitions, defined the construct as "any behavior performed through electronic or digital media by individuals or groups that repeatedly communicates hostile or aggressive messages intended to inflict harm or discomfort on others" (p. 278). It is notable that this definition includes three key components that can serve to distinguish cyberbullying from other forms of electronic deviance: (1) the behavior is repetitive, (2) the messages are intentional, and (3) the messages are uncomfortable or harmful for the recipient. Another closely related definition by Smith et al. (2008) states that cyberbullying is "an aggressive, intentional act carried out by a group or individual, using electronic forms of contact, repeatedly and over time against a victim who cannot easily defend him or herself" (p. 376). The unique, additional aspect of cyberbullying provided by this definition is the vulnerability of the victim.

Cyberbullying can be distinguished from traditional face-to-face bullying due to its unique features that are enabled by technology use. For example, for face-to-face bullying to be repetitive, the perpetrator would engage in repetitive harmful behaviors. In contrast, one act of cyberbullying can be experienced repeatedly by the target and observers, such as posting a harmful video online (which can then be viewed repetitively) or rereading an e-mail (Dooley, Pyzalski, & Cross, 2009). Additionally, traditional bullying can be characterized by a power imbalance, with the perpetrator typically having more physical or psychological power than the target. In contrast, a victim can be vulnerable to cyberbullying because the perpetrator may gain power by having better information technology (IT) skills or by becoming anonymous by using unknown e-mail accounts, online IDs, or phone numbers (Dooley et al., 2009). Furthermore, while a target can escape traditional bullying by avoiding the perpetrator, cyberbullying can occur anytime and anywhere that technology is accessed (Dooley et al., 2009). Also, cyberbullying can hypothetically be observed by a limitless audience by sharing or forwarding messages or photos online (Dooley et al., 2009). Interestingly, a potential advantage for a target of cyberbullying is the ability to keep permanent records of cyberbullying behaviors by saving messages like e-mails (D'Cruz & Noronha, 2013). These could be used as evidence of cyberbullying behavior when the target needs to bring the cyberbullying to the attention of an outside party, such as human resources.

Building upon these definitions of cyberbullying and the features that distinguish cyberbullying from traditional bullying, researchers have recently developed comprehensive definitions of *workplace cyberbullying*. Farley et al. (2016) defined workplace cyberbullying as:

> a situation where over time, an individual is repeatedly subjected to perceived negative acts conducted through technology (e.g., phone, email, web sites and social media) which are related to their work context. In this situation the target of workplace cyberbullying has difficulty defending him or herself against these actions.
>
> *(p. 295)*

In this definition, intent to harm has been omitted because it can be difficult to clearly determine a perpetrator's intent in an electronic context (Farley et al., 2016). Similarly, Vranjes, Baillien, Vandebosch, Erreygers, and De Witte (2017) defined workplace cyberbullying as:

> all negative behavior stemming from the work context and occurring through the use of [Information and Communication Technologies] ICTs, which is either (a) carried out repeatedly and over a period of time or (b) conducted at least once but forms an intrusion into someone's private life, (potentially) exposing it to a wide online audience. This behavior leaves the target feeling helpless and unable to defend.
>
> *(p. 326)*

Notably, this definition clarifies that cyberbullying can be a single act that, through wide audience exposure, may be similar to a repetitive act of cyberbullying. If these two very similar definitions of workplace cyberbullying are synthesized, workplace cyberbullying can be conceptualized as *negative, technology-mediated behaviors that are repetitively experienced by a vulnerable target within the work context.* Some characteristic behaviors of workplace cyberbullying may include (1) person-related behaviors such as gossiping online, (2) work-related behaviors such as withholding important information, and (3) intrusive behaviors enabled by 24/7 digital technologies such as obtaining embarrassing personal information and sharing it widely (Vranjes et al., 2018).

Several constructs used to describe aggressive workplace behaviors are related to workplace bullying, including social undermining, incivility, abusive supervision, and interpersonal conflict (Hershcovis, 2011). Although some researchers argue that these terms could be lumped together with bullying under the umbrella of workplace aggression, others argue that there are features of each behavior that can serve to distinguish them as unique constructs, such as the behavior's intent, intensity, frequency, perceived invisibility, and the perpetrator-victim relationship (Hershcovis, 2011). When specifically examining related constructs in the cyber domain, cyber incivility and cyberharassment stand out as related but potentially different workplace behaviors when compared to cyberbullying.

Cyber incivility is defined as "rude/discourteous behaviors occurring through Information and Communication Technologies (ICTs) such as e-mail or text messages" (Giumetti et al., 2012, p. 148). Cyber incivility differs from cyberbullying in that, with cyber incivility, the intent to harm is ambiguous and the behavior is of lower intensity (Hershcovis, 2011). Cyberharrassment is a broader term, referring to a cluster of behaviors using technology to menace someone (Durkin & Patterson, 2011). Cyberharrassment is of stronger intensity than cyberbullying, and the intent to harm is clear; cyberharrassment behaviors might include electronic communications that are sexist, racist, threatening, or frightening (Whitty & Carr, 2006).

Because cyberbullying is an emerging construct within workplace aggression, the following sections review research on the prevalence, correlates, and measures of workplace cyberbullying and omit studies specific to cyber incivility or cyberharrassment. However, because clear definitions and measures of workplace cyberbullying were developed after much of this research was conducted, there may be overlap between the reviewed research on cyberbullying and related constructs. Furthermore, because research on workplace cyberbullying is a relatively small body of literature, I reference research on traditional face-to-face bullying in the workplace to generate practical implications and future research directions.

Prevalence of Cyberbullying in the Workplace

A first step toward understanding the effects of cyberbullying on workers is to describe the prevalence of this phenomenon across cultures. When examining the prevalence of workplace cyberbullying, researchers have also aimed to describe common cyberbullying behaviors and the status of perpetrators and their targets.

Limited studies have examined the prevalence of workplace cyberbullying in the United States (US). In a survey of 3,699 US adults, 20.1% reported that most of their cyberbullying experiences were in adulthood, with 72.7% of this subsample reporting that the perpetrator of the cyberbullying was a coworker (Kowalski, Toth, & Morgan, 2018). In a survey of 107 working undergraduate students in the US, 30.8% reported experiencing cyberbullying at least once per month, with non-Whites reporting more cyberbullying than Whites (Kowalski, Giumetti, Schroeder, & Reese, 2012). Additionally, cyberbullying was more common for workers who reported that the Internet was essential for their work as compared to the workers for whom the Internet was non-essential. Among those who reported cyberbullying, the most commonly reported cyberbullying behaviors were being addressed in unprofessional terms (60.6%), having someone show a lack of interest in one's statements or opinions (51.5%), and condescension (36.4%). The most common sources of cyberbullying were a coworker (54.5%), customer or client (45.5%), supervisor (42.4%), stranger (27.3%), and subordinate (24.2%), and the most common mediums were text message (57.6%), e-mail (45.5%), and instant message (27.3%) (Kowalski et al., 2012).

Research examining the prevalence of cyberbullying in European countries is more comprehensive than the US research. In a sample of 649 office employees at a Fortune 500 company in the United Kingdom (UK), 9.2% of respondents reported experiencing bullying via e-mail, with work-related insults and intimidation from direct managers and peers being the most common (Baruch, 2005). In a sample of 158 trainee medical doctors in the UK, 46.2% reported experiencing at least one instance of cyberbullying (Farley, Coyne, Sprigg, Axtell, & Subramanian, 2015). Fellow trainees were the most common perpetrators (35.6%) followed by consultants (26.0%), managers (13.7%), nurses (4.1%), and patients or relatives (1.4%). Across three samples of employees working in higher education in the UK, 80–88% experienced a cyberbullying act in the past six months, and 14–20% were classified as cyberbullying targets, defined as experiencing one negative behavior at least weekly over six months (Coyne, Farley et al., 2017). The targets most commonly reported having views or opinions ignored (52–58%), exposure to unmanageable workload (42–58%), being given tasks with unreasonable or impossible targets or deadlines (40–59%), being ordered to do work through electronic means below your level of competence (47%), and being ignored or excluded (40–41%). In a sample of 3,371 Swedish working adults, 9.7% were classified as cyberbullying targets (one negative behavior weekly over six months), with men and supervisors being exposed to more cyberbullying behaviors than females and non-supervisors (Forssell, 2016). The most frequent cyberbullying behavior in this study was being ignored via e-mail or text message followed by having work-related information withheld, and the most common medium for cyberbullying was e-mail. Similarly, in a sample of working adults from Sweden, men reported experiencing more cyberbullying acts than women (Jönsson, Muhonen, Forssell, & Bäckström, 2017).

A couple of studies have also examined the prevalence of workplace cyberbullying in Australia and New Zealand. In a sample of 103 male members of the Australian Manufacturing Worker's Union, 10.7% had been cyberbullied by e-mail or phone (Privitera & Campbell, 2009). The most common cyberbullying behaviors were having information withheld that affected work performance and being ordered to do work below the worker's competence level. In a sample of over 2,000 working adults in New Zealand, 2.8% had been cyberbullied, using a more stringent classification criteria of experiencing two or more negative acts weekly for at least six months (Gardner et al., 2016). Managerial employees were most likely to experience cyberbullying.

Overall, across this small body of research, prevalence estimates of workplace cyberbullying ranged from about 3% to 20% depending on how cyberbullying was defined and measured. This is similar to the estimated 11% to 18% of employees that have experienced face-to-face workplace bullying (Nielsen, Matthiesen, & Einarsen, 2010). Thus far, workplace cyberbullying prevalence has been measured from the perspective of the targets and not the perpetrators. Workplace cyberbullying appears to consist of a variety of behaviors that originate from individuals with more, equal, or less power than the target and that occur through a variety of ICTs. With workplace cyberbullying established as a prevalent phenomenon, it is important to understand features of employees and organizations that are associated with workplace cyberbullying.

Correlates of Workplace Cyberbullying

The workplace cyberbullying literature is dominated by correlational, survey-based research. In this section, I summarize person-related and work-related variables associated with workplace cyberbullying. It is important to keep in mind throughout this review of the research that causality is difficult to establish due to a lack of experimental methods. Whereas researchers might make a theoretical argument that a variable such as mental health is an outcome of experiencing workplace cyberbullying, it is also possible that an individual's mental health could make them more likely to experience or perceive workplace cyberbullying.

Workplace cyberbullying has been associated with several person-related variables, including a worker's health, emotions, and personality. For instance, experiencing cyberbullying at work predicted a small decrease in mental well-being six months later for a sample of working European adults in the public sector (Vranjes et al., 2018). Workplace cyberbullying was also positively associated with burnout (Kowalski et al., 2012), depression (Kowalski et al., 2018), and anxiety (Baruch, 2005). In a sample of working adults in New Zealand, experiencing a greater frequency of cyberbullying behaviors was associated with poorer physical health (Gardner et al., 2016). In a study of undergraduate workers, experiencing cyberbullying was positively correlated with feeling scared, ashamed, embarrassed, helpless, irritated, and angry (Kowalski et al., 2012). Using a qualitative approach, aspects of targets' personalities (e.g., vulnerability) and perpetrators' personalities (e.g., anger management problems) were described as possible correlates of workplace cyberbullying (Heatherington & Coyne, 2014).

Additionally, workplace cyberbullying has been associated with several work-related variables, including employees' attitudes and actions related to the job or organization. Experiencing cyberbullying has been correlated with decreased job satisfaction (Baruch, 2005; Kowalski et al., 2018). A cyberbullied employee is also more likely to be searching for a job or intending to quit (Baruch, 2005; Kowalski et al., 2012), and they report increased counterproductive work behaviors (CWBs) (Kowalski et al., 2018) and decreased job performance (Baruch, 2005). Some situational and organizational factors (e.g., reorganization) may be associated with workplace cyberbullying as well (Heatherington & Coyne, 2014). For example, greater perceived organizational support and greater effectiveness of organizational responses were associated with less cyberbullying (Gardner et al., 2016). Moving beyond these simple correlates of workplace cyberbullying, in the next section, I summarize theoretical mediators and moderators of the relationships.

Mediators and Moderators of Relationships with Workplace Cyberbullying

Recently, research has expanded beyond simple correlations to propose and test possible mediators and moderators of the relationships between workplace cyberbullying and theorized predictors and outcomes. These studies allow for a more in-depth investigation of how person-related and work-related factors work in combination to predict the experience or outcomes of workplace cyberbullying.

One mediation model examined how relationships with coworkers influenced perceptions of the organization and subsequent employee outcomes (Muhonen, Jönsson, & Bäckström, 2017). In this study of Swedish working adults, the authors found that cyberbullying victimization was associated with less social support from colleagues and superiors. In turn, this reduced social support was associated with a poorer social organizational climate, which was subsequently associated with lower employee engagement, well-being, health, and greater intention to quit.

More commonly, mediation models of workplace cyberbullying build upon the idea that one's affect or emotions can influence perceptions of the organization, which in turn could influence one's experience of cyberbullying. For instance, in a sample of working adults in Taiwan, positive affect was positively associated with perceived organization innovation climate (e.g., "At work, I can use my own ideas"; Hong, Lin, Hwang, Hu, & Chen, 2014). Subsequently, perceived organization innovation climate was negatively associated with psychological responses to being cyberbullied (e.g., "When I am cyberbullied, I feel very frustrated"). These psychological outcomes were positively associated with cyberbullying experiences. Similar to studying positive affect, Snyman and Loh (2015) found that experiencing cyberbullying was positively associated with stress, and this relationship was partially mediated by optimism in a sample of white collar workers.

In another model, Coyne, Farley, and colleagues (2017) have used disempowerment theory (Kane & Montgomery, 1998) to suggest that a cyberbullying victim may interpret cyberbullying as violating his/her dignity which produces negative affect, and negative affect in turn negatively impacts his/her attitudes and behaviors. In a sample of trainee medical doctors in the UK, both cyberbullying and self-blame were positively associated with mental strain, and these relationships were mediated by negative affect (Farley et al., 2015). Additionally, in this sample of trainee medical doctors, cyberbullying and perpetrator blame were negatively associated with job satisfaction, and this relationship was mediated by interactional injustice, which reflects being treated with less respect and dignity at work. Furthermore, in a series of three studies of higher education employees in the UK, cyberbullying was positively associated with mental strain and negatively associated with job satisfaction, and these relationships were mediated by state negative affect (Coyne, Farley et al., 2017). Moreover, the association between cyberbullying and job satisfaction was mediated by interactional justice. However, the model suggested by disempowerment theory with sequential mediation of cyberbullying outcomes by interactional justice and negative affect was not supported. This suggests that each theorized outcome of workplace cyberbullying may have a different mediator or unique combinations of mediators (Coyne, Farley et al., 2017).

Finally, Vranjes et al. (2017) have proposed an Emotion Reaction model of workplace cyberbullying. In this model, stressors related to the job, team, and organization are theorized to elicit emotions such as anger, fear, or sadness. In turn, these emotions elicit cyberbullying perpetration or victimization. Perceived control over one's work-related stressors is theorized to moderate the relationship between stressors and emotions, and regulating one's emotions via coping strategies like reappraisal or suppression is theorized to moderate the links between stressors, emotions, and cyberbullying. As future research aims to test the Emotion Reaction model and other models of workplace cyberbullying, researchers should aim to use reliable and valid measures of workplace cyberbullying, which I summarize in the following section.

Measures of Workplace Cyberbullying

When workplace cyberbullying emerged as a construct, there were initially no scales to measure it directly. A common choice was to use a modified version of the Negative Acts Questionnaire (NAQ) or the Negative Acts Questionnaire Revised (NAQ-R; Einarsen, Hoel, & Notelaers, 2009). For example, Privitera and Campbell (2009) modified the NAQ-R by asking participants to report the frequency with which the bullying behaviors were experienced by e-mail, by SMS, and by phone. The NAQ-R is a 22-item scale with three subscales: personal bullying, work-related bullying, and physically intimidating forms of bullying. An example item from the NAQ-R's work-related factor is "Someone withholding information which affects your performance." Response options are never, now and then, monthly, weekly, and daily. The overall measure has excellent internal reliability (α=0.90). Validity of the scale was established with significant correlations between the NAQ-R and measures of related variables, including health, work performance, turnover intentions, organizational climate, and stress from relationships with colleagues.

Other authors have chosen to use their own, previously unvalidated measures of workplace cyberbullying. For example, Gardner et al. (2016) developed a measure of cyberbullying which uses a list of 20 negative acts such as "I have received rude, insulting or offensive online communications by people at work," with response options ranging from 1 = *never* to 5 = *daily*. Fortunately, the measurement of workplace cyberbullying has been advanced by the recent development and validation of scales intended to measure this construct specifically. These include the Cyber Negative Acts Questionnaire (CNAQ), the Workplace Cyberbullying Measure (WCM), the Inventory of Cyberbullying Acts at Work (ICA-W), and the Cyberbullying Questionnaire (CBQ).

The Cyber Negative Acts Questionnaire (CNAQ; Farley et al., 2015) is a modified version of the Negative Acts Questionnaire Revised (NAQ-R; Einarsen et al., 2009). Farley et al. (2015) used 19 of the items from the NAQ-R to make the CNAQ which asks how frequently participants experience the bullying behaviors through eight forms of technology, including: (1) text messaging, (2) pictures, photographs or video clips, (3) telephone calls, (4) e-mail, (5) chat rooms, (6) instant messaging, (7) websites, and (8) social networking websites. The CNAQ has high internal reliability (α=0.85). Coyne, Farley et al. (2017) conducted an exploratory factor analysis (EFA) of the CNAQ and reduced it to 16 items that comprise two factors: work-related cyberbullying and person-related cyberbullying.

The Workplace Cyberbullying Measure (WCM) is a 17-item measure with two subscales that were established through EFA and confirmatory factor analysis (CFA): work-related cyberbullying and person-related cyberbullying (Farley et al., 2016). Participants are asked how often over the last six months they experienced each work-related act through different technologies (e.g., text message, e-mail). An example item from the work-related cyberbullying factor is "been unfairly blamed for work problems." Response options are "never," "now and then," "at least monthly," "at least weekly," and "daily." The WCM also includes a self-labeling definition item which asks participants to state whether they have been cyberbullied at work over the last six months. The response options are "No," "Yes, now and then," "Yes, monthly," "Yes, weekly," and "Yes, almost daily." The WCM has high internal reliability (α=0.93). The WCM is strongly correlated with measures of traditional workplace bullying and cyber-aggression, which provides support for convergent validity. Additionally, the WCM is moderately correlated with ICT hassles and learning expectations, providing support for divergent validity of the measure. It also explains additional variance in emotional exhaustion over and above traditional bullying and cyber-aggression, suggesting that the WCM taps into some unique aspects of cyberbullying (Farley et al., 2016).

The Inventory of Cyberbullying Acts at Work (ICA-W) is a 10-item measure of cyberbullying in the workplace with three subscales established through EFA and CFA: work-related, person-related, and intrusion (Vranjes et al., 2018). An example item from the ICA-W's work-related subscale is "Your emails, phone calls or messages are ignored at work." Participants respond to the items on a 5-point Likert scale with the following labels: 1 = *never*, 2 = *one time*, 3 = *monthly*, 4 = *weekly*, and 5 = *daily*. The overall scale has high internal reliability (α=0.81) with good internal reliability for each subscale: person-related (α = 0.78), work-related (α = 0.72), and intrusion (α =0.78). Convergent validity of the scale was established with significant correlations between the ICA-W and measures of related constructs, such as role conflicts, job insecurity, interpersonal conflicts, and a one-item measure of cyberbullying.

The Cyberbullying Questionnaire (CBQ) consists of 20 items measuring cyberbullying behaviors in the workplace, and the Cyberbullying Questionnaire short version (CBQ-S) contains seven of those items (Jönsson et al., 2017). Exploratory structural equation modeling (ESEM) indicated one factor. Participants are asked to report how often they experienced the behaviors related to their work over the past six months through eight different technologies (text messaging, pictures/photos or video clips, phone calls, email, chat rooms, instant messaging, websites, and social networking websites). An example behavior on both the CBQ and the CBQ-S is "Rude messages have been sent to you via digital media." Participants respond on a 5-point scale: 1 = *never*, 2 = *now and then*, 3 = *monthly*, 4 = *weekly*, 5 = *daily*. The CBQ and CBQ-S have high internal reliability in both Swedish and US samples (α = 0.96 and 0.88, respectively). Additionally, criterion validity was established with negative correlations between cyberbullying, work engagement, and well-being, and a positive correlation between cyberbullying and intention to quit.

When choosing a measure of workplace cyberbullying to use in future studies, researchers should aim to use a reliable and valid measure of the construct. The WCM, ICA-W, and CBQ/CBQ-S have been validated and have strong reliability. When examining similarities in factor structure, the CNAQ, WCM, and ICA-W have work-related and person-related factors. Importantly, both the WCM and the ICA-W underwent EFA and CFA to establish their factor structure. The ICA-W differs from the other scales with the addition of the intrusion factor, which includes items such as "Somebody takes over your identity," making it an appropriate measure for studies in which studying intrusion may be particularly relevant. The WCM stands out as a possible top choice for measuring workplace cyberbullying due to its demonstrated ability to tap into unique aspects of workplace cyberbullying that go beyond traditional bullying and cyberaggression. Across all of the measures, the full versions are similar in length (10–20 items), and the CBQ-S is a shorter version (seven items) that could be used if survey length and participant burden are concerns for a certain research study. One last point to note is that the measures summarized here only examine workplace cyberbullying from the perspective of the target, indicating a need for future research to develop measures of workplace cyberbullying perpetration.

Directions for Future Research

Workplace cyberbullying research is in its infancy and small in scope, leaving numerous avenues for future research. First, workplace cyberbullying has only recently been clearly defined as negative, technology-mediated behaviors that are repetitively experienced by a vulnerable target within the work context (Farley et al. 2016; Vranjes et al., 2018). This conceptual definition should be used as the foundation for future investigations of the construct with an eye toward examining how cyberbullying compares to other forms of cyberaggression. For example, cyberbullying has been shown to differ from traditional bullying and cyberaggression (Farley et al., 2016), and it would be helpful to further explore how cyberbullying is distinct from cyber incivility. This movement toward a consistent definition of the construct will be aided by reliable and valid measures of workplace cyberbullying (Farley et al., 2015; Farley et al., 2016; Jönsson et al.,

2017; Vranjes et al., 2018). Future work with these measures should more clearly define the frequency with which the behaviors need to be experienced to be considered a target of cyberbullying. Past research has defined being a cyberbullying target as experiencing one to two negative behaviors at least weekly over the past six months (Coyne, Farley et al., 2017; Gardner et al., 2016), but an approach that considers the unique aspects of repetition (e.g., repeatedly watching a video or reading an e-mail) needs to be considered. Additionally, the existing measures of workplace cyberbullying focus primarily on the experience of the victim; thus, more effort could be directed toward developing measures of the perpetrator's and bystander's motives and behaviors. Also, given that workplace norms can vary across cultures, the workplace cyberbullying measures should be cross-culturally translated and validated. Then these measures could be used to more consistently study cyberbullying prevalence across different cultures, job types, and work contexts. This would be particularly helpful for examining potential cross-cultural differences in the power differential between targets and perpetrators.

Second, a host of variables could be studied in relation to workplace cyberbullying. Given the limited findings regarding gender differences in workplace cyberbullying, future studies could further explore this relationship to determine if men are experiencing workplace cyberbullying more often than women (Forssell, 2016; Jönsson et al., 2017). Studies examining the link between workplace cyberbullying and physical health are also quite limited, and the introduction of psychophysiological measures of the stress response (e.g., blood pressure, heart rate variability) could serve to help explain decreases in physical health (Giumetti et al., 2013). Future research could also aim to explore variables that have been associated with traditional workplace bullying, such as symptoms of post-traumatic stress disorder, organizational commitment, and sickness absence (Nielsen & Einarsen, 2012; Nielsen, Tangen, Idsoe, Matthiesen, & Mageroy, 2015; Nielsen, Indregard, & Overland, 2016). Other authors have suggested investigating the relationships between cyberbullying in the workplace and trait anger, narcissism, approval of aggression, job dissatisfaction, interpersonal conflicts, behavioral ethics, counterproductive workplace behaviors (CWBs), emotional intelligence (EI), different types of aggression, upward cyberbullying from low to high status individuals, and the "dark triad" personality traits of psychopathy, Machiavellianism, and narcissism (Keskin, Akgün, Ayar, & Kayman, 2016; Madan, 2014; Salazar, 2017; Schimmel & Nicholls, 2013). Proposed mediation and moderation models such as the Emotion Reaction model (Vranjes et al., 2017) should be tested, and new models of workplace cyberbullying might be developed and tested as well (Monks et al., 2009).

Third, the lack of studies that employ an experimental design is quite apparent in this body of research, limiting the ability to draw cause and effect conclusions. However, this is understandable because it may be ethically unsound to expose individuals to workplace cyberbullying within their real work contexts due to the negative mental and physical stress that could result. Laboratory studies of mock work situations may be one way to successfully study variables that cause or can result from workplace cyberbullying, as has been done in the workplace cyber incivility literature (Giumetti et al., 2013). While laboratory studies will suffer from decreased external validity, they can allow for more control over extraneous variables and improved internal validity. Using vignettes of workplace cyberbullying is another alternative to real world cyberbullying. Recently, Coyne, Gopaul, and colleagues (2017) studied witnesses' feelings toward cyberbullies and their targets. Interestingly, they found that working adults responding to bullying vignettes were less likely to feel sympathy for a bullying target and more likely to support the bullying perpetrator for work-related cyberbullying as opposed to personal bullying offline.

Finally, as it appears that workplace cyberbullying may have a plethora of negative individual and organizational outcomes, it is imperative that future research examine the effectiveness of interventions to reduce workplace cyberbullying. Due to the absence of studies examining workplace cyberbullying interventions, research examining the effectiveness of traditional bullying interventions in the workplace and cyberbullying in other contexts such as schools can be used to guide future research directions. For instance, in a review of interventions for traditional workplace bullying, Escartín (2016) identified approaches that effectively reduced workplace bullying or its correlates, including therapy for bullying victims, a zero-tolerance bullying program, and cognitive rehearsal training. Escartín (2016) suggests that future bullying intervention research use waiting-list control groups, use mixed-method approaches, measure outcomes at more than two time points, expand beyond European nations, and explore the optimal length of interventions. A review of school bullying interventions has shown that longer duration and greater intensity interventions were the most effective (Ttofi & Farrington, 2011), suggesting that duration and intensity are important considerations for workplace cyberbullying interventions. Additionally, the cultural, racial, and ethnic context in which an intervention is implemented and tested should be considered. Past school bullying research has found that interventions in more homogenous samples were more effective than interventions in more heterogenous samples (Evans, Fraser, & Cotter, 2014).

Practical Implications

As researchers continue to expand our understanding of workplace cyberbullying, its correlates, and the effectiveness of intervention programs, organizations should aim to draw upon this body of research to guide the prevention of workplace cyberbullying and to aid those experiencing negative effects resulting from workplace cyberbullying. First, organizations can develop clear and visible zero-tolerance policies for cyberbullying behavior, with clear definitions and descriptions of workplace cyberbullying, while maintaining freedom of expression for employees (Escartín, 2016; Piotrowski, 2012; Sarkar, 2015; West, Foster, Levin,

Edmison, & Robibero, 2014). Although developing clear organizational policies for appropriate electronic communication is essential, it is likely that employees may not follow company policy, which necessitates other processes for preventing cyberbullying (Whitty & Carr, 2006). Another possibility is that human resources could aim to screen out potentially aggressive or biased candidates during the selection process (Sarkar, 2015). Furthermore, intervention programs could increase managers' awareness of the signs and symptoms of cyberbullying and help them to respond appropriately to instances of cyberbullying, with the goal of reducing future occurrences (Piotrowski, 2012; Sarkar, 2015). When implementing cyberbullying interventions, the intervention facilitators should be respected and trusted by employees, the organization should be committed to the program, and the climate should be positive (Escartín, 2016). Additionally, mentorship and team-building programs could aim to improve relationships among employees (Escartín, 2016; West et al., 2014).

When considering how to help individuals who have already experienced cyberbullying in the workplace, it is informative to know what a target of workplace cyberbullying does in response to the incidents. Kowalski et al. (2018) found that, after experiencing workplace cyberbullying, US workers were most likely to not do anything (64.3%), followed by report the behavior (17.7%), save the evidence (17.0%), ask the person to stop (14.4%), bully back (8.5%), block/avoid contact (6.2%), and make fun of the perpetrator (5.6%). Similarly, working undergraduate students who experienced cyberbullying were also most likely to do nothing (36.3%) followed by ask the person to stop (30.3%), tell somebody or report it (15.2%), and save the evidence (15.2%) (Kowalski et al., 2012). In a qualitative study of workplace cyberbullying, workers who were targets of cyberbullying coped by avoiding or confronting the perpetrator, controlling the communication medium with the perpetrator, or seeking revenge (Heatherington & Coyne, 2014). Due to the negative outcomes associated with workplace cyberbullying, taking no action or aggressive action is less than ideal. It may be necessary to provide employees with the training and resources they need to act appropriately in response to cyberbullying. To that end, organizations should have an established process and committee for handling cyberbullying complaints confidentially and legally (Escartín, 2016; Piotrowski, 2012). Also, stress reduction or therapy programs could be provided for affected employees (Escartín, 2016; Sarkar, 2015).

Conclusion

In summary, important recent advancements in the workplace cyberbullying literature include the establishment of a clear conceptual definition and the validation of workplace cyberbullying measures. The body of literature examining the prevalence, correlates, mediators, and moderators of workplace cyberbullying is small, leaving the field wide open for future research. Importantly, it is clear that workplace cyberbullying is associated with many negative person-related and work-related factors, which provides the impetus for the development and evaluation of workplace cyberbullying interventions to prevent the occurrence of this behavior and to mitigate its adverse outcomes. As these interventions are explored, organizations can seek to develop policies and procedures to increase awareness and management of workplace cyberbullying.

References

Baruch, Y. (2005). Bullying on the net: Adverse behavior on e-mail and its impact. *Information & Management, 42*, 361–371. doi:10.1016/j.im.2004. 02. 001

Coyne, I., Farley, S., Axtell, C., Sprigg, C., Best, L., & Kwok, O. (2017). Understanding the relationship between experiencing workplace cyberbullying, employee mental strain and job satisfaction: A disempowerment approach. *The International Journal of Human Resource Management, 28*(7), 945–972. doi:10.1080/09585192.2015.1116454

Coyne, I., Gopaul, A., Campbell, M., Pankasz, A., Garland, R., & Cousans, F. (2017). Bystander responses to bullying at work: The role of mode, type, and relationship to target. *Journal of Business Ethics*, 1–15. doi:10.1007/s10551-017-3692-2https://link.springer.com/article/10.1007/s10551-017-3692-2

D'Cruz, P., & Noronha, E. (2013). Navigating the extended reach: Target experiences of cyberbullying at work. *Information and Organization, 23*, 324–343. doi:10.1016/j.infoandorg.2013.09.001

Dooley, J. J., Pyzalski, J., & Cross, D. (2009). Cyberbullying versus face-to-face bullying: A theoretical and conceptual review. *Journal of Psychology, 217*(4), 182–188. doi:10.1027/0044-3409.217. 4. 182

Durkin, K., & Patterson, D. (2011). Cyberbullying, cyberharassing, and cyberstalking. In C. D. Bryant (Ed.), *Routledge handbook of deviant behavior* (pp. 450–455). New York, NY: Routledge.

Einarsen, S., Hoel, H., & Notelaers, G. (2009). Measuring exposure to bullying and harassment at work: Validity, factor structure and psychometric properties of the Negative Acts Questionnaire-Revised. *Work & Stress, 23*(1), 24–44. doi:10.1080/02678370902815673

Escartín, J. (2016). Insights into workplace bullying: Psychosocial drivers and effective interventions. *Psychology Research and Behavior Management, 9*, 157–169. doi:10.2147/PRBM.S91211

Evans, C. B. R., Fraser, M. W., & Cotter, K. L. (2014). The effectiveness of school-based bullying prevention programs: A systematic review. *Aggression and Violent Behavior, 19*, 532–544. doi:10.1016/j.avb.2014.07.004

Farley, S., Coyne, I., Axtell, C., & Sprigg, C. (2016). Design, development and validation of a workplace cyberbullying measure, the WCM. *Work & Stress, 30*(4), 293–317. doi:10.1080/02678373.2016.1255998

Farley, S., Coyne, I., Sprigg, C., Axtell, C., & Subramanian, G. (2015). Exploring the impact of workplace cyberbullying on trainee doctors. *Medical Education, 49*, 436–443. doi:10.1111/medu.12666

Forssell, R. (2016). Exploring cyberbullying and face-to-face bullying in working life – Prevalence, targets and expressions. *Computers in Human Behavior, 58*, 454–460. doi:10.1016/j.chb.2016.01.003

Gardner, D., O'Driscoll, M., Cooper-Thomas, H. D., Roche, M., Bentley, T., Catley, B., …Trenberth, L. (2016). Predictors of workplace bullying and cyber-bullying in New Zealand. *International Journal of Environmental Research and Public Health, 13*, 1–14. doi:10.3390/ijerph13050448

Giumetti, G. W., Hatfield, A. L., Scisco, J. L., Schroeder, A. N., Muth, E. R., & Kowalski, R. M. (2013). What a rude e-mail! Examining the differential effects of incivility versus support on mood, energy, engagement, and performance in an online context. *Journal of Occupational Health Psychology, 18*(3), 297–309. doi:10.1037/a0032851

Giumetti, G. W., McKibben, E. S., Hatfield, A. L., Schroeder, A. N., & Kowalski, R. M. (2012). Cyber incivility @ work: The new age of interpersonal deviance. *Cyberpsychology, Behavior, and Social Networking, 15*(3), 148–154.

Heatherington, W., & Coyne, I. (2014). Understanding individual experiences of cyber-bullying encountered through work. *International Journal of Organization Theory and Behavior, 17*(2), 163–192.

Hershcovis, M. S. (2011). "Incivility, social undermining, bullying…oh my!": A call to reconcile constructs within workplace aggression research. *Journal of Organizational Behavior, 32*, 499–519. doi:10.1002/job

Hong, J., Lin, C., Hwang, M., Hu, R., & Chen, Y. (2014). Positive affect predicting worker psychological response to cyber-bullying in the high-tech industry in Northern Taiwan. *Computers in Human Behavior, 30*, 307–314. doi:10.1016/j.chb.2013.09.011

Jönsson, S., Muhonen, T., Forssell, R. C., & Bäckström, M. (2017). Assessing exposure to bullying through digital devices in working life: Two versions of a Cyberbullying Questionnaire (CBQ). *Psychology, 8*, 477–494. doi:10.4236/psych.2017.83030

Kane, K., & Montgomery, K. (1998). A framework for understanding disempowerment in organizations. *Human Resource Management, 37*, 263–275. doi:10.1002/(SICI)1099-050X(199823/24)37:3/4<263::AID-HRM8>3.0.CO;2-U

Keskin, H., Akgün, A. E., Ayar, H. & Kayman, S. S. (2016). Cyberbullying victimization, counterproductive work behaviours and emotional intelligence at workplace. *Procedia – Social and Behavioral Sciences, 235*, 281–287. doi:10.1016/j.sbspro.2016.11doi:031

Kowalski, R. M., Giumetti, G. W., Schroeder, A. N., & Reese, H. H. (2012). Cyber-bullying among college students: Evidence from multiple domains of college life. In L. A. Wankel & C. Wankel (Eds.), *Misbehavior online in higher education* (pp. 293–321). Bingley, UK: Emerald Publishing Group Limited.

Kowalski, R. M., Toth, A., & Morgan, M. (2018). Bullying and cyberbullying in adulthood and the workplace. *The Journal of Social Psychology, 158*(1), 64–81. doi:10.1080/00224545.2017.1302402

Madan, A. O. (2014). Cyber aggression / cyber bullying and the dark triad: Effect on workplace behavior / performance. *International Journal of Social, Behavioral, Educational, Economic, Business and Industrial Engineering, 8*(6), 1740–1745. Retrieved from http://scholar.waset.org/1999.10/9998533

Monks, C. P., Smith, P. K., Naylor, P., Barter, C., Ireland, J. L., & Coyne, I. (2009). Bullying in different contexts: Commonalities, differences and the role of theory. *Aggression and Violent Behavior, 14*, 146–156. doi:10.1016/j.avb.2009. 01. 004

Muhonen, T., Jönsson, S., & Bäckström, M. (2017). Consequences of cyberbullying behaviour in working life: The mediating roles of social support and social organizational climate. *International Journal of Workplace Health, 10*(5), 376–390. doi:10.1108/IJWHM-10-2016-0075

Nielsen, M. B., & Einarsen, S. (2012). Outcomes of exposure to workplace bullying: A meta-analytic review. *Work & Stress, 26*(4), 309–332. doi:10.1080/02678373.2012.734709

Nielsen, M. B., Indregard, A. R., & Overland, S. (2016). Workplace bullying and sickness absence: A systematic review and meta-analysis of the research literature. *Scandinavian Journal of Work and Environmental Health, 42*(5), 359–370. doi:10.5271/sjweh.3579

Nielsen, M. B., Matthiesen, S. B., & Einarsen, S. (2010). The impact of methodological moderators on prevalence rates of workplace bullying. A meta-analysis. *Journal of Occupational and Organizational Psychology, 83*, 955–979. doi:10.1348/096317909X481256

Nielsen, M. B., Tangen, T., Idsoe, T., Matthiesen, S. B., & Mageroy, N. (2015). Post-traumatic stress disorder as a consequence of bullying at work and at school. A literature review and meta-analysis. *Aggression and Violent Behavior, 21*, 17–24. doi:10.1016/j.avb.2015.01.001

Piotrowski, C. (2012). From workplace bullying to cyberbullying: The enigma of e-harassment in modern organizations. *Organization Development Journal, 30*(4), 44–53.

Privitera, C., & Campbell, M. A. (2009). Cyberbullying: The new face of workplace bullying? *Cyberpsychology & Behavior, 12*(4), 395–400. doi:10.1089=cpb.2009.0025

Purcell, K., & Rainie, L. (2014). *Technology's impact on workers*. Pew Research Center. Retrieved from www.pewinternet.org/2014/12/30/technologys-impact-on-workers/

Salazar, L. R. (2017). Workplace bullying in digital environments: Antecedents, consequences, prevention, and future directions. In B. Christiansen & H. C. Chandan (Eds.), *Handbook of research on organizational culture and diversity in the modern workforce* (pp. 132–154). Hershey, PA: IGI Global. doi:10.4018/978-1-5225-2250-8.ch007

Sarkar, A. (2015). Step-by-step to stopping the cyber-bully: How organizations can help to tackle the menace. *Human Resource Management International Digest, 23*(7), 31–33. doi:10.1108/HRMID-07-2015-0129

Schimmel, K. & Nicholls, J. (2013). Workplace cyber bullying: A research agenda. In J. Lipinksi & L. M. Crothers (Eds.), *Bullying in the workplace: Causes, symptoms, and remedies* (pp. 223–236). New York, NY: Routledge.

Smith, P. K., Mahdavi, J., Carvalho, M., Fisher, S., Russell, S., & Tippett, N. (2008). Cyberbullying: Its nature and impact in secondary school pupils. *Journal of Child Psychology and Psychiatry, 49*(4), 376–385. doi:10.1111/j.1469-7610.2007.01846.x

Snyman, R., & Loh, J. M. I. (2015). Cyberbullying at work: The mediating role of optimism between cyberbullying and job outcomes. *Computers in Human Behavior, 53*, 161–168. doi:10.1016/j.chb.2015.06.050

Tokunaga, R. S. (2010). Following you home from school: A critical review and synthesis of research on cyberbullying victimization. *Computers in Human Behavior, 26*(3), 277–287. doi:10.1016/j.chb.2009.11.014

Ttofi, M. M., & Farrington, D. P. (2011). Effectiveness of school-based programs to reduce bullying: A systematic and meta-analytic review. *Journal of Experimental Criminology, 7*, 27–56. doi:10.1007/s11292-010-9109-1

Vranjes, I., Baillien, E., Vandebosch, H., Erreygers, S. & De Witte, H. (2017). The dark side of working online: Towards a definition and an Emotion Reaction model of workplace cyberbullying. *Computers in Human Behavior, 69*, 324–334. doi:10.1016/j.chb.2016.12.055

Vranjes, I., Baillien, E., Vandebosch, H., Erreygers, S. & De Witte, H. (2018). When workplace bullying goes online: Construction and validation of the Inventory of Cyberbullying Acts at Work (ICA-W). *European Journal of Work and Organizational Psychology, 27*(1), 28–39. doi:10.1080/1359432X.2017.1363185

West, B., Foster, M., Levin, A., Edmison, J., & Robibero, D. (2014). Cyberbullying at work: In search of effective guidance. *Laws, 3*, 598–617. doi:10.3390/laws3030598

Whitty, M. T., & Carr, A. N. (2006). New rules in the workplace: Applying object-relations theory to explain problem Internet and email behaviour in the workplace. *Computers in Human Behavior, 22*(2), 235–250. doi:10.1016/j.chb.2004.06.005

7

CYBERBULLYING IN THE WORKPLACE

Cross-Cultural Issues

Erin M. Richard, Julianna J. Walsh, and Zhiqing E. Zhou

Organizational research has seen an increased amount of attention aimed at understanding the phenomenon of workplace bullying (Gloor, 2014; Van den Brande, Baillien, DeWitte, Elst, & Godderis, 2016). Such attention is well deserved as bullying has been linked to important work-related outcomes, such as difficulty concentrating, lower self-efficacy, poor job attitudes, increased illness, higher absenteeism, reduced productivity, and higher turnover intentions (Djurkovic, McCormack, & Casimir, 2004; Hoel & Cooper, 2003; Keashly & Jagatic, 2003; Moayed, Daraiseh, Shell, & Salem, 2006; Tepper, 2000). Exponential improvements in technology over the past several decades have also created a new conduit for bullying in organizations: work-related information and communications technologies (W-ICTs), such as email and text messaging. Communication via W-ICT is one of the most common forms of communication in organizations (Brown, Duck, & Jimmieson, 2014; Vidgen, Sims, & Powell, 2011), yet the nature of communication via W-ICT has been proposed to increase the likelihood of incivility and bullying (Giumetti, McKibben, Hatfield, Schroeder, & Kowalski, 2012; Privitera & Campbell, 2009). For example, behavioral norms are less salient when communicating online, leading to an online disinhibition effect whereby individuals behave differently (and often more aggressively) than they would in face-to-face settings (Suler, 2004). Additionally, W-ICT lacks many of the nonverbal cues available in face-to-face communication (e.g., tone of voice, body language). This is particularly true of the leaner, text-based forms of W-ICT (e.g., email). As a result, messages may be perceived as more intensely negative than intended by the sender (Byron, 2008), leading to exchanges that become increasingly aggressive over time (Andersson & Pearson, 1999; Friedman & Currall, 2003). Thus, given the popularity of W-ICT, workplace cyberbullying is a topic with which organizations will have to contend for the foreseeable future.

Cyberbullying refers to intentional aggressive behavior from one or a group of perpetrators that occurs repeatedly and over time through electronic forms of communication (Smith et al., 2008). While this definition was originally developed for the educational context, it has since been integrated with definitions of workplace bullying in order to put forth the following defining features of workplace cyberbullying: (1) unwanted aggressive behaviors, (2) that are enacted in a work-related context, (3) with repeated and long-term occurrence, (4) targeted at victims with a lack of power and/or ability to defend themselves, and (5) manifested through work-related information and communications technologies (W-ICTs) (e.g., Coyne et al., 2017; Olweus, 1993; Vranjes, Baillien, Vandebosch, Erreygers, & DeWitte, 2017).

Although there has been increasing research attention on cyberbullying at work (e.g., Coyne et al., 2017; Vranjes et al., 2017; also see Chapters 6 and 8 of this book), the literature in this area is still in its infancy, and, as a result, little to no research has examined workplace cyberbullying from a cross-cultural perspective. However, research on cultural differences in workplace bullying as well as research on cultural differences in communication suggest that workplace cyberbullying may indeed vary substantially between cultures. The goal of this chapter is to stimulate research on this topic by reviewing literature on cultural differences in both workplace bullying and computer-mediated communication and discussing the implications of those two bodies of research for viewing cyberbullying through a cultural lens. We start by reviewing research and theory that have examined workplace bullying from a cultural perspective.

Workplace Bullying: Cultural Perspectives

Cultural values play an important role in employees' perceptions of and reactions to work-related events like bullying (Gelfand, Erez, & Aycan, 2007). Yet despite the increased attention paid to the antecedents and consequences of workplace bullying over the past 20 years, researchers have just begun to examine the role of culture in understanding workplace bullying (Escartín, Zapf, Arrieta, & Rodríguez-Carballeira, 2011; Jacobson, Hood, & Van Buren, 2014). Recent developments in this line of research suggest that culture influences not only the nature or form of workplace bullying, but also its prevalence, associated meanings, and outcomes.

Two commonly used frameworks in cross-cultural research are Hofstede's (1980) national cultural values and the Global Leadership and Organizational Behavior Effectiveness (GLOBE) research program's value dimensions (House, Hanges, Javidan, Dorfman, & Gupta, 2004). Among the four national cultural values in Hofstede's (1980) framework (power distance, individualism, uncertainty avoidance, and masculinity), power distance has been the most commonly studied value dimension when it comes to workplace bullying (e.g., Loh,

Restubog, & Zagenczyk, 2010), likely due to the power imbalance component of most bullying definitions. Among the nine cultural dimensions in the GLOBE framework, some of them (e.g., humane orientation, performance orientation, and future orientation; Power et al., 2013) have been directly tested in the workplace bullying context, and others (e.g., assertiveness, power distance, and in-group collectivism) have been proposed to affect the form and prevalence of workplace bullying but remain untested (Jacobson et al., 2014). The following sections review research and theory that have examined the role of culture or cultural values in understanding workplace bullying. Specifically, we review how cultural variables relate to the definitions and terminology associated with the workplace bullying construct, prevalence rates, and outcomes of workplace bullying.

Cultural Differences in the Construct of Workplace Bullying

A major challenge in cross-cultural research on workplace bullying is that the definitions and terminology used to describe the phenomenon are also culturally dependent (Jacobson et al., 2014). The same behavior labeled as "bullying" in one culture may not be considered bullying in another culture. For example, Escartín et al. (2011) found differences in how workplace bullying is defined between Central American employees and Southern European employees. Central American participants tended to include both physical and psychological behaviors in their definition of workplace bullying, while Southern European participants considered workplace bullying to be mainly a psychological construct. Furthermore, bullying behavior was perceived differently across cultures depending on whether the perpetrator was a superior or a colleague. Central American participants equated bullying with mistreatment from a supervisor, while Southern European participants considered workplace bullying to also come from coworkers and subordinates. On the other hand, both Central American participants and Southern European participants considered direct (e.g., directly causing harm to the victims) and indirect (e.g., causing harm by hurting people or objects valued by the victims) behavior to be components of the definition of workplace bullying (Escartín et al., 2011).

D'Cruz, Paull, Omari, and Guneri-Cangarli (2016) used a qualitative method to compare target experiences of workplace bullying across cultures. They explored sources, manifestations, etiology, outcomes, coping, interventions, and bystander behaviors by applying a cross-cultural framework that combined both Hofstede's and GLOBE approaches. Surveying participants from Turkey, Australia, and India, they identified areas of convergence and divergence among the three countries. Example areas of convergence included behavioral manifestations of workplace bullying (person- and task-related behavior), adverse emotional and physical outcomes, and the belief that filing complaints was not a preferred option. In terms of differences, D'Cruz et al. (2016) found that Australian participants reported supervisors and peers as sources, but Indian and Turkish participants mainly considered supervisors as sources. D'Cruz et al. (2016) argued that the hierarchical, authority-ranking nature of Indian and Turkish societies (an indication of high power distance) and the egalitarian nature of Australian society (an indication of low power distance) might account for the differences.

Seo, Leather, and Coyne (2012) theorized that people of the Far East might view bullying in a different light than people of Western countries, and they, specifically, used South Korea to demonstrate how a country's history and culture might impact the peoples' attitude toward the concept. Seo et al. (2012) provide an explanation of how group orientation, conformity, and high power distance values lead South Koreans to view certain negative acts as bullying when the perpetrator was a colleague but not when the perpetrator was a superior. They also described how, under the philosophy and moral system of Confucianism, obedience and respect for seniors might lead to mistreatment by superiors being overlooked. Finally, Seo et al. (2012) described how cultural values can influence the vocabulary used to label mistreatment. They mention that South Korea's collectivist values influence the use of terms for bullying such that the terms imply the action of bullying is a group action.

In addition to the terms used to describe and define bullying, Jacobson et al. (2014) suggested that culture would impact the form in which workplace bullying is likely to manifest. For example, they proposed that covert bullying (in which the bullying is less visible and hostile intent is concealed) is likely to be more common than overt bullying (where the hostile intent is explicit) in cultures low on assertiveness, high on in-group collectivism, or low on power distance. Jacobson et al. (2014) also proposed that bullying would be more likely to take on a group-based form (compared to a more dyad-based form) in cultures low on assertiveness or high on in-group collectivism.

Cultural Differences in the Prevalence of Workplace Bullying

Researchers have suggested that the prevalence of workplace bullying also varies across cultures (Jacobson et al., 2014; Moayed et al., 2006). There are likely two main reasons for differences in prevalence rates. First, cultural differences in labeling certain behaviors as workplace bullying may lead to differences in prevalence rates across cultures. For example, the reported prevalence rate of workplace bullying was 3% in Denmark (Agervold, 2007) compared to 51% in Turkey (Bilgel, Aytac, & Bayram, 2006). Mikkelsen and Einarsen (2001) found a similarly low prevalence in Denmark (2–4% of their sample reported experiencing bullying in the workplace), but they found that those numbers increased when operationally defining bullying (i.e., occurring weekly for at least six months) or when asking if participants had witnessed others being bullied. This suggests that the operational definition and measurement of bullying need to be held constant when comparing prevalence rates across cultures.

Second, the prevalence of workplace bullying and other forms of mistreatment are likely influenced by cultural values. Mikkelsen and Einarsen (2001), for example, hypothesized that the low prevalence rates of workplace bullying in Denmark were due to commonly held feminine, individualistic, and low power distance cultural values (Einarsen, 2000; Hofstede, 1980). Similarly, Jacobson et al. (2014) have proposed that workplace bullying is likely to be more prevalent in cultures high on assertiveness, low on in-group collectivism, and high on power distance. To our knowledge, these propositions have yet to be tested empirically.

Other research has found that prevalence rates are higher in Northern and Western European countries than Southern and Eastern European countries (Arenas et al., 2015; Giorgi, Arenas, & Leon-Perez, 2011). Arenas et al. (2015) suggested that the higher rates of workplace bullying prevalence in Northern European countries could be attributed to more awareness and sensitivity about the problem in those countries compared to Southern European countries, such as Spain or Italy. Further, Seo et al. (2012) noted that a prevalence rate of only 5.7% has been found in South Korea, and they proposed that close social bonding as a result of collectivist values makes the occurrence of workplace bullying even less prevalent than in European countries (Seo et al., 2012). Such strong social ties might also reduce the likelihood of bullying being reported when it does occur.

One of the goals of a meta-analysis by Nielsen, Matthiesen, and Einarsen (2010) was to demonstrate how measurement methods and sampling techniques moderated the estimated prevalence rates of workplace bullying. Neilsen et al. found that research has reported lower prevalence rates in Scandinavian countries than in other European and Non-European countries. They also note a sampling bias towards Scandinavian countries due to the sheer number of studies conducted in that region and the number of studies including Scandinavian samples in their meta-analysis (more than a quarter). Therefore, they recommend interpreting general prevalence results with care because Scandinavian rates might be influencing overall prevalence rates. In addition, Nielsen et al. (2010) called for more studies to "standardize the definition and assessment of workplace bullying" (p. 325) so that results from studies in different cultures can be compared.

Cultural Differences in the Acceptance and Outcomes of Workplace Bullying

Not only has culture been examined as an influence on the definition and prevalence of workplace bullying but also as a lens that shapes how people construe and react to workplace bullying. Workplace bullying may simply be more accepted in some cultures than others (Salin, 2003). Loh et al. (2010) proposed that this difference might be attributed to differences in power distance. They argue that cultures with high power distance might be more likely to accept the power imbalance that accompanies bullying, such that the behavior will be more acceptable and have weaker effects in these cultures. By comparing samples from

Singapore and Austria, they found that the negative effects of workplace bullying on job satisfaction and workgroup identification were stronger for the sample from Austria (considered low power distance) than the sample from Singapore (considered high power distance).

Power et al. (2013) also examined how the acceptability of workplace bullying is related to cultural values using samples from 14 countries across six continents. Using three of the cultural practices examined by the GLOBE study (House et al., 2004), Power et al. (2013) found that humane orientation (which emphasizes caring and support from high authority figures) was negatively related to the acceptability of work-related bullying, while performance orientation (which emphasizes accomplishment) was positively related to the acceptance of bullying. Future orientation (which includes a focus on maintaining relationships) was found to negatively relate to the acceptability of workplace bullying.

Kernan, Watson, Chen, and Kim (2011) argued that cultural values could affect people's perception of justice after being abused. In addition, they suggested that cultural values could also impact employees' attributions for supervisor bullying, such that, in some cultures, the victims might make internal attributions for the abuse (i.e., blame themselves) and thus be more likely to accept the experience of supervisor bullying. Using a cultural framework by Schwartz (1994), the authors proposed that power values (that emphasize wealth and achievement), achievement values (that emphasize personal success), and benevolence values (that emphasize concern for close others in daily interactions) would moderate the effect of supervisor bullying on outcomes. Their results suggested that achievement values and benevolence values exacerbated the negative effects of supervisor bullying on employee job satisfaction and perceived organizational support, but, surprisingly, power values did not moderate the effects of supervisor bullying.

Finally, in addition to their effects on individual responses to workplace bullying, cultural values may also impact organizational responses. For example, in D'Cruz et al.'s (2016) comparison of Turkey, Australia, and India, the researchers found that Australian employees reported the existence of more formal intervention and coping programs in their organizations, possibly due to the highly egalitarian, low power distance values found in Australia.

Cultural Differences as a Basis for Mistreatment

Cultural differences can also impact workplace mistreatment from another angle. Simply belonging to different cultural groups can, at times, instigate intercultural conflict and make some employees targets of bullying in the workplace. Neuman and Baron (1998) discuss how workforce diversity can be a social determinant of workplace aggression when individuals, due to stereotyping or miscommunication, have trouble working with those who are dissimilar to themselves. According to the Selective Incivility Theory, individuals of different racial and ethnic backgrounds might be targeted more often for mistreatment in the workplace due to the prevalence of discriminatory attitudes (Cortina, 2008).

In general, research has supported the idea that minorities and out-group members are at higher risk of being bullied in the workplace. In Finland, Bergbom, Vartia-Vaaanen, and Kinnunen (2015) analyzed how much bullying immigrants experience as opposed to natives, and how that differs by immigrants' cultural distance. Cultural distance was described as cultural "dissimilarity" and determined by country of origin and native language(s). They did indeed find that, on average, immigrants experienced more bullying, but the least culturally distant group of immigrants did not experience any more bullying than natives experienced. On the other hand, the intermediate culturally distant group experienced almost three times more bullying than natives, and the most culturally distant group experienced almost eight times more bullying than natives (Bergbom et al., 2015). Bergbom et al.'s (2015) research suggests that predicting workplace mistreatment with respect to cultural background may have more to do with cultural distance than the immigrant classification.

Summary and Implications

The section above began to lay a foundation for future theoretical and empirical investigations of workplace cyberbullying by reviewing research and theory on cultural differences in workplace bullying in general. Some of these studies (Giorgi, Leon-Perez, & Arenas, 2015; Mikkelsen & Einarsen, 2001; Seo et al., 2012) were single-country studies that focused on how the historical background and cultural values of a nation can influence the prevalence of, mentality toward, and reaction to workplace bullying. A common theme across many of these articles was the call for more research analyzing workplace bullying in particular countries or cultures, asserting that not enough research has been conducted on workplace bullying in those particular cultures (e.g., Mikkelsen & Einarsen, 2001; Seo et al., 2012). Conversely, other studies (e.g., Arenas et al., 2015; Kernan et al., 2011; Loh et al., 2010) used multi-nation samples and compared different cultures on forms, prevalence, and reactions to workplace bullying, frequently drawing on cultural value frameworks (Hofstede, 1980; House et al., 2004; Schwartz, 1994) to explain such differences. Notably, these two approaches of examining workplace bullying reflect the distinction between the emic and etic perspectives in cultural research—two approaches that are ideally integrated to overcome each other's limitations (Morris, Leung, Ames, & Lickel, 1999).

The workplace bullying research reviewed above has several implications for future research on workplace cyberbullying. First, given that understanding of the nature of workplace bullying differs substantially across cultures (Mikkelsen & Einarsen, 2001), careful attention must be paid to operational definitions of cyberbullying before attempting to compare its prevalence across cultures. Second, the role of the perpetrator (e.g., supervisor, peer, subordinate) can substantially change how the same act is viewed from different cultural perspectives (Seo et al., 2012); therefore, the extent to which a message sent via W-ICT is interpreted as an instance of cyberbullying is likely to be dependent on the sender of the message, their role in the organization, and the interaction between that role and cultural values like power distance or assertiveness. Third, tolerance for cyberbullying in the workplace is likely to vary greatly across cultures based on values and socio-cultural norms (e.g., Ghosh, 2017), as will employee reactions (Giorgi et al., 2015) and organizational responses (D'Cruz et al., 2016) to cyberbullying. Such differences are important for understanding the need for and acceptance of workplace interventions to reduce cyberbullying within global organizations. Finally, because intercultural conflict and identity-based affective reactions are a potential cause of workplace bullying that cannot be overlooked (Bergbom et al., 2015; Cortina, Kabat-Farr, Leskinen, Huerta, & Magley, 2013; Welbourne, Gangadharan, & Sariol, 2015), viewing workplace cyberbullying through a cultural lens will require attention to cultural differences between employees within an organization as a potential antecedent to cyberbullying.

Role of Culture in Computer-Mediated Communication

Another area of scholarship that can be drawn upon to inform theory on cultural issues in workplace cyberbullying is research on work-related information and communications technologies (W-ICT)—particularly that examining cultural influences on W-ICT use and effectiveness. Due to the globalization of business, W-ICTs, such as email and text messages, have become a business necessity for coordinating and managing geographically dispersed employees (Olaniran, 2001). In spite of the fact that W-ICTs are intended to provide cost-savings and increase the pace of business in both local and multi-national organizations, W-ICTs also introduce challenges such as the frequent misperception of emotional intent and a higher likelihood of conflict escalation (e.g., Byron, 2008; Friedman & Currall, 2003). Adding to these challenges is the fact that researchers are just beginning to understand the cultural boundaries of W-ICT use and its effectiveness (Davis, Leas, & Dobelman, 2009; Richard & McFadden, 2016; Vignovic & Thompson, 2010). This dearth of research is unfortunate, given the conundrum that globalization simultaneously increases organizations' reliance on W-ICTs as well as the cross-cultural challenges associated with their implementation. Below, we review research and theory on cross-cultural differences that are particularly relevant to the use and effectiveness of W-ICTs, and we discuss their implications for workplace cyberbullying research.

Olaniran (2001) was among the first to encourage a better understanding of the cultural differences and implications associated with communication via W-ICTs. Drawing on social information processing theory (SIPT; Walther, 1992), Olaniran (2001) argued:

> If one accepts the idea that meanings are influenced by culture, then, perceptions of CMC [computer-mediated communication] media attributes and social interaction would reflect the nuances of cultural differences in norms and beliefs in multinational (intercultural) and multidomestic (crosscultural) organizations...
>
> *(p. 87)*

Such norms and beliefs have been characterized in a number of different ways in cross-cultural research. In the section below, we focus on two particular aspects of culture that we believe to be particularly relevant to understanding cross-cultural issues in workplace cyberbullying: (1) communication differences between high- vs. low-context cultures and (2) cultural differences related to the concept of face.

High-context vs. Low-context Cultures

The distinction between high-context and low-context cultures (Hall, 1976) has particular relevance for understanding cultural differences in communication via W-ICT. In high-context cultures, much of communication is tacit, rather than explicit, and employees rely heavily on nonverbal and contextual cues (e.g., silence, space between individuals, surroundings, nature of the relationship). On the other hand, employees in low-context cultures communicate more explicitly, placing more emphasis on the words themselves (Adair, Buchan, & Chen, 2009; Hall, 1959). Examples of countries with high-context communication styles include China, Japan, Korea, and Vietnam, whereas Germany, Scandinavia, Switzerland, and the United States have been associated with low-context communication (Ting-Toomey, 1985).

Olaniran (2001) pointed out the high degree of overlap between collectivism and dependence on context in communication, stating that "Characteristics of high-context cultures are suited to collectivistic cultural tendencies, whereas those of low context cultures are suited to individualistic cultural tendencies" (p. 85). The overlap between these cultural dimensions may help to explain some of the differences that have been found between individualist and collectivist cultures on several aspects of communication, such as the use of indirect vs. direct messages (e.g., Merkin, Taras, & Steel, 2014).

Because email communication lacks many of the nonverbal and contextual variables on which high-context cultures rely, researchers have suggested that email may be less acceptable to employees in these cultures (e.g., Olaniran, 2001; Peterson et al., 2010). According to Olaniran (2001), "it is imperative to determine how this tendency [for high-context communication] affects communication effectiveness in different media" (p. 86). Without the social context cues upon which high-context cultures typically depend, employees may find it particularly difficult to decipher the emotional intent behind a message (e.g., whether an email sender is being intentionally uncivil or aggressive). According to Davis et al. (2009):

> To [high-context] cultures, email is too impersonal. Communication between high- and low-context cultures can be very problematic. Information can be missed, nuances overlooked, humor or anger misinterpreted, or the status of the requester unacknowledged, resulting in poorer comprehension.
>
> *(p. 78)*

Because of their preference for social context in communication, individuals from high-context cultures might also be more likely to incorporate social cues (e.g., icons, electronic paralanguage and lexical surrogates, or parenthetical messages that express emotions) in their W-ICT messages (Olaniran, 2001). It is unclear how individuals from low-context cultures will interpret and respond to such cues, given that interpretation of these cues may be highly dependent on culture. For example, Western researchers have found that the smiley emoticon is often used in work-related email to soften statements that might otherwise sound too direct or harsh (Gacey & Richard, 2013). However, the interpretation of emoticons could differ substantially across cultures (Park, Barash, Fink, & Cha, 2013), leading to miscommunication during intercultural exchanges.

Cultural Differences in the Concept of Face

The concept of face also differs across cultures and has implications for the way in which individuals communicate. *Face* is a term often used to describe a construct similar to honor, respectability, or dignity, as exemplified in the expression "to save face." Goffman (1967) described the concept in the following manner:

> The term *face* may be defined as the positive social value a person effectively claims for himself by the lines others assume he has taken during a particular contact. Face is an image of self delineated in terms of approved social attributes—albeit an image that others may share, as when a person makes a good showing for his profession or religion by making a good showing for himself.
>
> *(p. 5)*

Brown and Levinson (1987) describe face as a resource that is "emotionally invested" and can be "lost, maintained, or enhanced, and must constantly be attended to in interaction" (p. 66).

Although the desire for face is believed to be universal (Brown & Levinson, 1987), the concept has been found to be qualitatively different between cultures. In many collectivist cultures, face is considered a construct that is shared by everyone in the interaction, and individuals are expected to behave in a manner that preserves the face of the dyad or group. Conversely, in most individualist cultures, face is conceptualized as belonging to an individual, and people typically focus on protecting their own face during interactions (Chang & Holt, 1994). For example, in the United States, an employee could save (individual) face by blaming a mistake on his or her interaction partner. However, in China, interaction partners are expected to consider each other's face in order to make an interaction go smoothly, as exemplified by the Chinese expression "everyone gets face" (Chang & Holt, 1994). Thus, blaming one's interaction partner, especially in front of others, would cause that person to lose face, and the entire dyad or group would lose face as a result.

In addition to cross-cultural differences in the nature of face, cultures also differ in the strategies they use to protect face. For example, requests and directives (e.g., requests to reschedule a meeting or extend a deadline; directives to edit a document) may be universally face-threatening in that they impose upon the autonomy of others. However, the strategies used by individuals to save face in the context of a request or directive are culturally driven. Olaniran (2001) gives the example of the Japanese culture, in which the word "no" is typically avoided out of concern for the face of the interaction partner. In Japan, even those in positions of power are likely to phrase negative responses indirectly (e.g., saying "it will be difficult" rather than "no"). This tendency could lead to ambiguity or misunderstanding when interacting with someone from a more direct culture because these individuals often perceive indirectness as a sign of dishonesty or submissiveness (Olaniran, 2001).

Richard and McFadden (2016) examined differences in email communication between U.S. and Chinese employees in the use of facework and indirectness when making requests via email. They found that, compared to their American counterparts, Chinese employees were more likely to use facework statements such as "I hope all is well" at the beginning of their emails, and they were more likely to explain the reasoning for their request before stating the request itself. Richard and McFadden (2016) then exposed Chinese and American employees to email requests that either followed or violated the norms of their own culture and found that Chinese employees had a stronger desire to do business with the sender of the email that included facework statements and placed reasoning before the request. American employees, on the other hand, reported higher levels of irritation with this type of email.

In a qualitative study exploring the challenges of W-ICT implementation in multinational organizations in the Middle East, Zaidman, Schwartz, and Te'eni (2008) found that the use of W-ICTs for certain types of messages could itself represent a threat to face. For example, an Israeli manager working at an Egyptian plant explained that his employees would feel offended if they were to receive written instructions from him via W-ICT because written instructions would send the message that he did not trust them. This example illustrates another point made by Olaniran (2001), who suggested that, in addition to the content of a message, the communication medium itself could become a symbol (e.g., of power or competence) based upon the unspoken norms of a culture.

Summary and Implications

In sum, cultures vary on a number of tendencies that may impact communication via W-ICT. Differences in high-context vs. low-context cultures may predict acceptance and use of W-ICT because of the relative lack of context cues available in the medium. Individuals from high- vs. low- context cultures also may differ in the cues they incorporate into their messages as well as their interpretation of messages from others. Further, cultural differences in the concept of face and differences in face-saving strategies such as directness and indirectness may introduce misunderstandings or other undesirable consequences during the use of W-ICTs for intercultural communication. Finally, the use of W-ICT itself may serve as a face-related cue that can assume different meanings across cultures. Differences between high- and low-context cultures as well as cultural differences related to face should, therefore, be carefully considered in future research on cyberbullying.

The topic of cross-cultural issues related to W-ICTs is relatively understudied given the electronically connected, global world of work. By reviewing the research that has been developed so far, we can discern two points of interest for understanding work-related cyberbullying. First, because cultural preferences for high-context vs. low-context communication will likely impact the way that individuals phrase their messages, expectations for the content and structure of W-ICT messages may be frequently violated during intercultural communication, which could increase perceptions of cyberbullying if individuals interpret the violation as a threat to face. Second, the use of W-ICT may not be appropriate across all situations in all cultures; if W-ICT is used in a situation considered inappropriate for the context, it may serve as an (intentional or unintentional) aggression cue that impacts perceptions of (and reactions to) cyberbullying.

A Way Forward: Suggestions for Future Research

Based on the research reviewed above, the next section will put forth a research agenda for studying cultural influences on the workplace cyberbullying phenomenon. Modeled roughly on Sender-Message-Receiver models of communication (e.g., Berlo, 1960; Shannon & Weaver, 1949), we suggest three components of the communication process that should be considered when examining cultural issues related to cyberbullying: cultural influences on the sender, cultural influences on the message, and cultural influences on the receiver (see Figure 7.1).

Cultural Influences on the Sender

We suggest that cultural values will impact the extent to which employees intentionally engage in workplace cyberbullying. First, employees are more likely to engage in workplace cyberbullying in cultures where bullying is considered

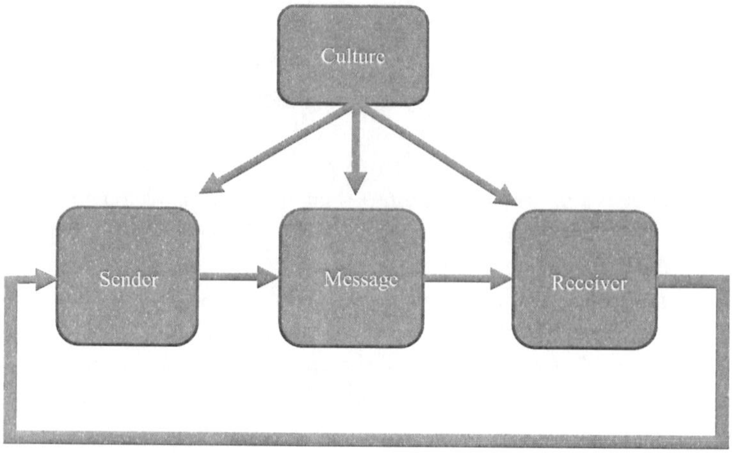

FIGURE 7.1 Cultural influences on workplace cyberbullying using the sender-message-receiver model of communication

more acceptable, such as those with high power distance (e.g., Singapore), low humane orientation (e.g., South Korea), high performance orientation (e.g., Canada), and low future orientation (e.g., Italy) (Einarsen, 2000; Loh et al., 2010; Power et al., 2013; Salin, 2003). Second, employees from cultures with a higher concern for protecting one's own face during an interaction and a lower concern for protecting mutual face (e.g., United States, Germany), may be more likely to engage in cyberbullying. On the other hand, employees who risk losing face when engaging in incivility or aggression (e.g., those from highly collective cultures) may be less likely to engage in cyberbullying—particularly against in-group members. Third, employees from cultures who value direct communication and see it as a sign of power (e.g., individualist, low-context cultures, such as the United States) may be more likely to enact cyberbullying to gain power and save face during negotiations or other forms of workplace conflict. Although cultural values are often assigned at the national level in cross-cultural research, we urge researchers to also examine cultural values at the individual level to account for within-nation variability in such values and better understand how individuals' cultural values shape cyberbullying behavior.

Cultural Influences on the Message

Because of cultural differences in preference for high- vs. low-context communication, employees will likely differ in the manner in which they construct W-ICT messages, which, in turn, should impact the likelihood that their message is perceived as cyberbullying. Within the message, senders from high-context cultures are likely to include more social context cues (Olaniran, 2001), such as the use of facework statements and indirect requests (i.e., presentation of reasoning before making a request; Richard & McFadden, 2016), whereas senders from low-context cultures are more likely to skip the niceties and directly state their intentions, requests, or directives.

We also propose that the extent to which bullying is considered physical versus psychological in a particular culture (Escartín et al., 2011) will influence message content. Individuals whose cultures place more emphasis on physical aggression when defining bullying may not consider *any* W-ICT interaction to be an instance of bullying because the interaction is not face-to-face. As a result, these individuals may feel more justified in sending aggressive messages via W-ICT because they do not believe they are engaging in bullying when there is a lack of physical threat. Methodologically, we suggest future research develop and use culture-invariant measures of cyberbullying behaviors so that cross-cultural comparisons of targets' interpretations of these behaviors can be conducted.

Cultural Influences on the Receiver

We propose that the cultural background of the message recipient will impact whether the W-ICT message is perceived as an instance of cyberbullying. The research we reviewed above suggested that cultures define bullying in different ways, leading to wide variation in whether a particular behavior is considered bullying by the target. We suggest that the use of W-ICTs serves to only increase the cultural variance in bullying perceptions by increasing the ambiguity of the message (Byron, 2008; Friedman & Currall, 2003). Further, the use of W-ICTs may introduce additional cross-cultural variance in bullying perceptions related to use of the W-ICT medium itself. For example, there may be many instances, like that mentioned by Zaidman et al. (2008), where a message that would typically be considered acceptable across cultures (instructions from a manager) may indeed become demeaning or insulting to individuals from particular cultures when communicated via W-ICT rather than face-to-face.

Recipient's threshold for determining whether an instance is considered cyberbullying can differ depending on the source (supervisor, colleague, subordinate) and the recipient's cultural beliefs about maintaining the status differential in that relationship (i.e., power distance). Additionally, the value for conformity to social norms, commonly an aspect of collectivistic societies, could influence the interpretation of a possible cyberbullying instance given the particular context and whether the message or behavior was in line with relevant cultural norms.

Another cultural difference taken from the literature in international business is the connectedness of a society, which specifically refers to the degree of Internet use (Berry, Guillén, & Zhou, 2010). It could be argued that unfamiliarity with the use of W-ICTs might inflate the possibility of miscommunication. The impact of connectedness on the perception of workplace cyberbullying could have unknown consequences. On one hand, unfamiliarity with the method of communication might decrease the likelihood that a recipient would perceive a message as uncivil due to a lack of knowledge of the norms associated with W-ICTs. On the other hand, the potential perceived bullying could be more salient to an individual unfamiliar with W-ICTs, and, with a lack of reference on how to respond, conflict could escalate quickly.

On that note, we propose that cultural variables will also influence the recipient's response to the message, which, in turn, may impact the sender's future behavior (consistent with the feedback loop included in many Sender-Message-Receiver models of communication; see Figure 7.1). Assuming that an employee considers a message to be an instance of bullying, the way in which that employee responds is likely driven by cultural values such as collectivism and power distance. For example, a high level of collectivism may prompt an individual to attempt to maintain harmony and, therefore, to ignore perceived cyberbullying as long as possible, whereas a high level of individualism may encourage employees to immediately report the incident or to respond to the sender with increased aggression. Under such circumstances, it is possible that the sender will retaliate with even greater aggression; thus, the severity of the incivility spiral or the escalation of conflict proposed in previous research (Andersson & Pearson, 1999; Friedman & Currall, 2003) may be determined by both the cultural background of both the sender and the receiver. To best capture these dynamic sender-receiver exchanges, we suggest future research use daily diary designs or weekly diary designs to examine how the targets of cyberbullying react to the experiences of cyberbullying differently depending on their cultural values. Longitudinal data will allow researchers to model cross-level relationships between cultural values (at the group or person level) and reactions to perceptions of cyberbullying (at the within-person or dyad level).

Finally, culture is also expected to influence whether individuals seek clarification of ambiguous messages that may or may not represent cyberbullying; however, the mechanisms through which culture influences such feedback seeking are unclear. For example, in cultures high in uncertainty avoidance (e.g., Italy, Korea), it is unclear whether concern for face will prevent the recipient from seeking clarification, or whether a strong desire to reduce uncertainty will encourage the recipient to do so.

Summary

With the wide use of computer-mediated communication in a globalized workforce, workplace cyberbullying is likely to become an increasingly prevalent phenomenon which could have detrimental effects on employees and organizations. We propose that it is critical to consider the role of culture in influencing how workplace cyberbullying is enacted and perceived, as well as how employees respond to perceived cyberbullying. While this line of research has not received sufficient attention, we believe future findings on these processes will have great practical implications for organizations that employ individuals from diverse cultural backgrounds as well as organizations who operate internationally.

References

Adair, W. L., Buchan, N., & Chen, X. P. (2009). Conceptualizing culture as communication in management and marketing research. In C. Nakata (Ed.), *Beyond Hofstede: Culture frameworks for global marketing and management* (pp. 146–180). New York, NY: Macmillan Palgrave.

Agervold, M. (2007). Bullying at work: A discussion of definitions and prevalence, based on an empirical study. *Scandinavian Journal of Psychology*, *48*(2), 161–172. doi:10.1111/j.1467-9450.2007.00585.x

Andersson, L. M., & Pearson, C. M. (1999). Tit for tat? The spiraling effect of incivility in the workplace. *The Academy of Management Review*, *24*(3), 452–471. doi:10.2307/259136

Arenas, A., Giorgi, G., Montani, F., Mancuso, S., Perez, J. F., Mucci, N., & Arcangeli, G. (2015). Workplace bullying in a sample of Italian and Spanish employees and its relationship with job satisfaction, and psychological well-being. *Frontiers in Psychology*, *6*, 1–10. doi:10.3389/fpsyg.2015.01912

Bergbom, B., Vartia-Vaananen, M., & Kinnunen, U. (2015). Immigrants and natives at work: Exposure to workplace bullying. *Employee Relations*, *37*(2), 158–175. doi:10.1108/ER-09-2014-0101

Berlo, D. K. (1960). *The process of communication*. New York, NY: Holt, Rinehart, & Winston.

Berry, H., Guillén, M. F., & Zhou, N. (2010). An institutional approach to cross-national distance. *Journal of International Business Studies*, *41*, 1460–1480. doi:10.1057/jibs.2010.28

Bilgel, N., Aytac, S., & Bayram, N. (2006). Bullying in Turkish white-collar workers. *Occupational Medicine*, *56*(4), 226–231. doi:10.1093/occmed/kqj041

Brown, R., Duck, J., & Jimmieson, N. (2014). E-mail in the workplace: The role of stress appraisals and normative response pressure in the relationship between e-mail stressors and employee strain. *International Journal of Stress Management*, *21*(4), 325–347. doi:10.1037/a0037464

Brown, P., & Levinson, S. (1987). *Politeness: Some universals in language use*. Cambridge: Cambridge University Press.

Byron, K. (2008). Carrying too heavy a load? The communication and miscommunication of emotion by email. *The Academy of Management Review*, *33*(2), 309–327. doi:10.2307/20159399

Chang, H. C., & Holt, R. (1994). A Chinese perspective on face as inter-relational concern. In S. Ting-Toomey (Ed.), *The challenge of facework: Cross-cultural and interpersonal issues* (pp. 95–132). Albany, NY: SUNY Press.

Cortina, L. (2008). Unseen injustice: Incivility as modern discrimination in organizations. *The Academy of Management Review*, *33*, 55–75. doi:10.2307/20159376

Cortina, L., Kabat-Farr, D., Leskinen, E., Huerta, M., & Magley, V. (2013). Selective incivility as modern discrimination in organizations. *Journal of Management*, *39*, 1579–1605. doi:10.1177/0149206311418835

Coyne, I., Farley, S., Axtell, C., Sprigg, C., Best, L., & Kwok, O. (2017). Understanding the relationship between experiencing workplace cyberbullying, employee mental strain and job satisfaction: A dysempowerment approach. *The International Journal of Human Resource Management*, *28*(7), 945–972. doi:10.1080/09585192.2015.1116454

D'Cruz, P., Paull, M., Omari, M., & Guneri-Cangarli, B. (2016). Target experiences of workplace bullying: Insights from Australia, India and Turkey. *Employee Relations*, *38*(5), 805–823. doi:10.1108/ER-06-2015-0116

Davis, A. S., Leas, P. A., & Dobelman, J. A. (2009). Did you get my E-mail? An exploratory look at intercultural business communication by E-mail. *Multinational Business Review*, *17*(1), 73–98. doi:10.1108/1525383x200900004

Djurkovic, N., McCormack, D., & Casimir, G. (2004). The physical and psychological effects of workplace bullying and their relationship to intention to leave: A test of the psychosomatic and disability hypotheses. *International Journal of Organization Theory and Behavior*, 7(4), 469–497. doi:10.1108/ijotb-07-04-2004-b001

Einarsen, S. (2000). Harassment and bullying at work: A review of the Scandinavian approach. *Aggression and Violent Behavior: A Review Journal*, *5*(4), 371–401. doi:10.1016/S1359-1789(98)00043–00043

Escartín, J., Zapf, D., Arrieta, C., & Rodríguez-Carballeira, Á. (2011). Workers' perception of workplace bullying: A cross-cultural study. *European Journal of Work and Organizational Psychology*, *20*(2), 178–205. doi:10.1080/13594320903395652

Friedman, R. A., & Currall, S. C. (2003). Conflict escalation: Dispute exacerbating elements of e-mail communication. *Human Relations*, *56*, 1325–1347. doi:10.2139/ssrn.459429

Gacey, H. J. & Richard, E. M. (2013, August). *Influence of emoticons on perceived negative affect and professionalism in work-related email*. Paper presented at the 73rd annual meeting of the Academy of Management, Orlando, FL.

Gelfand, M. J., Erez, M., & Aycan, Z. (2007). Cross-cultural organizational behavior. *Annual Review of Psychology*, *58*, 479–514. doi:10.1146/annurev.psych.58.110405.085559

Ghosh, R. (2017). Workplace incivility in Asia- How do we take a socio-cultural perspective? *Human Resource Development International*, *20*(4), 263–267. doi:10.1080/13678868.2017.1336692

Giorgi, G., Arenas, A., & Leon-Perez, J. M. (2011). An operative measure of workplace bullying: The negative acts questionnaire across Italian companies. *Industrial Health*, *49*(6), 686–695. doi:10.2486/indhealth.ms1287

Giorgi, G., Leon-Perez, J., & Arenas, A. (2015). Are bullying behaviors tolerated in some cultures? Evidence for a curvilinear relationship between workplace bullying and job satisfaction among Italian workers. *Journal of Business Ethics*, *131*(1), 227–237. doi:10.1007/s10551-014-2266-9

Giumetti, G. W., McKibben, E. S., Hatfield, A. L., Schroeder, A. N., & Kowalski, R. M. (2012). Cyber incivility @ work: The new age of interpersonal deviance. *Cyberpsychology, Behavior, and Social Networking*, *15*(3), 148–154. doi:10.1089/cyber.2011.0336

Gloor, J. L. (2014). Review of bullying and harassment in the workplace: Developments in theory, research, and practice, 2nd ed. *Academy of Management Learning & Education*, *13*(1), 145–148. doi:10.5465/amle.2014.0020

Goffman, E. (1967). *Interaction ritual: Essays on face-to-face interaction*. Oxford: Aldine.

Hall, E. T. (1959). *The silent language*. Garden City, NY: Doubleday.

Hall, E. T. (1976). *Beyond culture*. Garden City, NY: Anchor Press.

Hoel, H. & Cooper, C. (2003). Organizational effects of bullying: Bullying and emotional abuse in the workplace. In S. Einarsen, H. Hoel, D. Zapf & C. L. Cooper (Eds.), *Bullying and emotional abuse in the workplace: International perspectives in research and practice* (pp. 145–146). London: Taylor & Francis.

Hofstede, G. (1980). *Culture's consequences: International differences in work-related values.* Newbury Park, CA: Sage Publications.

House, R. J., Hanges, P. J., Javidan, M., Dorfman, P. W., & Gupta, V. (2004). *Culture, leadership, and organizations: The GLOBE study of 62 societies.* Thousand Oaks, CA: Sage Publications.

Jacobson, K. J. L., Hood, J. N., & Van Buren, H. J., III. (2014). Workplace bullying across cultures: A research agenda. *International Journal of Cross Cultural Management, 14*(1), 47–65. doi:10.1177/1470595813494192

Keashly, L., & Jagatic, K. (2003). By another name: American perspectives on workplace bullying. In S. Einarsen & H. Hoel & D. Zapf & C. L. Cooper (Eds.), *Bullying and emotional abuse in the workplace* (pp. 31–61). London, UK: Taylor & Francis.

Kernan, M. C., Watson, S., Chen, F. F., & Kim, T. G. (2011). How cultural values affect the impact of abusive supervision on worker attitudes. *Cross Cultural Management, 18*(4), 464–484. doi:10.1108/13527601111179528

Loh, J., Restubog, S. L. D., & Zagenczyk, T. J. (2010). Consequences of workplace bullying on employee identification and satisfaction among Australians and Singaporeans. *Journal of Cross-Cultural Psychology, 41*(2), 236–252. doi:10.1177/0022022109354641

Merkin, R., Taras, V., & Steel, P. (2014). State of the art themes in cross-cultural communication research: A systematic and meta-analytic review. *International Journal of Intercultural Relations, 38*, 1–23. doi:10.1016/j.ijintrel.2013.10.004

Mikkelsen, E. G., & Einarsen, S. (2001) Bullying in Danish work-life: Prevalence and health correlates. *European Journal of Work and Organizational Psychology, 10*(4), 393–413. doi:10.1080/13594320143000816

Moayed, F. A., Daraiseh, N., Shell, R., & Salem, S. (2006). Workplace bullying: A systematic review of risk factors and outcomes. *Theoretical Issues in Ergonomics Science*, 7(3), 311–327. doi:10.1080/14639220500090604

Morris, M. W., Leung, K., Ames, D., & Lickel, B. (1999). Views from inside and outside: Integrating emic and etic insights about culture and justice judgment. *Academy of Management Review, 24*(4), 781–796. doi:10.2307/259354

Neuman, J. H., & Baron, R. A. (1998). Workplace violence and workplace aggression: Evidence concerning specific forms, potential causes, and preferred targets. *Journal of Management, 24*(3), 391–419. doi:10.1177/014920639802400305

Nielsen, M. B., Matthiesen, S. B., & Einarsen, S. (2010). The impact of methodological moderators on prevalence rates of workplace bullying. A meta-analysis. *Journal of Occupational and Organizational Psychology, 83*(4), 955–979. doi:10.1348/096317909X481256

Olaniran, B. A. (2001). The effects of computer-mediated communication on transculturalism. In V. H. Milhouse, M. K. Asante & P. O. Nwosu (Eds.), *Transcultural realities: Interdisciplinary perspectives on cross-cultural relations* (pp. 83–105) Thousand Oaks, CA: Sage Publications.

Olweus, D. (1993) *Bullying at school: What we know and what we can do.* Oxford, UK: Blackwell.

Park, J., Barash, V., Fink, C., & Cha, M., (2013) *Emoticon style: Interpreting differences in emoticons across cultures.* Proceedings of the 7th International Conference on Weblogs and Social Media, ICWSM 2013. Retrieved from www.aaai.org/ocs/index.php/ICWSM/ICWSM13/paper/viewFile/6132/6386

Peterson, M. F., Thomason, S. J., Althouse, N., Athanassiou, N., Curri, G., Konopaske, R., … Rowney, J. A. (2010). Social structures and personal values that predict e-mail use: An international comparative study. *Journal of Global Information Management, 18*(2), 57–84. doi:10.4018/jgim.2010040103

Power, J. L., Brotheridge, C. M., Blenkinsopp, J., Bowes-Sperry, L., Bozionelos, N., Buzády, Z., … Nnedumm, A. U. O. (2013). Acceptability of workplace bullying: A comparative study on six continents. *Journal of Business Research, 66*(3), 374–380. doi:10.1016/j.jbusres.2011.08.018

Privitera, C. & Campbell, M. A. (2009). Cyberbullying: The new face of workplace bullying? *CyberPsychology & Behavior, 12*(4), 395–400. doi:10.1089/cpb.2009.0025

Richard, E. M., & McFadden, M. (2016). Saving face: Reactions to cultural norm violations in business request emails. *Journal of Business and Psychology, 31*(2), 307–321. doi:10.1007/s10869-015-9414-9

Salin, D. (2003). Ways of explaining workplace bullying: A review of enabling, motivating and precipitating structures and processes in the work environment. *Human Relations, 56* (10), 1213–1232. doi:10.1177/00187267035610003

Schwartz, S. H. (1994). Beyond individualism/collectivism: New cultural dimensions of values. In U. Kim, H. C. Triandis, Ç. Kâğitçibaşi, S.-C. Choi, & G. Yoon (Eds.), *Individualism and collectivism: Theory, method, and applications* (pp. 85–119). Thousand Oaks, CA: Sage Publications.

Seo, Y. N., Leather, P., & Coyne, I. (2012). South Korean culture and history: The implications for workplace bullying. *Aggression and Violent Behavior, 17*(5), 419–422. doi:10.1016/j.avb.2012.05.003

Shannon, C. E., & Weaver, W. (1949). *The mathematical theory of communication*. Urbana, Illinois: University of Illinois Press.

Smith, P. K., Mahdavi, J., Carvalho, M., Fisher, S., Russell, S., & Tippett, N. (2008). Cyberbullying: Its nature and impact in secondary school pupils. *Journal of Child Psychology and Psychiatry, 49*(4), 376–385. doi:10.1111/j.1469-7610.2007.01846.x

Suler, J. (2004). The online disinhibition effect. *Cyberpsychology and Behavior,* 7, 321–326. doi:10.1089/1094931041291295

Tepper, B. (2000). Consequences of abusive supervision. *The Academy of Management Journal, 43*(2), 178–190. doi:10.5465/1556375

Ting-Toomey, S. (1985). Toward a theory of conflict and culture. In W. Gudykunst, L. Stewart, & S. Ting-Toomey (Eds.), *Communication, culture, and organizational processes* (pp. 71–86). Beverly Hills, CA: Sage.

Van den Brande, W., d. B., Baillien, E., De Witte, H., Elst, T. V., & Godderis, L. (2016). The role of work stressors, coping strategies and coping resources in the process of workplace bullying: A systematic review and development of a comprehensive model. *Aggression and Violent Behavior, 29*, 61–71. doi:10.1016/j.avb.2016.06.004

Vidgen, R., Sims, J., & Powell, P. (2011). Understanding e-mail overload. *Journal of Communication Management, 15*(1), 84–98. doi:10.1108/13632541111105277

Vignovic, J. A., & Thompson, L. F. (2010). Computer-mediated cross-cultural collaboration: Attributing communication errors to the person versus the situation. *Journal of Applied Psychology, 95*(2), 265–276. doi:10.1037/a0018628

Vranjes, I., Baillien, E., Vandebosch, H., Erreygers, S., & De Witte, H. (2017). The dark side of working online: Towards a definition and an Emotion Reaction model of workplace cyberbullying. *Computers in Human Behavior, 69*, 324–334. doi:10.1016/j.chb.2016.12.055

Walther, J. B. (1992). Interpersonal effects in computer-mediated interaction: A relational perspective. *Communication Research, 19*(1), 52–90. doi:10.1177/009365092019001003

Welbourne, J. L., Gangadharan, A., & Sariol, A. M. (2015). Ethnicity and cultural values as predictors of the occurrence and impact of experienced workplace incivility. *Journal of Occupational Health Psychology, 20*(2), 205–217. doi:10.1037/a0038277

Zaidman, N., Schwartz, D. G., & Te'eni, D. (2008). Challenges to ICT implementation in multinationals. *Education, Business and Society: Contemporary Middle Eastern Issues, 1*(4), 267–277. doi:10.1108/17537980810929984

8

CYBERBULLYING IN THE WORKPLACE

Developmental Perspectives

Nicole L. Mowry and Gary W. Giumetti

Internet and email usage at work has increasingly become the norm in the past decade (Madden & Jones, 2008; Purcell & Rainie, 2014). With the rise of Internet use at work also comes an increase in time actually spent online, which may make workers more likely to experience various forms of misbehavior, including cyberbullying (Center for the Digital Future, 2017). Cyberbullying can be defined as "an aggressive, intentional act carried out by a group or individual, using electronic forms of contact, repeatedly and over time against a victim who cannot easily defend him or herself" (Smith et al., 2008, p. 376). While the increase in technology has been positive in some regards in the workplace, it has also led to the rise of cyberbullying in the workplace (Coyne, Farley et al., 2017; Farley, Coyne, Axtell, & Spring, 2016; Farley, Coyne, Sprigg, Axtell, & Subramanian, 2015). Unfortunately, cyberbullying could have some negative impacts on workers. For example, research has found that cyberbullying has a negative impact on both job satisfaction and mental strain (Farley et al., 2015).

Whereas technology is being adopted and integrated into the lives of all people, there are clear differences in the age groups that use it the most. Research shows that younger individuals use technology more than older individuals in daily life and at work (Madden & Jones, 2008; Pew Research Center, 2018a; Purcell & Rainie, 2014). Because different age groups use technology in different ways and at different rates, there may be differences in both the prevalence of cyberbullying across age groups at work, as well as the impact that cyberbullying has on people of different ages. However, to the authors' knowledge, there is no existing research that examines age as it relates to workplace cyberbullying.

This chapter will review the literature on age differences in cyberbullying in the workplace as well as draw conclusions based on the literature in a variety of related areas to create a more comprehensive picture of what this may look like in the workplace. First, we will explore the prevalence of technology use in the workplace, with a focus on how workers of different ages interact with it. Then, we will discuss existing research that has examined the relationship between age and cyberbullying followed by a discussion of how age might serve as a moderator of cyberbullying – outcomes relationships. Finally, we will discuss implications of these findings for future research and practice.

Technology Use in the Workplace

Throughout the past few decades, information and communications technologies (or ICTs) have been increasingly integrated into more jobs around the world. The use of ICTs in the workplace has been changing in both form and frequency through the years. For example, as of 2008, 62% of a nationally representative sample of US workers said they use the Internet or email at work about once per day or more and only 16% said they use social networking sites at work every few days or more often (Madden & Jones, 2008). In 2014, the percentage of US workers who said they use the Internet or email at work increased to 78% (Purcell & Rainie, 2014), and, in 2016, 24% indicated that they use social media sites at work (Olmstead, Lampe, & Ellison, 2016). In addition to more people accessing the Internet, email, and social media at work, the amount of time spent using the Internet at work has also increased over time. The Center for the Digital Future at USC reported that employed Internet users spent an average of 14.3 hours online per week in 2017, as compared with only 6.2 hours in 2003 (Center for the Digital Future, 2017). Taken together, these data suggest that a majority of the workforce is using ICTs at work and that ICT usage has been increasing over time.

Beyond the increased usage of the Internet and email at work, these digital tools have also changed the ways that employees perform their jobs as well as how co-workers interact with each other. For example, many workers feel that the Internet and email have enabled them to increase the number of people with whom they communicate outside of their company (Purcell & Rainie, 2014). Additionally, workers report that digital tools allow more flexibility in the hours worked, and that these tools have made them more productive (Purcell & Rainie, 2014). Burlacu, Truxillo, and Bauer (2017) comment that interactions between people are no longer face-to-face and groups of people may not work or live in the same location, with many workers being on virtual teams. A 2012 Society for Human Resource Management survey found that 46% of the organizations surveyed use virtual teams (Minton-Eversole, 2012). Whereas the use of technology can be beneficial due to the fact that it allows more people to connect and work on projects (Keyton, 2017), it can also lead to communication problems (Cascio & Montealegre, 2016). For example, Thompson and Coovert (2003) found that, compared to face-to-face teams, virtual teams have higher levels of confusion and lower levels of satisfaction and accuracy.

Increased technology use at work has also been linked with other negative outcomes beyond decreased satisfaction and accuracy. For example, increased technology use has been linked with increased perceptions of overload and stress (Barber & Santuzzi, 2015; Barley, Meyerson, & Grodal, 2011) as well as increased counterproductive workplace behaviors, such as cyberloafing and other forms of cyberdeviance (e.g., see Andreassen, Torsheim, & Pallesen, 2014; Charlier, Giumetti, Reeves, & Greco, 2017). Barley et al. (2011) found that the more time people spent reading and responding to their emails, the more overloaded they felt. During the three-day study, 60% of the participants reported that they checked their work email when they were at home. Respondents blamed email as the source of their stress, and Barley et al. (2011) identified two main anxieties that lie behind email usage – fear of falling behind in work and fear of missing out on important information. Relatedly, Barber and Santuzzi (2015) note that the heavy reliance on email for workplace communications can lead some individuals to feel pressure to respond quickly – a phenomenon that they call telepressure. These authors found that individuals who experienced telepressure were also more likely to report higher levels of burnout and absenteeism, and poorer sleep quality.

In addition to perceptions of feeling overloaded and pressured to respond quickly, increased technology availability and use at work has also been linked with various forms of workplace cyberdeviance. Workplace cyberdeviance is a term that refers to harmful employee behavior that is carried out using technology and that conflicts with an organization's goals (Charlier et al., 2017). Whereas there are a host of different cyberdeviant behaviors that employees may engage in, the two that have received the most research attention are cyberloafing (or using the Internet at work for personal things; Lim, 2002) and cyberaggression or cyberbullying. Andreasson et al. (2014) found that availability of social network sites at work was linked with increased cyberloafing, a finding that has been confirmed in a recent meta-analytic study (Mercado, Giordano, & Dilchert, 2017). In addition to cyberloafing, other research has suggested that ICT demands (such as being expected to stay current with ICTs at work) are linked with workplace cyberbullying (Farley et al., 2016). Overall, the findings indicate that technology use in the workplace has been increasing, and its use has been linked with both positive and negative outcomes for employees. In the next section, we will take a look at whether the use of technology may differ depending on the age of employees.

Age Differences in Technology Use

Evidence suggests that there are age differences in the use of technology at work. More specifically, findings typically show that younger workers use a greater number of digital tools and use those tools more often than older workers. Additionally, there are differences in willingness to adopt new technology at work as well as differences in how technology influences opinions of co-workers (Burlacu et al., 2017; Morris & Venkatesh, 2000; Olmstead et al., 2016; Van Dijk

& Hacker, 2003). In this section, we review research that has examined age differences in technology use at work to help set the stage for a discussion of how age might relate to cyberbullying experiences at work.

Among US adults, the Pew Research Center has found that 94% of younger adults (ages 18–29) own a smartphone, as compared to 73% of adults aged 50–64 and 46% of adults aged 65 and older (Pew Research Center, 2018a). Additionally, nearly all younger adults (ages 18–49) are using the Internet (~98%), but only 87% of adults aged 50–64, and 66% of adults over the age of 65 reported using the Internet (Pew Research Center, 2018b). Whereas these data are for all adults (and not limited to only those who are working), other data from the Pew Research Center paint a similar picture. Specifically, Madden and Jones (2008) reported that only 60% of employed adults over the age of 65 were using the Internet at work, as compared to 90% of workers aged 18 to 49. In a more recent survey, the Pew Research Center asked online adults how important the Internet was to their job, and 69% of workers over the age of 60 indicated that it was very important or somewhat important, as compared to 78% of workers under the age of 60 (Purcell & Rainie, 2014). These data suggest that, over time, the rate of Internet use among older workers has increased. However, there still appear to be age differences in Internet use at work, with younger workers using it more than older workers do.

Some of the possible reasons for age differences in technology use may be differences in skill levels, attitudes toward technology, and personality. Early research on the "digital divide" found that 73% of Dutch adults aged 18–34 had reasonable or good digital skills (e.g., using word processing software, the Internet, and email), whereas only 33% of people aged 65+ had reasonable or good skills (Van Dijk & Hacker, 2003). Other early research found that older workers had more negative attitudes toward using technology than younger workers (Morris & Venkatesh, 2000). More recent research on the digital divide found that older adults (over the age of 65) adapt to new technology less easily, have less comfort with current technology, and also have higher frustration with technology than younger adults (age 18–44; Volkom, Stapley, & Amaturo, 2014). Other research looking at factors predicting use of technology found that older adults tended to have higher computer anxiety and lower levels of self-efficacy, which both led to lower levels of technology adoption (Czaja et al., 2006).

Research also suggests that technology impacts younger and older workers in different ways. For example, 23% of workers aged 18 to 29 stated that social media information has positively impacted their opinions of colleagues while only 9% of older employees aged 50 to 64 have experienced this. There is also, however, sometimes a negative impact that information learned from social media can have on professional opinions of others. It was found that 29% of young workers (aged 18 to 29) have seen something online that negatively impacted their opinion of a colleague, and only 9% of older individuals (aged 50 to 64) have stated that this has happened (Olmstead et al., 2016). Burlacu et al. (2017) report that older workers have increasingly been using technology in the workplace and their views of technology have changed over time from feeling anxious about technology use to becoming more comfortable with it. This is supported by recent evidence from the Pew Research Center, which shows that older adults were more likely to own a smartphone in 2017 than in 2013, as well as more likely to use the Internet, tablet computers, and social media sites (Anderson & Perrin, 2017). However, as noted above, there is still an age difference in ICT use at work, with a greater number of younger workers using ICTs at work than older workers.

Implications of Age Differences in Technology Use for Cyberbullying

The previous section noted that younger adults are more likely to own and use digital tools than older adults. This increased time spent using digital tools may make younger adults more susceptible to cyberbullying. Within the youth cyberbullying literature, many studies have found that greater technology use is linked with a greater likelihood of cyberbullying (e.g., see Bauman, 2010; Beran, Rinaldi, Bickham, & Rich, 2012). This makes sense because, if an individual is spending more time online, there is a greater chance that he/she may be exposed to a possible perpetrator of cyberbullying. Meta-analytic evidence from the youth cyberbullying literature has also supported this linkage, with frequency of Internet use being positively correlated with both cyberbullying perpetration (corrected correlation = 0.20) and cyberbullying victimization (corrected correlation = 0.17) (Kowalski, Giumetti, Schroeder, & Lattanner, 2014).

The positive correlation between the use of digital tools and cyberbullying that is described above continues to be supported when looking at studies on the prevalence of cyberbullying in younger vs. older adults. Nationwide surveys of adults have found age differences in cyberbullying prevalence. For example, the Center for the Digital Future found that, among older adults (over 55 years old), 6% reported being bullied or harassed online as compared to 20% of younger adults (ages 18 to 34; Center for the Digital Future, 2017). Additionally, the Pew Research Center reported that 67% of younger adults (ages 18 to 29 years old) have been the target of harassment online as compared to 20% of adults ages 50 and older (Duggan, 2017). It is important to note that data for both of these studies came from samples of all adults in the US. Thus, they describe the prevalence of cyberbullying and harassment generally, rather than cyberbullying in the workplace among employed adults specifically. Therefore, we turn our attention to research conducted in the workplace in the next section.

Bullying and Cyberbullying in the Workplace

The relationship between cyberbullying in the workplace and age is a relatively new topic of research. That being said, there are many studies on related topics that have been performed and can support claims about how cyberbullying in the workplace will affect individuals in different age groups in different ways. There are two main categories of studies that will be discussed: the first are studies that looked at bullying in general in the workplace, with some consideration of age, and the second are studies that focused on cyberbullying in the workplace as a whole.

Bullying in the Workplace

Bullying is not uncommon in the workplace. A study by Hoel, Cooper, and Faragher (2001) found that more than 10% of their participants had experienced workplace bullying in the past six months alone. Of these individuals, almost 75% of them reported that the bullying they endured was from a person in a supervisory or managerial position. For two-thirds of the bullied workers, it had been a long-term occurrence, happening for more than one year. This estimate is on the lower end of estimations of workplace bullying, as Ariza-Montes, Leal-Rodríguez, and Leal-Millán (2015) reported that the likelihood of workplace bullying in their sample was almost 75%.

Meta-analytic evidence suggests that prevalence rates for workplace bullying range from 5% to 28%, depending on the region of the world and the method used to assess bullying (Nielsen, Matthiesen, & Einarsen, 2010). Studies in Scandinavia that used a self-labeling measure of bullying and included a definition of bullying had the lowest rates of bullying (5%), whereas studies in non-European countries that used the self-labeling measure of bullying and did not include the definition of bullying reported the highest rates of bullying on average (28%) (Nielsen et al., 2010).

Bullying and age. When examining age and workplace bullying, Vartia (1996) found that bullied individuals cite age as a reason for bullying 22% of the time (e.g., because he/she is the oldest or youngest employee). There are contradictory findings as to which groups are the most vulnerable to workplace bullying in general. Some studies suggest that younger and older workers are the least likely to be bullied (Notelaers, Vermunt, Baillien, Einarsen, & Witte, 2011), whereas other studies suggest that younger and older workers are more vulnerable than middle-aged workers (Ariza-Montes et al., 2015; López-Carbarcos, Vázquez-Rodríguez, & Gieure, 2017; Olafsson & Jóhannsdóttir, 2004). Evidence for the former pattern comes from Notelaers et al. (2011), who found that workers aged 34–54 were up to 1.7 times more likely to be bullied in the workplace than younger (under 25 years old) or older workers (over age 54).

Other literature contrasts these findings and suggests that younger and/or older workers are more likely to be bullied (Ariza-Montes et al., 2015; Lopez-Carbarcos et al., 2017; Olafsson & Jóhannsdóttir, 2004). The risk of younger workers being bullied can be explained because they are new to the workplace and are more likely to be pushed around because it is a rite of passage (Lopez-Carbarcos et al., 2017), and, as noted above, they may be spending more time online than older workers. Relatedly, meta-analytic research on the related construct of abusive supervision has found a negative relationship between subordinate age and abusive supervision, suggesting that younger workers are more likely to experience abusive supervision (Zhang & Bednall, 2016). Older workers, it has been theorized, endure bullying due to increased passivity due to their older age, which can be representative of their lack of belief that the workplace will be able to properly handle bullying (Lopez-Carbarcos et al., 2017; Olafsson & Jóhannsdóttir, 2004). It has also been found that not only are older workers bullied more often, but they are also more aware of this bullying as there is a positive correlation between individuals considering themselves bullied and age (Ariza-Montes et al., 2015). Overall, the mixed findings suggest that more research is needed in this area to determine which group of individuals is more at risk of being bullied.

Cyberbullying in the Workplace

The literature discussed above focused solely on traditional bullying in the workplace. There is additional research on cyberbullying in the workplace that can supplement these findings. There are a variety of ways cyberbullying can manifest in a workplace. For example, the Cyber Negative Acts Questionnaire (CNAQ) measures variables such as having one's opinions ignored, being given unreasonable tasks, being ignored or excluded, and being given an unmanageable workload. Farley et al. (2015) found that 46.2% of participants, doctors over six months into their training, had experienced cyberbullying at least one time, and that cyberbullying was negatively related to job satisfaction, and mental strain, while controlling for gender, age, and general job stress. In a study by Coyne, Farley et al. (2017), 87.5% of employees from three UK universities reported experiencing cyberbullying. Coyne, Farley et al. (2017) also found that cyberbullying was related to increased mental strain and decreased job satisfaction. Additionally, Farley et al. (2016) reported that cyberbullying was linked with increased emotional exhaustion, even after controlling for cyberaggression and traditional bullying.

Cyberbullying and age. Regarding the relationship between age and cyberbullying, existing research is somewhat mixed on the degree of relationship between these two variables. For example, Kowalski, Toth, and Morgan (2018) found a small but significant negative relationship (r = -0.13, p <0.001) between age and cyberbullying. The significance of this relationship, however, may be influenced by the large sample size upon which it was based (n = 3548). Also, Farley et al. (2016) and Coyne, Farley et al. (2017) reported that there was a small positive (although nonsignificant) relationship between age and frequency of cyberbullying. It is important to note that the age range in the latter two studies was restricted, which may make it more difficult to find a relationship.

Research on the related construct of cyber incivility (that is, rude or discourteous messages that are transmitted via ICTs; Giumetti, McKibben, Hatfield,

Schroeder, & Kowalski, 2012) has largely found a small negative (although non-significant) relationship between cyber incivility and age, ranging from -0.06 to -0.14 (Giumetti, 2016; Giumetti et al., 2012; Giumetti, Saunders, Brunette, DiFrancesco, & Graham, 2016; Park, Fritz, & Jex, 2015). However, one study by Krishnan (2016) found a small positive (although non-significant) relationship between cyber incivility and age. Research by Ford (2013) on the related construct of virtual harassment (that is, intentionally harmful behaviors that occur via ICTs), found a small, but significant negative relationship (-0.16, $p < 0.05$) between age and virtual harassment.

The evidence from the traditional bullying literature suggests that the relationship may be curvilinear, with younger and older workers experiencing more cyberbullying than middle-aged adults (e.g., see Ariza-Montes et al., 2015; Lopez-Carbarcos et al., 2017; Olafsson & Jóhannsdóttir, 2004), or with middle-aged adults experiencing more cyberbullying than younger and older adults (Notelaers et al., 2011). This possibility was tested using data from Giumetti, Allison, and Kowalski (2018). Specifically, we created a quadratic age term by squaring age and used this quadratic age term in a hierarchical polynomial regression to predict cyber incivility from supervisors and cyber incivility from coworkers. Results revealed that the quadratic age term significantly predicted supervisor cyber incivility victimization ($\beta = -0.13$, $t(235) = -1.98$, $p < 0.05$). Examining a plot of this non-linear relationship revealed an inverted U-shape, with younger and older workers reporting less frequent cyber incivility from supervisors, and middle-aged workers reporting more cyber incivility from supervisors. We also re-analyzed data from Giumetti (2016) and found a similar pattern of results. However, this pattern of results was not confirmed after re-analyzing data from Giumetti et al. (2016), nor data from Kowalski et al. (2018).

Taken together, these findings suggest that the statistical relationship between age and cyberbullying is still unclear. The existing research suggests that the linear correlation between cyberbullying and age is small and non-significant. Research on related constructs of cyber incivility and virtual harassment has reported similar findings. However, when examined using polynomial regression to test for a non-linear relationship, we found a significant inverted U-shaped relationship between age and cyber incivility. Future research should continue to explore the possible non-linear relationship of age with cyberbullying and related constructs to help us gain a clearer picture of how these two variables are related.

Age as a Moderator of Cyberbullying-Outcome Relationships

One additional way that age might relate to cyberbullying is that age may serve as a moderator of the relationship between cyberbullying and employee outcomes. That is, the relationship between experiencing cyberbullying victimization and a variety of outcomes, such as job-related outcomes (e.g., job satisfaction, task and contextual performance, work motivation, and withdrawal) and emotion-related outcomes (e.g., irritability, burnout, and depression), may depend on the age of the participant. There are two possible ways in which age may interact with cyberbullying-outcome relationships. One possibility is that older workers may be more strongly impacted by cyberbullying experiences than younger workers. The second possibility is that older workers may be less strongly impacted by cyberbullying experiences than younger workers. We will consider each of these possibilities in turn, including possible theoretical reasons for each pattern, and existing evidence from related research.

On the one hand, older workers may be impacted more strongly than younger workers as a result of experiencing cyberbullying at work. For example, older workers might experience more withdrawal and burnout than younger workers as a result of exposure to high levels of workplace cyberbullying. According to Socioemotional Selectivity Theory (SST; Carstensen, 2006), adults give more weight to emotionally laden goals as the amount of time remaining in life decreases. When applied to the workplace, this theory suggests that emotion-related experiences at work will be more important the more future working time is limited. That is, older workers are expected to be more sensitive to situations that threaten their well-being, and they are expected to also place more value on social interactions and goals (Carstensen, Isaacowitz, & Charles, 1999; Kooij, De Lange, Jansen, Kanfer, & Dikkers, 2011). The Decremental Theory of aging also predicts a similar pattern. This theory argues that a number of mental (e.g., increase in illness and dependency) and physical (e.g., decreases in energy and agility) changes may occur as one ages (Giniger, Dispenzieri, & Eisenberg, 1983). These changes may negatively impact a worker's health and coping resources, resulting in stronger stressor-outcome relationships as individuals age. Thus, both the Socioemotional Selectivity Theory and the Decremental Theory of aging suggest that older workers may be more negatively impacted by interpersonal mistreatment such as cyberbullying at work than younger workers.

Some support for this general idea exists in the traditional bullying and mistreatment literature. For example, Kakarika, González-Gómez, and Dimitriades (2017) found that age moderated the relationship between workplace bullying and perceptions of psychological contract breach (or the extent to which the organization has broken its promises to the employee). Specifically, older females had a stronger positive relationship between workplace bullying and perceptions of psychological contract breach than younger females and both younger and older males. In addition, Cheng (2012) found that older adults experienced more hurt feelings and a more negative mood after being rejected than did younger participants.

On the other hand, older workers may be less negatively impacted than younger workers by cyberbullying in the workplace. One reason for this pattern of results might be that older workers are better able to cope with mistreatment as they get older, perhaps due to becoming more emotionally competent (Gross et al., 1997), more emotionally stable (Carstensen, Pasupathi, Mayr, & Nesselroade, 2000), or more effectively using coping resources (Shirom, Gilboa, Fried, & Cooper, 2008).

Support for this idea was found in a meta-analysis by Zhang and Liao (2015), who found that older workers' emotional exhaustion was less negatively impacted by abusive supervision than younger workers. Additionally, Mauno, Ruokolainen, and Kinnunen (2013) found that older age buffered the negative relationship between workload and job satisfaction, as well as between work-family conflict and life satisfaction. Further, Shirom et al. (2008) found meta-analytically that age moderated the relationship between role ambiguity and performance, such that this relationship was weaker among older samples. It is important to note, however, that the available studies for either of these possible forms of the interaction between age and cyberbullying-outcome relationships have not examined workplace cyberbullying. Thus, we hope that future research will help us to determine if either of these patterns (or neither) is supported by evidence. We turn to other directions for future research in the next section.

Future Research

Based on the literature reviewed above, we can recommend a number of different directions for future research. First, more research is needed that looks at the use of ICTs at work. Specifically, it would be informative to know when and how often different forms of communication are used (such as text messaging, chat, social media, and email), and how their use may differ by age (as well as other demographic groups) and by occupation. Recognizing that unlimited Internet use at work is likely to detract from productivity, most organizations have created acceptable Internet use policies (Young, 2010). Given this, researchers should examine the extent to which these policies impact use of ICTs at work. Relatedly, more research is needed that looks at how workplace policies and training related to online communication impact rates of cyberbullying, and whether there may be age differences in policy acceptance or compliance.

Beyond policies, researchers could also examine the effectiveness of prevention and intervention strategies. For example, researchers could adapt school-based cyberbullying programs (e.g., see Cross et al., 2016) and determine whether they may be effective at reducing the likelihood of cyberbullying victimization at work. Current recommendations from human resources (HR) are to provide training and education for staff members and managers about cyberbullying and interpersonal mistreatment (Wright, 2016). Researchers could examine the effectiveness of these HR programs. Existing research on one such program called Civility, Respect, and Engagement in the Workplace (or CREW) suggests that such an intervention can be effective at improving the quality of the work environment, and reducing interpersonal mistreatment (Leiter, Day, Oore, & Spence Laschinger, 2012). The key features of the CREW program include weekly meetings between coworkers and a facilitator to discuss effective ways of communicating with one another, and working through structured exercises to break out of dysfunctional ways of communicating (Leiter, Laschinger, Day, &

Oore, 2011). In between the weekly meetings, participants complete activities to help them commit to practicing and recognizing civility in their work environment. Evidence suggests that the CREW intervention was effective at reducing incivility and distress, and boosting civility, respect, job satisfaction, and management trust both immediately after the six month program (Leiter et al., 2011), and after a one year follow-up (Leiter et al., 2012). More research on similar interventions is needed.

Whereas existing cyberbullying research suggests that there is no linear relationship between cyberbullying and employee age, future research is needed that examines other possible forms of this relationship. As noted above, research on workplace bullying suggests that both younger and older workers might be more likely to experience traditional bullying than middle-aged workers (e.g., see Ariza-Montes et al., 2015; Lopez-Carbarcos et al., 2017; Ólafsson & Jóhannsdóttir, 2004). This suggests that the form of the relationship might be U-shaped. Thus, future researchers should check for this possible curvilinear relationship between age and cyberbullying. In addition to the shape of the relationship, researchers should also take care to select a sample of employees that represent the full age range of adults (e.g., from 18 to 65 +). This will help to avoid problems of range restriction and help to provide a clearer picture of the linkage between age and workplace cyberbullying across the lifespan.

Existing research has helped us to understand some of the negative consequences of experiencing cyberbullying at work, including decreased satisfaction and increased mental strain (Coyne, Farley et al., 2017; Farley et al., 2015), as well as decreased perceptions of interactional justice and increased emotional exhaustion (Farley et al, 2016). However, less is known about the possible antecedents of workplace cyberbullying. That is, what factors might predict whether someone is likely to perpetrate or be a victim of workplace cyberbullying? Whereas we know that frequency of internet use is linked with cyberbullying among youth samples (e.g., see Kowalski et al., 2014), less is known about other possible antecedents among working adults. Research on other forms of interpersonal mistreatment and deviance have found evidence for several individual difference antecedents, including moral disengagement (e.g., Claybourn, 2011; Valle, Kacmar, Zivnuska, & Harting, 2018), anger (Khan, Quratulain, & Crawshaw, 2013), and narcissism (Palmer, Komarraju, Carter, & Karau, 2017). Additionally, a number of situational antecedents of workplace harassment have been uncovered in previous research, including family-to-work conflict (Courtright, Gardner, Smith, McCormick, & Colbert, 2016), low social support and high work demands (Rodwell, Demir, & Flower, 2013), poor leadership quality (Hauge, Skogstad, & Einarsen, 2007) and a climate for organizational justice (Rubino et al., 2018).

Future research should not only explore whether these antecedents predict exposure to workplace cyberbullying, but also examine the extent to which age might interact with these variables. For example, are older workers more likely to seek out and be influenced by social support (e.g., Carstensen et al., 1999), and, thus, might older workers be less likely to engage in perpetration of cyberbullying or better able to cope with victimization? Additionally, given evidence that suggests that anger tends to be lower among older adults (Zimprich & Mascherek, 2012), might we expect that a possible linkage between anger and cyberbullying perpetration will be weaker among older adults?

Finally, more research is needed on bystanders or witnesses of workplace cyberbullying. That is, when a co-worker is copied on several emails that are harassing and abusive to his/her co-worker, what happens to the witness? Existing research on the role of bystanders/witnesses of traditional workplace bullying has focused on two issues: factors that predict whether the witness intervenes or helps out; and the psychological and physical toll of witnessing bullying. Research on the former has uncovered a number of variables that make it more likely for the witness to help out, including self-efficacy and severity of the incident (Hellemans, Dal Cason, & Casini, 2017), being friends with the target of bullying (Coyne, Gopaul et al., 2017), and perceptions of organizational safety and supervisory support (MacCurtain, Murphy, O'Sullivan, MacMahon, & Turner, 2018). Research on the psychological and physical toll of witnessing workplace bullying has found that witnesses tend to have lower job satisfaction than non-involved employees (Hauge et al., 2007) as well as higher anxiety (Hansen et al., 2006) and higher mental stress reactions (Vartia, 2001). We recommend that future researchers extend these findings from the traditional bullying realm to the realm of cyberbullying. In addition, we recommend that researchers examine how the age of the witness/bystander relates to the likelihood of intervening and to the experience of negative outcomes from witnessing workplace cyberbullying.

In summary, the research presented above paints a picture from which one can draw assumptions about the relationship between age and cyberbullying in the workplace. However, more direct research on age and cyberbullying needs to occur. From the information gathered above, it is clear that there is a gap in the literature with regard to the impact that cyberbullying can have on different age groups in the workplace. Identifying the groups that are most at risk and better understanding the consequences of maltreatment will enable employers and HR representatives to make positive changes in their workplace to better prevent and provide assistance to those who are dealing with cyberbullying.

References

Anderson, M., & Perrin, A. (2017, May). *Tech adoption climbs among older adults*. Retrieved from www.pewinternet.org/2017/05/17/tech-adoption-climbs-among-older-adults/

Andreassen, C. S., Torsheim, T., & Pallesen, S. (2014). Predictors of use of social network sites at work: A specific type of cyberloafing. *Journal of Computer-Mediated Communication, 19*(4), 906–921. doi:10.1111/jcc4.12085

Ariza-Montes, A., Leal-Rodríguez, A. L., & Leal-Millán, A. G. (2015). A comparative study of workplace bullying among public and private employees in Europe. *Journal of Occupational and Environmental Medicine, 57*(6), 695–700. doi:10.1097/JOM.0000000000000437

Barber, L. K., & Santuzzi, A. M. (2015). Please respond ASAP: Workplace telepressure and employee recovery. *Journal of Occupational Health Psychology, 20*(2), 172–189. doi:10.1037/a0038278

Barley, S., Meyerson, D., & Grodal, S. (2011). E-mail as a source and symbol of stress. *Organization Science, 22*(4), 887–906. doi:10.1287/orsc.1100.0573

Bauman, S. (2010). Cyberbullying in a rural intermediate school: An exploratory study. *The Journal of Early Adolescence, 30*(6), 803–833. doi:10.1177/0272431609350927

Beran, T. N., Rinaldi, C., Bickham, D. S., & Rich, M. (2012). Evidence for the need to support adolescents dealing with harassment and cyber-harassment: Prevalence, progression, and impact. *School Psychology International, 33*(5), 562–576. doi:10.1177/0143034312446976

Burlacu, G., Truxillo, D. M., & Bauer, T. N. (2017). Employee age differences in using Internet-based tools at work. In G. Hertel, D. L. Stone, R. D. Johnson, & J. Passmore (Eds.), *The Wiley Blackwell handbook of the psychology of the Internet at work* (pp. 449–479). Hoboken, NJ: Wiley-Blackwell. doi:10.1002/9781119256151.ch20

Carstensen, L. L. (2006). The influence of a sense of time on human development. *Science, 312*(5782), 1913–1915. doi:10.1126/science.1127488

Carstensen, L. L., Isaacowitz, D. M., & Charles, S. T. (1999). Taking time seriously: A theory of socioemotional selectivity. *American Psychologist, 54*(3), 165–181. doi:10.1037/0003-066X.54. 3. 165

Carstensen, L. L., Pasupathi, M., Mayr, U., & Nesselroade, J. R. (2000). Emotional experience in everyday life across the adult life span. *Journal of Personality and Social Psychology, 79*(4), 644–655. doi:10.1037/0022-3514.79.4.644

Cascio, W. & Montealegre, R. (2016). How technology is changing work and organizations. *Annual Review of Organizational Psychology and Organizational Behavior, 3*, 349–375. doi:1146/annurev-orgpsych-041015-062352

Center for the Digital Future. (2017). *The 2017 digital future report*. Retrieved from www.digitalcenter.org/wp-content/uploads/2018/04/2017-Digital-Future-Report-2.pdf

Charlier, S. D., Giumetti, G. W., Reeves, C. J., & Greco, L. M. (2017). Workplace cyberdeviance. In G. Hertel, D. L. Stone, R. D. Johnson, & J. Passmore (Eds.), *The Wiley Blackwell handbook of the psychology of the Internet at work* (pp. 131–156). Hoboken, NJ: Wiley-Blackwell. doi:10.1002/9781119256151.ch7

Cheng, Y. (2012). *Age differences in emotional reactions to social rejection*. (Unpublished doctoral dissertation). North Carolina State University, Raleigh, NC.

Claybourn, M. (2011). Relationships between moral disengagement, work characteristics and workplace harassment. *Journal of Business Ethics, 100*(2), 283–301. doi:10.1007/s10551-010-0680-1

Courtright, S. H., Gardner, R. G., Smith, T. A., McCormick, B. W., & Colbert, A. E. (2016). My family made me do it: A cross-domain, self-regulatory perspective on antecedents to abusive supervision. *Academy of Management Journal, 59*(5), 1630–1652. doi:10.5465/amj.2013.1009

Coyne, I., Farley, S., Axtell, C., Sprigg, C., Best, L., & Kwok, O. (2017). Understanding the relationship between experiencing workplace cyberbullying, employee mental strain and job satisfaction: A dysempowerment approach. *The International Journal of Human Resource Management, 28*(7), 945–972. doi:10.1080/09585192.2015.1116454

Coyne, I., Gopaul, A., Campbell, M., Pankász, A., Garland, R., & Cousans, F. (2017). Bystander responses to bullying at work: The role of mode, type and relationship to target. *Journal of Business Ethics*, doi:10.1007/s10551-017-3692-2

Cross, D., Shaw, T., Hadwen, K., Cardoso, P., Slee, P., Roberts, C., & ... Barnes, A. (2016). Longitudinal impact of the Cyber Friendly Schools program on adolescents' cyberbullying behavior. *Aggressive Behavior, 42*(2), 166–180. doi:10.1002/ab.21609

Czaja, S. J., Charness, N., Fisk, A. D., Hertzog, C., Nair, S. N., Rogers, W. A., & Sharit, J. (2006). Factors predicting the use of technology: Findings from the center for research and education on aging and technology enhancement (CREATE). *Psychology and Aging, 21*(2), 333–352. doi:10.1037/0882-7974.21.2.333

Duggan, M. (2017). *Online harassment 2017*. Pew Research Center. Retrieved from www.pewinternet.org/2017/07/11/online-harassment-2017/

Farley, S., Coyne, I., Axtell, C., & Sprigg, C. (2016). Design, development and validation of a workplace cyberbullying measure, the WCM. *Work & Stress, 30*(4), 293–317. doi:10.1080/02678373.2016.1255998

Farley, S., Coyne, I., Sprigg, C., Axtell, C., & Subramanian, G. (2015). Exploring the impact of workplace cyberbullying on trainee doctors. *Medical Education, 49*(4), 436–443. doi:10.1111/medu.12666

Ford, D. P. (2013). Virtual harassment: Media characteristics' role in psychological health. *Journal of Managerial Psychology, 28*(4), 408–428. doi:10.1108/JMP-12-2012-0398

Giniger, S., Dispenzieri, A., & Eisenberg, J. (1983). Age, experience, and performance on speed and skill jobs in an applied setting. *Journal of Applied Psychology, 68*, 469–475.

Giumetti, G. W. (2016, April). *Development and validation of the Cyber-Incivility at Work Scale*. In D. Ward & E. Eatough (Co-chairs), *Novel workplace stressors and their implications for employee health*. Symposium presented at the 31st annual meeting of the Society for Industrial-Organizational Psychology, Anaheim, CA.

Giumetti, G. W., Allison, B. A., & Kowalski, R. M. (2018). *Cyber-incivility predicts incremental variance in turnover intentions, burnout, and commitment above face-to-face incivility: A two-wave panel study*. Unpublished manuscript, Quinnipiac University, Hamden, CT.

Giumetti, G. W., McKibben, E. S., Hatfield, A. L., Schroeder, A. N., & Kowalski, R. M. (2012). Cyber incivility @ work: The new age of interpersonal deviance. *Cyberpsychology, Behavior, and Social Networking, 15*(3), 148–154. doi:10.1089/cyber.2011.0336

Giumetti, G. W., Saunders, L. A., Brunette, J. P., DiFrancesco, F. M., & Graham, P. G. (2016). Linking cyber incivility with job performance through job satisfaction: The buffering role of positive affect. *Psi Chi Journal of Psychological Science, 21*, 230–240. Retrieved from www.psichi.org/page/214JNWinter2016

Gross, J. J., Carstensen, L. L., Pasupathi, M., Tsai, J., Götestam Skorpen, C., & Hsu, A. C. (1997). Emotion and aging: Experience, expression, and control. *Psychology and Aging, 12*(4), 590–599. doi:10.1037/0882-7974.12. 4. 590

Hansen, Å. M., Hogh, A., Persson, R., Karlson, B., Garde, A. H., & Ørbæk, P. (2006). Bullying at work, health outcomes, and physiological stress response. *Journal of Psychosomatic Research, 60*(1), 63–72. doi:10.1016/j.jpsychores.2005. 06. 078

Hauge, L. J., Skogstad, A., & Einarsen, S. (2007). Relationships between stressful work environments and bullying: Results of a large representative study. *Work & Stress, 21*(3), 220–242. doi:10.1080/02678370701705810

Hellemans, C., Dal Cason, D., & Casini, A. (2017). Bystander helping behavior in response to workplace bullying. *Swiss Journal of Psychology, 76*(4), 135–144. doi:10.1024/1421-0185/a000200

Hoel, H., Cooper, C. L., & Faragher, B. (2001). The experience of bullying in Great Britain: The impact of organizational status. *European Journal of Work and Organizational Psychology, 10*(4), 443–465. doi:10.1080/13594320143000780

Kakarika, M., González-Gómez, H. V., & Dimitriades, Z. (2017). That wasn't our deal: A psychological contract perspective on employee responses to bullying. *Journal of Vocational Behavior, 100*, 43–55. doi:10.1016/j.jvb.2017.doi:02.005

Keyton, J. (2017). Communication in organizations. *Annual Review of Organizational Psychology and Organizational Behavior, 4*, 501–526. doi:10.1146/annurev-orgpsych-032516-113341

Khan, A. K., Quratulain, S., & Crawshaw, J. R. (2013). The mediating role of discrete emotions in the relationship between injustice and counterproductive work behaviors: A study in Pakistan. *Journal of Business and Psychology, 28*(1), 49–61. doi:10.1007/s10869-012-9269-2

Kooij, D. M., de Lange, A. H., Jansen, P. W., Kanfer, R., & Dikkers, J. E. (2011). Age and work-related motives: Results of a meta-analysis. *Journal of Organizational Behavior, 32*(2), 197–225. doi:10.1002/job.665

Kowalski, R. M., Giumetti, G. W., Schroeder, A. N., & Lattanner, M. R. (2014). Bullying in the digital age: A critical review and meta-analysis of cyberbullying research among youth. *Psychological Bulletin, 140*(4), 1073–1137. doi:10.1037/a0035618

Kowalski, R. M., Toth, A., & Morgan, M. (2018). Bullying and cyberbullying in adulthood and the workplace. *The Journal of Social Psychology, 158*(1), 64–81. doi:10.1080/00224545.2017.1302402

Krishnan, S. (2016). Electronic warfare: A personality model of cyber incivility. *Computers in Human Behavior, 64*, 537–546. doi:10.1016/j.chb.2016. 07. 031

Leiter, M. P., Day, A., Oore, D. G., & Spence Laschinger, H. K. (2012). Getting better and staying better: Assessing civility, incivility, distress, and job attitudes one year after a civility intervention. *Journal of Occupational Health Psychology, 17*(4), 425–434. doi:10.1037/a0029540

Leiter, M. P., Laschinger, H. S., Day, A., & Oore, D. G. (2011). The impact of civility interventions on employee social behavior, distress, and attitudes. *Journal of Applied Psychology, 96*(6), 1258–1274. doi:10.1037/a0024442

Lim, V. K. G. (2002). The IT way of loafing on the job: Cyberloafing, neutralizing and organizational justice. *Journal of Organizational Behavior, 23*(5), 675–694. doi:10.1002/job.161

López-Carbarcos, M., Vázquez-Rodríguez, P., & Gieure, C. (2017). Gender and age differences in the psychosocial risk factors of workplace bullying. *Psychology & Marketing, 34*(11), 1023–1030. doi:10.1002/mar.21041

MacCurtain, S., Murphy, C., O'Sullivan, M., MacMahon, J., & Turner, T. (2018). To stand back or step in? Exploring the responses of employees who observe workplace bullying. *Nursing Inquiry, 25*(1), e12207. doi:10.1111/nin.12207

Madden, M., & Jones, S. (2008, September). *Networked workers*. Retrieved from www.pewinternet.org/2008/09/24/networked-workers/

Mauno, S., Ruokolainen, M., & Kinnunen, U. (2013). Does aging make employees more resilient to job stress? Age as a moderator in the job stressor–well-being relationship in three Finnish occupational samples. *Aging & Mental Health, 17*(4), 411–422. doi:10.1080/13607863.2012.747077

Mercado, B. K., Giordano, C., & Dilchert, S. (2017). A meta-analytic investigation of cyberloafing. *The Career Development International, 22*(5), 546–564. doi:10.1108/CDI-08-2017-0142

Minton-Eversole, T. (2012). *Virtual teams used most by global organizations, survey says*. Retrieved from www.shrm.org/resourcesandtools/hr-topics/organizational-and-employee-development/pages/virtualteamsusedmostbyglobalorganizations,surveysays.aspx

Morris, M., & Venkatesh, V. (2000). Age difference in technology adoption decisions: Implications for a changing work force. *Personnel Psychology, 53*(2), 375–403. doi:10.1111/j.1744–6570.2000.tb00206.x

Nielsen, M. B., Matthiesen, S. B., & Einarsen, S. (2010). The impact of methodological moderators on prevalence rates of workplace bullying: A meta-analysis. *Journal of Occupational and Organizational Psychology, 83*(4), 955–979. doi:10.1348/096317909X481256

Notelaers, G., Vermunt, J., Baillien, E., Einarsen, S., & De Witte, H. (2011). Exploring risk groups workplace bullying with categorical data. *Industrial Health, 49*, 73–88. doi:10.2486/indhealth.ms1155

Ólafsson, R. F., & Jóhannsdóttir, H. L. (2004). Coping with bullying in the workplace: The effect of gender, age and type of bullying. *British Journal of Guidance & Counselling, 32*(3), 319–333. doi:10.1080/03069880410001723549

Olmstead, K., Lampe, C., & Ellison, N. B. (2016, June). *Social media and the workplace*. Retrieved from www.pewinternet.org/2016/06/22/social-media-and-the-workplace/

Palmer, J. C., Komarraju, M., Carter, M. Z., & Karau, S. J. (2017). Angel on one shoulder: Can perceived organizational support moderate the relationship between the Dark Triad traits and counterproductive work behavior? *Personality and Individual Differences, 110*, 31–37. doi:10.1016/j.paid.2017. 01. 018

Park, Y., Fritz, C., & Jex, S. M. (2015). Daily cyber incivility and distress: The moderating roles of resources at work and home. *Journal of Management, 44*, 2535–2557. doi:10.1177/0149206315576796

Pew Research Center. (2018a). *Mobile fact sheet*. Retrieved from www.pewinternet.org/fact-sheet/mobile/

Pew Research Center. (2018b). *Internet/broadband fact sheet*. Retrieved from www.pewinternet.org/fact-sheet/internet-broadband/

Purcell, K., & Rainie, L. (December, 2014). *Technology's impact on workers*. Retrieved from www.pewInternet.org/2014/12/30/technologys-impact-on-workers/

Rodwell, J., Demir, D., & Flower, R. L. (2013). The oppressive nature of work in healthcare: Predictors of aggression against nurses and administrative staff. *Journal of Nursing Management, 21*(6), 888–897. doi:10.1111/jonm.12086

Rubino, C., Avery, D. R., McKay, P. F., Moore, B. L., Wilson, D. C., Driel, M. S., & ... McDonald, D. P. (2018). And justice for all: How organizational justice climate deters sexual harassment. *Personnel Psychology, 71*, 519–544. doi:10.1111/peps.12274

Shirom, A., Gilboa, S. S., Fried, Y., & Cooper, C. L. (2008). Gender, age and tenure as moderators of work-related stressors' relationships with job performance: A meta-analysis. *Human Relations, 61*(10), 1371–1398. doi:10.1177/0018726708095708

Smith, P. K., Mahdavi, J., Carvalho, M., Fisher, S., Russell, S., & Tippett, N. (2008). Cyberbullying: Its nature and impact in secondary school pupils. *Journal of Child Psychology and Psychiatry, 49*(4), 376–385. doi:10.1111/j.1469-7610.2007.01846.x

Thompson, L. F., & Coovert, M. D. (2003). Teamwork online: The effects of computer conferencing on perceived confusion, satisfaction and postdiscussion accuracy. *Group Dynamics: Theory, Research, and Practice*, 7(2), 135–151. doi:10.1037/1089-2699.7.2.135

Valle, M., Kacmar, K. M., Zivnuska, S., & Harting, T. (2018). Abusive supervision, leader-member exchange, and moral disengagement: A moderated-mediation model of organizational deviance. *The Journal of Social Psychology*, doi:10.1080/00224545.2018.1466776

Van Dijk, J., & Hacker, K. (2003). The digital divide as a complex and dynamic phenomenon. *The Information Society, 19*, 315–326. doi:10.1080/01972240390227895

Vartia, M. (1996). The sources of bullying—Psychological work environment and organizational climate. *European Journal of Work and Organizational Psychology, 5*(2), 203–214. doi:10.1080/13594329608414855

Vartia, M. A. (2001). Consequences of workplace bullying with respect to the well-being of its targets and the observers of bullying. *Scandinavian Journal of Work, Environment & Health, 27*(1), 63–69. doi:10.5271/sjweh.588

Volkom, M., Stapley, J. C., & Amaturo, V. (2014). Revisiting the digital divide: Generational differences in technology use in everyday life. *North American Journal of Psychology, 16*(3), 557–574.

Wright, A. D. (2016, May 13). *What HR can do about cyberbullying in the workplace.* Retrieved from www.shrm.org/resourcesandtools/hr-topics/technology/pages/what-hr-can-do-about-cyberbullying-in-the-workplace.aspx

Young, K. (2010). Policies and procedures to manage employee Internet abuse. *Computers in Human Behavior, 26*(6), 1467–1471. doi:10.1016/j.chb.2010. 04. 025

Zhang, Y., & Bednall, T. C. (2016). Antecedents of abusive supervision: A meta-analytic review. *Journal of Business Ethics, 139*(3), 455–471. doi:10.1007/s10551-015-2657-6

Zhang, Y., & Liao, Z. (2015). Consequences of abusive supervision: A meta-analytic review. *Asia Pacific Journal of Management, 32*(4), 959–987. doi:10.1007/s10490-015-9425-0

Zimprich, D., & Mascherek, A. (2012). Measurement invariance and age-related differences of trait anger across the adult lifespan. *Personality and Individual Differences, 52*(3), 334–339. doi:10.1016/j.paid.2011. 10. 030

9

CYBERBULLYING IN ROMANTIC RELATIONSHIPS

A Review of Research in the United States

Penny A. Leisring

Imagine your significant other encouraging you through text messages to kill yourself. That is what 18-year-old Conrad Roy III experienced in the days leading up to his death by suicide in Massachusetts (LeBlanc, 2017). Seventeen-year-old Michelle Carter sent text messages over several days to her boyfriend, Roy, who was considering killing himself. Within one of her many text messages she wrote, "The time is right and you're ready, you just need to do it!" (LeBlanc, 2017). Roy's body was found in his truck in a Kmart parking lot, and he died from self-inflicted carbon-monoxide poisoning (Brockington, 2017). Carter was convicted of involuntary manslaughter in 2017 and was sentenced to serve 15 months in jail (Sanchez, Lance, & Levenson, 2017).

Consider also the case of 18-year-old Jessica Logan from Ohio. Logan's ex-boyfriend distributed a nude photo of Logan to hundreds of people after the couple's romantic relationship ended. Logan hanged herself in her home in 2008 after being bullied by peers who saw the photo (Celizik, 2009). These cases illustrate some of the ways in which emotional pain can be caused through digital means by current and former romantic partners.

Cyberbullying will be referred to in this chapter as *cyber abuse*. As Wolford-Clevenger and colleagues (2016) point out, the term "cyber abuse" is inclusive in that "cyber" reflects the wide range of information and communication technologies that can be used, and "abuse" is a broad term that encompasses the many types of victimization by romantic partners. Text messaging, email, and social media platforms make it easy for people to perpetrate abuse toward their romantic partners and ex-partners (Bennett, Guran, Ramos, & Margolin, 2011; Leisring & Giumetti, 2014). These acts can range from swearing and insulting or calling a partner names, to more severe acts such as making threats or publicly humiliating one's partner (Leisring & Giumetti, 2014). People also use information and communication technologies such as location sharing applications to monitor and stalk current and former romantic partners and to sexually coerce them (Bufis, Leisring, & Brinkmann, 2007; Southworth, Dawson, Fraser, & Tucker, 2005; Zweig, Dank, Yahner, & Lachman, 2013). Gone are the days that abuse stops when people are physically apart. Due to mobile technology like cell phones, abuse can occur 24 hours per day and messages can be reread over and over, which may contribute to their negative ramifications. This chapter examines the phenomenon of cyber abuse within romantic relationships in the United States. I will also review prevalence and methods with which various cyber forms of abuse and cyberstalking occur in the context of romantic relationships. I will also discuss the correlates of cyber abuse and cyberstalking within the context of romantic relationships. I will provide suggestions for victims of partner cyber abuse as well as cyber abuse prevention strategies. In addition, I will provide suggested directions for future research.

Methods and Prevalence of Cyber Abuse in Romantic Relationships

There are many varied ways with which technology can be used to abuse and monitor romantic partners. Several measures of cyber abuse have been published that examine a broad array of cyber abuse behaviors (see Chapter 10, this volume for a review; Bennett et al., 2011; Hamby, 2013; Leisring & Giumetti, 2014; Smith-Darden, Kernsmith, Victor, & Lathrop, 2017). Cyber abuse measures all assess slightly different modes of abuse and some assess victimization only, perpetration only, or both victimization and perpetration. This chapter will focus on four types of cyber abuse in romantic relationships: emotional/psychological abuse, intrusion/monitoring behaviors, exclusionary acts, and sexual coercion.

Emotional/Psychological Abuse

This type of abuse occurs when a person uses texts, emails, or social media to send mean, insulting, or hostile messages to another person. This may include name calling, swearing, making threats, or using all capital letters to "shout" at one's partner (Bennett et al., 2011; Leisring & Giumetti, 2014). Threats may be vague warnings regarding harm to one's partner, their possessions, or to the partner's family or friends (Tokunaga & Aune, 2017). Threats can also be specific involving bodily harm or damage to one's reputation (Tokunaga & Aune, 2017). Perpetrators may also threaten through technology to harm themselves (e.g., as a consequence if the victim were to end the relationship) (Marganski & Melander, 2018). Emotional abuse can also involve humiliating one's partner or sabotaging their professional or social reputation by posting/sending out embarrassing photos or stories that may be true or false about their partner to others (Bennett et al., 2011; Tokunaga & Aune, 2017).

Cyber forms of emotional abuse appear to be extremely common among dating partners. In one of the first studies of cyber abuse between dating partners, 25% of youth between 13 and 18 years of age reported that their romantic partners called them names, put them down, or said "really mean" things to them via technology (Picard, 2007). Furthermore, 10% of the teens in that study reported that their partners had made physical threats toward them using a cell phone or computer (Picard, 2007). Leisring and Giumetti (2014) used a more comprehensive measure of cyber psychological abuse and found that 93% of the college participants in their study had experienced at least one act of cyber dating abuse during their current romantic relationship. Marganski and Melander (2018) found that 73% of college students had been victimized by intimate partner cyber abuse in the past year. Wolford-Clevenger and colleagues (2016) found that 30% of the college students in their sample had specifically received an angry or insulting text message from their partner in the past year. In two samples of adults recruited through Amazon's Mechanical Turk, it was found that 29–32% of respondents reported having experienced psychological forms of cyber abuse in the past six months (Watkins, Maldonado, & DiLillo, 2016). Prevalence rates seem to vary somewhat based on the time frame in question and the specific victimization experiences being examined. However, studies of adolescents, college students, and adults all find that emotional/psychological forms of cyber abuse are quite common in romantic relationships.

Intrusion/Monitoring Behaviors

Sometimes the terms "cyber dating abuse" and "cyberstalking" have been used interchangeably (Marcum, Higgins, & Nicholson, 2017). Cyberstalking/monitoring is certainly one method by which cyber abuse can be perpetrated. Monitoring can include a range of behaviors that initially may be interpreted as an expression of care or concern (e.g., repeatedly checking in to see where one's partner is; Draucker & Martsoff, 2010). These behaviors may increase in frequency and make the victim uncomfortable (Reed, Tolman, & Ward, 2017). Victims may be required by their partners to send pictures proving their current location or activities (Hamby, 2013; Wolford-Clevenger et al., 2016). Victims may receive excessive unwanted messages, calls, and emails (Bennett et al., 2011). Victims may also be pressed to share passwords for their computers, phones, email accounts, and social media accounts (Smith-Darden et al., 2017), and partners may monitor their activities online to see whom they have been interacting with (Watkins et al., 2016). In some cases, high school girls have reported creating fake social networking profiles to monitor their boyfriend's social networking activities (Lucero, Weisz, Smith-Darden, & Lucero, 2014). Perpetrators may also install GPS tracking devices on their partner's cell phone and/or they may install key logging devices on their victim's computer which provide information about everything the victim types (Tokunaga & Aune, 2017).

Reed and colleagues (2017) found that 53% of adolescents in their sample experienced cyber forms of monitoring and controlling behaviors perpetrated by their dating partners. Thirty-eight percent of college students admitted to monitoring their current partners' behavior on social media accounts (Shorey, Cornelius, & Strauss, 2015). Almost 20% of college students reported that their romantic partners checked or read their emails or text messages without permission (Wolford-Clevenger et al., 2016), and almost 16% of college students have indicated that their partner forced them to reveal their passwords to their cell phone and social media accounts (Marganski & Melander, 2018). Almost 5% of college students reported that their partners required them to send pictures so that they could check up on their current location (Wolford-Clevenger et al., 2016). Watkins and colleagues (2016) found that cyber stalking victimization in the past six months was reported by 43–45% of their adult participants. Because invasive behaviors like using GPS tracking systems or key-logging devices require advanced computer and technology skills, it has been suggested that they are probably the least common types of cyberstalking (Tokunaga & Aune, 2017), and exact prevalence rates of these types of victimization are unclear.

Exclusion

This occurs when a partner is dropped from a friend list or blocked from contact on one's social media or messaging programs (Bennett et al., 2011). It also can involve a partner intentionally ignoring communications from one's partner to hurt the partner's feelings (Watkins et al., 2016). This may be the cyber equivalent of stomping out of a room or house, which is one of the items on a traditional face-to-face measure of psychological abuse (Straus, Hamby, Boney-McCoy, & Sugarman, 1996). Studies on cyber abuse have not always included attention to this particular form of cyber abuse. However, it appears that it may be a particularly common form since Marganski and Melander (2018) found that 47% of college students indicated that their partners had purposefully ignored their communications through technology. It is currently unclear whether victims find this form of cyber abuse any less distressing than other forms. We do know from research with married couples that disengaging behaviors (e.g., remaining silent during face-to-face interactions with one's partner) are associated with decreased relationship satisfaction over time (Barry & Lawrence, 2013), so exclusionary behaviors in a cyber context may also be harmful to relationships.

Sexual Coercion

This type of cyber abuse involves cyber communication of a sexual nature. In some cases, a person is pressured to send sexually explicit messages, images, or videos to their partner (Smith-Darden et al., 2017). The texts or images may at times be shared publicly to embarrass the victim. Other forms of sexual cyber abuse occur when the victim is sent unwanted sexual images by their partner or when one's partner sends texts or emails to pressure the person into engaging in unwanted sexual acts. Some measures of cyber partner abuse include subscales that examine sexual forms of cyber abuse (Watkins et al., 2016; Zweig et al., 2013). Zweig and colleagues (2013) found that rates of sexual cyber abuse victimization were lower than rates of non-sexual forms of cyber abuse victimization, yet 11% of students in Grades 7 to 12 in their study reported being victimized by sexual forms of cyber abuse. Rates were even higher in the study by Reed and colleagues (2017). Thirty-two percent of the adolescents in their sample reported cyber forms of sexual coercion victimization. Girls had higher rates of cyber sexual victimization than boys in both of these studies (Reed et al., 2017; Zweig et al., 2013).

Shorey and colleagues (2015) found that 1.9% of college students reported that their current partners sent them pornographic images when they did not want them to. A similar rate (2.4%) of respondents in an ethnically diverse group of sixth graders reported sending unwanted sexual images to their partners (Peskin et al., 2017). Sexual forms of cyber partner abuse also occur in adult relationships. In two samples of adults, 14–18% of respondents indicated that they were victimized by sexual forms of cyber abuse in the past six months (Watkins et al., 2016).

Correlates of Cyber Abuse in Romantic Relationships

Research has begun to examine whether the correlates and consequences of cyber forms of partner abuse are similar to the correlates and consequences of traditional partner abuse. What has emerged is a pattern where many dysfunctional characteristics found to be associated with traditional offline abuse in prior literature are indeed also associated with cyber forms of abuse. Aspects of cyber abusive behavior have been found to be associated with jealousy, anxious attachment, anger/hostility, poor emotional regulation, low self-control, and alcohol use (Kellerman, Margolin, Borofsky, Baucom, & Iturralde, 2013; Marcum, Higgins, & Poff, 2016; Marcum et al., 2017; Reed, Tolman, & Safyer, 2015; Van Ouytsel et al., 2017; Watkins et al., 2016; Wright, 2015; Zweig et al., 2013). The following experiences and characteristics are also associated with the perpetration of cyber forms of partner abuse and thus may set the stage for cyber abuse to occur: deviant peer associations, bullying experiences, family risk factors, a history of adverse child experiences, poor relationship satisfaction, increased time on social networking sites, and non-cyber relationship abuse (Kellerman et al., 2013; Leisring & Giumetti, 2014; Leisring, Giumetti, Vélez, & Scotto, 2017; Marcum et al., 2017; Smith-Darden et al., 2017; Van Ouytsel et al., 2017; Watkins et al., 2016; Yahner, Dank, Zweig, & Lachman, 2015). The following variables have also been found to correlate with cyber abuse and they may be consequences of cyber abuse: substance use, depression, anxiety, fear, and anger (Bennett et al., 2011; Lindsay, Booth, Messing, & Thaller, 2016; Zweig et al.,

2013; Zweig, Lachman, Yahner, & Dank, 2014). Teens in Michigan who were interviewed as part of a small qualitative study often reported that jealousy and distrust in relationships occurred as a result of cyber abuse (Lucero et al., 2014). It has been suggested that cyber abuse may lead to worse consequences than offline forms of psychological abuse because in many cases the abusive communications (e.g., texts, emails) can be reread (Melander, 2010).

Research studies on cyber abuse in the United States have been mainly cross-sectional. However, cyber abuse victimization, cyber abuse perpetration, and physical abuse victimization predicted cyber abuse victimization one year later in a sample of adolescents (Temple et al., 2016). Also, anxious attachment among adolescents predicted cyber abuse perpetration one year later (Wright, 2015). Additional longitudinal studies that examine correlates of cyber abuse would help to clarify which factors play a causal role and which result from cyber abuse experiences. It is clear, however, from multiple studies that cyber abuse is related to non-cyber forms of abuse and that its correlates are also similar to those of non-cyber forms of abuse (Leisring & Guimetti, 2014; Temple et al., 2016; Watkins et al., 2016; Wolford-Clevenger et al., 2016). Thus, it appears that cyber abuse is simply another method by which abuse occurs in romantic relationships. This idea that cyber abuse is an extension of traditional forms of abuse was supported by a national study of abuse and cyber abuse among teens (Korchmaros, Ybarra, Langhinrichsen-Rohling, Boyd, & Lenhart, 2013). Korchmaros and colleagues (2013) found that psychological abuse in face-to-face and telephone contexts was more common than abuse in online and texting contexts. Dating abuse via texting and in online contexts was especially common among teens who had perpetrated abuse face-to-face or via telephone calls. Cyber forms of dating abuse have also been found to be associated with reproductive coercion and contraception non-use in teen girls (Dick et al., 2014).

Suggestions for Individuals (and Parents)

There are concrete steps that can be taken to reduce one's likelihood of being a victim of cyber abuse by one's current or former romantic partners. People should pay close attention to their privacy settings on social media and to the material that they post about themselves. For example, if they do not want an ex-partner to know that they are dating someone new, then they should refrain from posting information online about their new relationship. They should also be aware that posting pictures of themselves with their new partner may increase feelings of jealousy in an ex-partner. Settings on social media should be arranged so that only one's friends can see information about them and so that friends cannot tag them in posts and pictures without their approval. Passwords for social media should be complex with letters, numbers, and special characters, and they should be changed regularly and kept private.

Cyber victimization often occurs after the dissolution of romantic relationships (Hoff & Mitchell, 2009). Thus, particular care should be taken before breaking up with one's partner (Dardis & Gidycz, 2017). Dardis and Gidycz recommend changing passwords before ending one's relationship. Reed and colleagues (2017) examined responses to digital abuse and some victims "blocked" their ex-partners on social media and blocked them from calling or texting on their cell phones. People may want to also consider blocking the friends or family members of an ex-partner on social media to reduce the likelihood that information gets communicated to one's ex-partner by others. If there has been a history of abuse in one's relationship, victims may also want to delete or change their email or social media accounts or change usernames as well as passwords (Tokunaga & Aune, 2017). Installing antivirus software may be warranted to keep abusers from compromising one's computer or gaining access to private information (Tokunaga & Aune, 2017). This is particularly true if the ex-partner's abuse included intrusion and monitoring behaviors that had given them prior access to the victim's technology.

Parents should check in regularly with their children about the health of their romantic relationships and parents should be aware that, if cyber abuse is taking place, other forms of abuse may also be occurring (Temple et al., 2016). Since 15% of sixth graders reported perpetrating some form of cyber dating abuse (Peskin et al., 2017), attention by parents is warranted at an early age. Rueda, Lindsay, and Williams (2014) suggest that parental boundaries that allow parents to observe their teen's technology-based communications can alert parents to unhealthy dating relationship characteristics and can facilitate important parent-child discussions. Smith-Darden and colleagues (2017) found that parental involvement appears to serve a protective function against the perpetration of cyber abuse in middle school and high school students. In their study, they looked at parental involvement as a combined factor involving consistently monitoring adolescent behavior (not necessarily cyber behaviors), establishing rules, communicating, and bonding emotionally with one's child. Future research should establish which components of parental involvement are more important in preventing cyber abuse (Smith-Darden et al., 2017).

Clinicians working with victims of cyber abuse should recommend that victims document their victimization, for example by taking a screen shot or photo of threatening messages (Wolford-Clevenger et al., 2016). Such documentation will be helpful if victims pursue legal assistance and protection or assistance through Title IX in educational settings. Finn and Atkinson (2009) developed a technology safety project for victims of partner violence and clinicians regarding methods for the safe and private use of technology. Their program also addresses ways in which technology can be used to connect victims with community resources. Tips for the safe use of technology should be a standard part of safety planning for victims of partner abuse (Wick et al., 2017).

Suggestions for Cyber Abuse Prevention Programming

Since the rates of cyber abuse are high among youth and college students, educational institutions can and should play a large role in the prevention of such abuse. Given the overlap between cyber and non-cyber forms of partner abuse, a focus on cyber abuse should be included in institutional endeavors to prevent and address intimate partner violence. Wolford-Clevenger and colleagues (2016) suggest that cyber abuse be included in school policies regarding interpersonal violence and that victims be provided with resources. Assessment of cyber abuse should be included in school climate surveys assessing traditional forms of dating abuse and school personnel, like nurses, should have visible pamphlets and posters about cyber abuse (Van Ouytsel, Walrave, Ponnet, & Temple, 2016; Van Ouytsel et al., 2017).

Youth may not recognize the seriousness of behaviors that constitute cyber abuse (Lucero et al., 2014). Prevention programs should include material to help individuals distinguish between caring and possessive/abusive actions (e.g., excessive texting) and they should teach technology safety (e.g., never share passwords). A model program that covers healthy and unhealthy relationships is "the fourth R" (Van Ouytsel et al., 2016). This program has been implemented in Canada and Alaska and includes parent workshops as well as school-based curricula for middle and high school students. Information about this program can be found at https://youthrelationships.org/hrpp. Another prevention program, "Moms and Teens for Safe Dates" was developed specifically for mothers who are victims of domestic violence and their teenage children (Foshee et al., 2015). This interactive program prevented cyber abuse perpetration specifically in adolescents who had been exposed to high levels of domestic violence. Unfortunately, no effects of the program on cyber abuse victimization were found.

Miller and colleagues (2015) conducted a cluster randomized controlled trial to examine the effectiveness of a brief educational intervention provided in high school health centers. Results indicated that students in the intervention group reported reduced rates of cyber abuse victimization at the three-month follow-up compared to those in the control condition. This program called the school health center healthy adolescent relationship program (SHARP) is worthy of further study.

Marcum and colleagues (2017) suggest that high schools and colleges should provide basic information to students including the following: "1) what behaviors constitute cyberstalking; 2) the frequency of the occurrence in current relationships; 3) the legal and social repercussions of participating in the behavior; and 4) psychological and emotional responses by victims to the behaviors" (p. 385). Many institutions are implementing bystander prevention programming such as "Know your Power," "Green Dot," and "Scream Theater" for intimate partner violence (Coker et al., 2011; McMahon, Postmus, Warrener, & Koenick, 2014; Potter, 2012). The bystander approach may be particularly fruitful for the prevention of cyber abuse given that cyber forms of abuse are often taking place in "public" social media forums (Temple et al., 2016). Also, Alexy, Burgess, Baker, and Smoyak (2005) found that 75% of college students who were victims of cyberstalking, often by former romantic partners, told friends about their experiences. Thus, friends may be in a unique position to intervene in that they are more likely to be told about abuse that is occurring than family members (Alexy et al., 2005).

Given research on risk factors associated with cyber abuse, prevention programming may be especially fruitful if it targets youth who use substances (Stuart, O'Farrell, & Temple, 2009), youth with a history of four or more adverse childhood experiences (Smith-Darden et al., 2017), or anxiously attached women (Reed et al., 2015). Since cyber abuse seems to be an extension of traditional abuse in adolescents (Korchmaros et al., 2013), cyber abuse may decrease as a result of prevention programs for partner abuse in general. However, adding information about cyber abuse to existing violence prevention efforts seems wise. Sexual forms of cyber abuse may need their own prevention content. The Texas School Safety Center at Texas State University has developed an online educational prevention program called "before you text" that addresses "sexting" in youth (Texas School Safety Center, n.d.). Youth and adults need to be made aware of the psychological and legal consequences of sharing sexually explicit images. Adolescents who have shared nude digital images have been prosecuted under child pornography laws in some states (Judge, 2012).

Conclusion

Stonard and colleagues have described relationship violence as a "continuum of abusive behaviors that may be experienced or performed in person and/or through electronic means" (Stonard, Bowen, Lawrence, & Price, 2014, p. 413). This chapter has illustrated the various ways in which people can perpetrate abuse toward their current and former romantic partners through electronic means (i.e., cyber abuse). Cyber abuse can involve insults and threats, public humiliation, exclusion, monitoring and controlling behaviors, as well as sexual coercion. It would be ideal to identify subtypes of abuse that may have different risk factors and outcomes. For example, Preddy (2015) suggests that it may be useful to distinguish public forms of cyber aggression from private ones. This is in line with the findings by Leisring and Giumetti (2014) suggesting two different factors of cyber psychological abuse where threats and public humiliation were a separate factor distinct from behaviors characterized as mild forms of cyber psychological abuse (e.g., name calling and swearing). Research is needed to determine which cyber abuse acts cause the most fear and emotional distress and which are most closely associated with physical forms of partner violence (Wolford-Clevenger et al., 2016). It is quite possible that cyber abuse of a sexual nature such as digital sexual coercion or publicly distributing nude pictures (i.e., revenge pornography/nonconsensual pornography) may have a particularly deleterious effect on victims (Citron & Franks, 2014).

Research investigating the risk factors that make perpetration of cyber abuse more likely is warranted. Given their association with other forms of partner violence, mate retention tactics, jealousy, and substance abuse deserve additional attention in future studies of cyber abuse (Brem, Spiller, & Vandehey, 2015; Kellerman et al., 2013; Van Ouytsel et al., 2017). Longitudinal research would also greatly add to the literature by clarifying potential causal relations as most research in the area thus far has been cross-sectional. Marganski and Melander (2018) point out that longitudinal studies are needed to determine whether cyber abuse tends to precede other forms of partner abuse in romantic relationships. Thus far, temporal relationships between cyber abuse and other forms of partner violence in the United States have only been examined in the study by Temple and colleagues (2016). Researchers and clinicians looking to conduct an assessment of cyber abuse should include one of the various cyber abuse measures that exist (Hamby, 2013; Leisring & Giumetti, 2014; Watkins et al., 2016; Zweig et al., 2013), or, at the very least, they should use a measure of intimate partner violence that contains at least one item of cyber abuse. The short form of the revised Composite Abuse Scale (CAS-SF; Ford-Gilboe et al., 2016) includes the item "Harassed me by phone, text, email or using social media."

Cyber forms of dating abuse have been perpetrated by 15% of sixth graders (Peskin et al., 2017) and cyber abuse seems to increase in frequency in high school and college (Leisring & Giumetti, 2014; Smith-Darden et al., 2017). Ninety-three percent of college students indicated that they had perpetrated or been victimized by emotional forms of cyber abuse in their current romantic relationship (Leisring & Giumetti, 2014). Cyber abuse also occurs in adult romantic relationships (Leisring et al., 2017; Watkins et al., 2016) and it often co-occurs with physical abuse and face-to-face psychological abuse (Leisring & Giumetti, 2014; Temple et al., 2016; Watkins et al., 2016; Wolford-Clevenger et al., 2016). When cyber abuse occurs in the context of a physically abusive relationship, it may make victims feel more vulnerable (Melander, 2010).

This chapter has focused on research conducted in predominantly heterosexual relationships. However, one large study examining experiences of cyber dating abuse in 7–12th grade students in New York found that rates of cyber dating abuse victimization and perpetration were higher among gay, lesbian, and transgender students compared to heterosexual students (Dank, Lachman, Zweig, & Yahner, 2014). Future work should further examine cyber abuse in same-sex romantic relationships.

Like traditional forms of partner abuse (Langhinrichsen-Rohling, 2010; Straus & Gelles, 1990), cyber abuse is often bi-directional in nature (Kellerman et al., 2013; Leisring & Giumetti, 2014; Reed, Tolman, & Ward, 2016; Temple et al., 2016). Thus, it is common for individuals to both perpetrate and be a victim of cyber forms of partner abuse. Findings regarding gender have been mixed and deserve more attention in the literature. Some studies have failed to find any gender differences in the victimization of some forms of cyber abuse (e.g., Wolford-Clevenger et al., 2016). However, it appears that females may be victimized by sexual forms of cyber abuse at higher rates than males (Reed et al., 2017; Zweig et al., 2013), and women may find cyber abuse to be more distressing than men (Bennett et al., 2011). A focus on cyber abuse should be included in prevention and intervention efforts for intimate partner violence. Hopefully, youth, adults, parents, school personnel, researchers, and clinicians can simultaneously work to prevent cyber abuse and to reduce its impact on victims.

References

Alexy, E. M., Burgess, A. W., Baker, T., & Smoyak, S. A. (2005). Perceptions of cyber-stalking among college students. *Brief Treatment and Crisis Intervention, 5*, 279–289. doi:10.1093/brief-treatment/mhi020

Barry, R. A., & Lawrence, E. (2013). "Don't stand so close to me": An attachment perspective of disengagement and avoidance in marriage. *Journal of Family Psychology, 27*(3), 484–494. doi:10.1037/a0032867

Bennett, D. C. Guran., E. L., Ramos, M. C., & Margolin, G. (2011). College students' electronic victimization in friendships and dating relationships: Anticipated distress and associations with risky behaviors. *Violence and Victims, 26*(4), 410–429. doi:10.1891/0886-6708.26.4.410

Brem, M. J., Spiller, L. C., & Vandehey, M. A. (2015). Online mate-retention tactics on Facebook are associated with relationship aggression. *Journal of Interpersonal Violence, 30* (16), 2831–2850. doi:10.1177/0886260514554286

Brockington, A. (2017, June 16). *Michelle Carter found guilty of encouraging boyfriend's suicide with text messages*. Retrieved from www.nbcnews.com/news/us-news/michelle-carter-found-guilty-encouraging-boyfriend-s-suicide-text-messages-n773306

Bufis, V. M., Leisring, P. A., & Brinkmann, J. L. (2007, October). *The use of technological advancements in the perpetration of unwanted pursuit behaviors*. Poster presented at the 47th Annual Meeting of the New England Psychological Association, Danbury, CT.

Celizik, M. (2009, March 6). *Her teen committed suicide over "sexting."* Retrieved from www.today.com/parents/her-teen-committed-suicide-over-sexting-2D80555048

Citron, D. K., & Franks, M. A. (2014). Criminalizing revenge porn. *Wake Forest Law Review, 49*, 345–391. Retrieved from https://digitalcommons.law.umaryland.edu/fac_pubs/1420/

Coker, A. L., Cook-Craig, P. G., Williams, C. M., Fisher, B. S., Clear, E. R., Garcia, L. S., & Hegge, L. M. (2011). Evaluation of green dot: An active bystander intervention to reduce sexual violence on college campuses. *Violence Against Women, 17*, 777–796. doi:10.1177/107780121141026

Dank, M., Lachman, P., Zweig, J. M., & Yahner, J. (2014). Dating violence experiences of lesbian, gay, bisexual, and transgender youth. *Journal of Youth and Adolescence, 43*(5), 846–857. doi:10.1007/s10964-013-9975-8

Dardis, C. M., & Gidycz, C. A. (2017). Reconciliation or retaliation? An integrative model of postrelationship in-person and cyber unwanted pursuit perpetration among undergraduate men and women. *Psychology of Violence*. Advance online publication. doi:10.1037/vio0000102

Dick, R. N., McCauley, H. L., Jones, K. A., Tancredi, D. J., Goldstein, S., Blackburn, S., … Miller, E. (2014). Cyber dating abuse among teens using school-based health centers. *Pediatrics*, *134*(6), e1560–e1576. doi:10.1542/peds.2014-0537

Draucker, C. B., & Martsolf, D. S. (2010). The role of electronic communication technology in adolescent dating violence. *Journal of Child and Adolescent Psychiatric Nursing*, *23*(3), 133–142. doi:10.1111/j.1744-6171.2010.00235.x

Finn, J., & Atkinson, T. (2009). Promoting the safe and strategic use of technology for victims of intimate partner violence: Evaluation of the technology safety project. *Journal of Family Violence*, *24*(1), 53–59. doi:10.1177/1077801209346723

Ford-Gilboe, M., Wathen, C. N., Varcoe, C., MacMillan, H. L., Scott-Storey, K., Mantler, T., … Perrin, N. (2016). Development of a brief measure of intimate partner violence experiences: The Composite Abuse Scale (Revised)—Short Form (CAS R-SF). *BMJ Open*, *6*(12), 1–13. doi:10.1136/bmjopen-2016-012824

Foshee, V. A., Benefield, T., Dixon, K. S., Chang, L. Y., Senkomago, V., Ennett, S. T., … Bowling, J. M. (2015). The effects of Moms and Teens for Safe Dates: A dating abuse prevention program for adolescents exposed to domestic violence. *Journal of Youth and Adolescence*, *44*(5), 995–1010. doi:10.1007/s10964-015-0272-6

Hamby, S. (2013). *The Partner Cyber Abuse Questionnaire: Preliminary psychometrics of technology based intimate partner violence*. Paper presented at the Southeastern Psychological Association Conference, Atlanta, GA.

Hoff, D. L., & Mitchell, S. N. (2009). Cyberbullying: Causes, effects, and remedies. *Journal of Educational Administration*, *47*, 652–665. doi:10.1108/09578230910981107

Judge, A. M. (2012). “Sexting” among US adolescents: Psychological and legal perspectives. *Harvard Review of Psychiatry*, *20*(2), 86–96. doi:10.3109/10673229.2012.677360

Kellerman, I., Margolin, G., Borofsky, L. A., Baucom, B. R., & Iturralde, E. (2013). Electronic aggression among emerging adults: Motivations and contextual factors. *Emerging Adulthood*, *1*(4), 293–304. doi:10.1177/2167696813490159

Korchmaros, J. D., Ybarra, M. L., Langhinrichsen-Rohling, J., Boyd, D., & Lenhart, A. (2013). Perpetration of teen dating violence in a networked society. *Cyberpsychology, Behavior, and Social Networking*, *16*(8), 561–567. doi:10.1089/cyber.2012.0627

Langhinrichsen-Rohling, J. (2010). Controversies involving gender and intimate partner violence in the United States. *Sex Roles*, *62*(3–4), 179–193. doi:10.1007/s11199-009-9697-2

LeBlanc, P. (2017, June 8). *The text messages that led up to teen's suicide*. Retrieved from www.cnn.com/2017/06/08/us/text-message-suicide-michelle-carter-conrad-roy/index.html

Leisring, P.A. & Giumetti, G.W. (2014). Sticks and stones may break my bones, but abusive text messages also hurt: Development and validation of the cyber psychological abuse (CPA) scale. *Partner Abuse*, *5*(3), 323–334. doi:10.1891/1946-6560.5.3.323

Leisring, P.A., Giumetti, G.W., Vélez, C., & Scotto, D. (2017, November). *#ImOuttaHere: Linking cyber psychological abuse with relationship outcomes in adult romantic partners*. Poster presented at the 51st annual convention of the Association for Behavioral and Cognitive Therapies, San Diego, CA.

Lindsay, M., Booth, J. M., Messing, J. T., & Thaller, J. (2016). Experiences of online harassment among emerging adults: Emotional reactions and the mediating role of fear. *Journal of Interpersonal Violence*, *31*(19), 3174–3195. doi:10.1177/0886260515584344

Lucero, J. L., Weisz, A. N., Smith-Darden, J., & Lucero, S. M. (2014). Exploring gender differences: Socially interactive technology use/abuse among dating teens. *Journal of Women and Social Work*, *29*(4), 478–491. doi:10.1177/0886109914522627

Marcum, C. D., Higgins, G. E., & Nicholson, J. (2017). I'm watching you: Cyberstalking behaviors of university students in romantic relationships. *American Journal of Criminal Justice, 42*(2), 373–388. doi:10.1007/s12103-016-9358-2

Marcum, C. D., Higgins, G. E., & Poff, B. (2016). Exploratory investigation on theoretical predictors of the electronic leash. *Computers in Human Behavior, 61*, 213–218. doi:10.1016/j.chb.2016. 03. 010

Marganski, A., & Melander, L. (2018). Intimate partner violence victimization in the cyber and real world: Examining the extent of cyber aggression experiences and its association with in-person dating violence. *Journal of Interpersonal Violence, 33*(7), 1071–1095. doi:10.1177/0886260515614283

McMahon, S., Postmus, J. L., Warrener, C., & Koenick, R. A. (2014). Utilizing peer education theater to encourage bystander intervention with sexual violence. *Journal of College Student Development, 55*(1), 78–85. doi:10.1353/csd.2014.0001

Melander, L. A. (2010). College students' perceptions of intimate partner cyber harassment. *Cyberpsychology, Behavior, and Social Networking, 13*, 263–268. doi:10.1089/cyber.2009.0221

Miller, E., Goldstein, S., McCauley, H. L., Jones, K. A., Dick, R. N., Jetton, J., … Tancredi, D. J. (2015). A school health center intervention for abusive adolescent relationships: A cluster RCT. *Pediatrics, 135*(1), 76–85. doi:10.1542/peds.2014-2471

Peskin, M. F., Markham, C. M., Shegog, R., Temple, J. R., Baumler, E. R., Addy, R. C., … & Emery, S. T. (2017). Prevalence and correlates of the perpetration of cyber dating abuse among early adolescents. *Journal of Youth and Adolescence, 46*(2), 358–375. doi:10.1007/s10964-016-0568-1

Picard, P. (2007). *Tech abuse in teen relationships study*. Chicago, IL: Teen Research Unlimited. Retrieved from www.loveisrespect.org/wp-content/uploads/2009/03/liz-claiborne-2007-tech-relationship-abuse.pdf

Potter, S. J. (2012). Using a multi-media social marketing campaign to increase active bystanders on the college campus. *Journal of American College Health, 60*(4), 282–295. doi:10.1080/07448481.2011.599350

Preddy, T. M. (2015). *Assessment and investigation of electronic aggression in the romantic relationships of emerging adults* (Doctoral dissertation). Retrieved from http://trace.tennessee.edu/cgi/viewcontent.cgi?article=4846&context=utk_graddiss

Reed, L. A., Tolman, R. M., & Safyer, P. (2015). Too close for comfort: Attachment insecurity and electronic intrusion in college students' dating relationships. *Computers in Human Behavior, 50*, 431–438. doi:10.1016/j.chb.2015.03.050

Reed, L. A., Tolman, R. M., & Ward, L. M. (2016). Snooping and sexting: Digital media as a context for dating aggression and abuse among college students. *Violence Against Women, 22*(13), 1556–1576. doi:10.1177/1077801216630143

Reed, L. A., Tolman, R. M., & Ward, L. M. (2017). Gender matters: Experiences and consequences of digital dating abuse victimization in adolescent dating relationships. *Journal of Adolescence, 59*, 79–89. doi:10.1016/j.adolescence.2017. 05. 015

Rueda, H. A., Lindsay, M., & Williams, L. R. (2015). "She posted it on Facebook" Mexican American adolescents' experiences with technology and romantic relationship conflict. *Journal of Adolescent Research, 30*(4), 419–445. doi:10.1177/0743558414565236

Sanchez, R., Lance, N., & Levenson, E. (2017, August 3). *Woman sentenced to 15 months in texting suicide case*. Retrieved from www.cnn.com/2017/08/03/us/michelle-carter-texting-suicide-sentencing/index.html.

Shorey, R. C., Cornelius, T. L., & Strauss, C. (2015). Stalking in college student dating relationships: A descriptive investigation. *Journal of Family Violence, 30*(7), 935–942. doi:10.1007/s10896-015-9717-7

Smith-Darden, J. P., Kernsmith, P. D., Victor, B. G., & Lathrop, R. A. (2017). Electronic displays of aggression in teen dating relationships: Does the social ecology matter? *Computers in Human Behavior, 67*, 33–40. doi:10.1016/j.chb.2016. 10. 015

Southworth, C., Dawson, S., Fraser, C., & Tucker, S. (2005). A high-tech twist on abuse: Technology, intimate partner stalking, and advocacy. *Violence Against Women Online Resources*. Retrieved from www.acesdv.org/wp-content/uploads/2014/06/NNEDV_HighTechTwist_PaperAndApxA_English08.pdf

Stonard, K. E., Bowen, E., Lawrence, T. R., & Price, S. A. (2014). The relevance of technology to the nature, prevalence and impact of adolescent dating violence and abuse: A research synthesis. *Aggression and Violent Behavior, 19*(4), 390–417. doi:10.1016/j.avb.2014. 06. 005

Straus, M. A., & Gelles, R. J. (1990). *Physical violence in American families: Risk factors and adaptations to violence in 8,145 families*. New Brunswick, NJ: Transaction Publishers.

Straus, M. A., Hamby, S. L., Boney-McCoy, S., & Sugarman, D. B. (1996). The revised conflict tactics scales (CTS2) development and preliminary psychometric data. *Journal of Family Issues, 17*(3), 283–316. doi:10.1177/019251396017003001

Stuart, G. L., O'Farrell, T. J., & Temple, J. R. (2009). Review of the association between treatment for substance misuse and reductions in intimate partner violence. *Substance Use & Misuse, 44*(9–10), 1298–1317. doi:10.1080/10826080902961385

Temple, J. R., Choi, H. J., Brem, M., Wolford-Clevenger, C., Stuart, G. L., Peskin, M. F., & Elmquist, J. (2016). The temporal association between traditional and cyber dating abuse among adolescents. *Journal of Youth and Adolescence, 45*(2), 340–349. doi:10.1007/s10964-015-0380-3

Texas School Safety Center. (n.d.). *"Before you text" Sexting Prevention Course*. Retrieved from https://txssc.txstate.edu/tools/courses/before-you-text/

Tokunaga, R. S., & Aune, K. S. (2017). Cyber-defense: A taxonomy of tactics for managing cyberstalking. *Journal of Interpersonal Violence, 32*(10), 1451–1475. doi:10.1177/0886260515589564

Van Ouytsel, J., Walrave, M., Ponnet, K., & Temple, J. R. (2016). Digital forms of dating violence: What school nurses need to know. *NASN School Nurse, 31*(6), 348–353. doi:10.1177/1942602X16659907

Van Ouytsel, J., Torres, E., Choi, H. J., Ponnet, K., Walrave, M., & Temple, J. R. (2017). The associations between substance use, sexual behaviors, bullying, deviant behaviors, health, and cyber dating abuse perpetration. *The Journal of School Nursing, 33*(2), 116–122. doi:10.1177/1059840516683229

Watkins, L. E., Maldonado, R. C., & DiLillo, D. (2016). The Cyber Aggression in Relationships Scale: A new multidimensional measure of technology-based intimate partner aggression. *Assessment, 25*(5), 608–626. doi:10.1177/1073191116665696

Wick, S. E., Nagoshi, C., Basham, R., Jordan, C., Kim, Y. K., Nguyen, A. P., & Lehmann, P. (2017). Patterns of cyber harassment and perpetration among college students in the United States: A test of routine activities theory. *International Journal of Cyber Criminology, 11*(1), 24–38. doi:10.5281/zenodo.495770

Wolford-Clevenger, C., Zapor, H., Brasfield, H., Febres, J., Elmquist, J., Brem, M., … Stuart, G. L. (2016). An examination of the Partner Cyber Abuse Questionnaire in a college student sample. *Psychology of Violence, 6*(1), 156–162. doi:10.1037/a0039442

Wright, M. F. (2015). Cyber aggression within adolescents' romantic relationships: Linkages to parental and partner attachment. *Journal of Youth and Adolescence*, *44*(1), 37–47.

Yahner, J., Dank, M., Zweig, J. M., & Lachman, P. (2015). The co-occurrence of physical and cyber dating violence and bullying among teens. *Journal of Interpersonal Violence*, *30* (7), 1079–1089. doi:10.1177/0886260514540324

Zweig, J. M., Dank, M., Yahner, J., & Lachman, P. (2013). The rate of cyber dating abuse among teens and how it relates to other forms of teen dating violence. *Journal of Youth and Adolescence*, *42*(7), 1063–1077. doi:10.1007/s10964-013-9922-8

Zweig, J. M., Lachman, P., Yahner, J., & Dank, M. (2014). Correlates of cyber dating abuse among teens. *Journal of Youth and Adolescence*, *43*(8), 1306–1321. doi:10.1007/s10964-013-0047-x

10

CYBERBULLYING IN ROMANTIC RELATIONSHIPS

Cross-Cultural Issues

Esther Calvete, Manuel Gámez-Guadix, and Erika Borrajo

Abuse in romantic relationships is a severe problem that affects many couples around the world. Some studies indicate prevalence rates as high as 83% (Sánchez, Muñoz-Fernández, & Ortega-Ruiz, 2015; Wolford-Clevenger et al., 2016). Abuse in romantic relationships includes numerous modalities, such as psychological or emotional abuse, physical abuse, and sexual abuse. In recent decades, the popularity and easy access to new technologies among adolescents and young people have created new platforms on which abuse and aggression in dating relationships can be manifested.

Cyber dating abuse or cyber abuse in romantic relationships (CARR) has been described as monitoring, controlling, harassing or otherwise abusing a romantic partner via technology (Temple et al., 2016). There is some debate about whether CARR is a different phenomenon from traditional dating abuse (Cutbush, Williams, Miller, Gibbs, & Clinton-Sherrod, 2012; Temple et al., 2016; Zweig, Dank, Yanher, & Lachman, 2013). Some studies have examined the incremental impact of CARR over and above offline abuse on outcomes. For instance, Leisring and Giumetti (2014) found that CARR predicted unique variance in stress over physical abuse but not over offline psychological abuse. Morevoer, Zweig et al. (2013) found that almost all cyber abuse victims in romantic relationships also experienced offline psychological abuse. This overlap could suggest that CARR is just psychological dating abuse through new technologies. However, although forms of offline and online psychological abuse co-occur in relationships, there is some evidence to suggest that CARR and offline psychological abuse are different problems. First, cyber abuse also includes sexual forms of abuse (Jaen-Cortés, Rivera-Aragón, Reidl-Martínez, & García Méndez, 2017; Zweig et al., 2013), and thus it goes beyond psychological abuse. Second, some of the characteristics of cyber abuse are so specific that they make it a phenomenon in its own right. For example, CARR can be permanently manifested on the Internet and abusive messages and images can be forwarded by third parties, implying some revictimization (Stonard, Bowen, Lawrence, & Price, 2014). Once an image, video, or information is spread on the Internet by the partner or former partner, it can remain in cyberspace indefinitely (Gámez-Guadix, Almendros, Borrajo, & Calvete, 2015). It is almost impossible to delete some contents that have been disseminated via the Internet, as these contents can be stored by many people. This public nature of cyber abuse, which implies that aggression can be widespread and reach many people, can make humiliation especially harmful to the victim (Peskin et al., 2017). Finally, online victimization and harassment are primarily indirect, rather than face-to-face (Smith, 2012). The aggressor does not see the victim's reaction immediately, which can facilitate insensitivity and a lack of empathy towards the victim.

As with face-to-face abuse, CARR can take on multiple forms. Unfortunately, the study of these forms of CARR and their main characteristics has been hampered by the multiplicity of measures and methodologies used for their evaluation. This problem is especially evident when adopting an international perspective. The lack of homogeneity and the different questionnaires used make it difficult to establish valid conclusions about the magnitude of CARR. This chapter describes the main measures developed to assess CARR, as well as the incidence of this phenomenon among young people and adolescents in several countries. Finally, gender differences in victimization and perpetration and their reciprocity are reviewed.

Measurement of Cyber Abuse in Romantic Relationships

Table 10.1 presents a list of 35 different measures, obtained after performing searches on PROQUEST, SCOPUS, and Google Scholar. Various search terms such as "cyber dating abuse," "cyber dating violence," "online dating abuse," "online dating violence," "digital dating violence," and "cyber harassment" were used to perform this search.

Of the 35 measures included in Table 10.1, 20 have been developed in the US, nine in Europe, three in Mexico, two in Australia, and one in Canada. Most of the measures are very recent. Specifically, 19 of 35 (54%) have been developed between 2015 and 2017. Another notable aspect is that there are few adaptations of the existing measures to different languages. Some exceptions are the Online Interpersonal Violence and Abuse measure, which was used in five European countries (Bulgaria, Cyprus, England, Italy, and Norway; Barter et al., 2017), the Cyberdating Q-A, which was translated and used in Italian by Sánchez, Muñoz, Nocentini, Ortega-Ruiz, and Menesini (2014), and the Cyber Dating Abuse scale (Zweig et al., 2013), which was translated and used in Spanish by Sánchez, Muñoz-Fernández, and Vega-Gea (2017). In addition, some items of the Cyber Dating Abuse Questionnaire (Borrajo, Gámez-Guadix, Pereda, & Calvete, 2015),

TABLE 10.1 Measures of Cyber Abuse in Romantic Relationships

Authors	*Measure name*	*Country*	*Type*	*Items/Dimensions & Response format*	*Psychometric Evidence*	*Facet of CARR*	*Sample*
Barter et al. (2017)	Online Interpersonal Violence and Abuse	Bulgaria, Cyprus, England, Italy, Norway	B	6 items that assess 4 main ways in which new technologies could be used to inflict interpersonal violence and abuse: Emotional abuse (3) Controlling behavior (1) Surveillance (1) Isolation (1). Response format: 4-point scale: *never, once, a few times*, and *often*.	α = .76 - .86	Victimization	*N* = 3,299 young people who had been in a relationship Age range = 14–17
Bennett et al. (2011)	Electronic Victimization	US	C	It includes one form for victimization by friends and another for victimization by a partner Each of them with the following dimensions: Hostility (7 items) Intrusion (7 items) Humiliation (5 items) Exclusion (3 items) Response format: 5-point Likert scale of frequency in the last year Degree of anticipated emotional distress if the event were to occur	α = .73 - .77	Victimization	*N* = 437 (68% female) Age range = 18–22 years

Borrajo, Gámez-Guadix, Pereda, & Calvete (2015)	Cyber Dating Abuse Questionnaire	Spain	C	20 parallel items Direct aggression (11) Monitoring / control (9) Response format: 1 (Never) - 5 (very often) The questionnaire assesses the context in which these behaviors occurred (e.g., *jealousy, game / discussions*)	EFA and CFA α = .73 - .84 for perpetration, α = .81 -.87 for victimization	Victimization Perpetration	*N* = 788 young people (77.3% women) Age range = 18–30 years.
Burke et al. (2011)	Controlling Partner Inventory	US	C	18 parallel items Photos, Camera, GPS, Spyware (7) Excessive communication (4) Threats (3) Control behaviors (4) Response format: 0 (*never*) - 4 (*4 or more times*) It includes reviews of the appropriateness of these behaviors.	EFA Content and face validity established by expert researchers in the field. α = .90 for the total scale.	Perpetration Victimization Opinion on the appropriateness of these behaviors	*N* = 804 (67.1% females) Age range = 18–23 years

(Continued)

TABLE 10.1 (Cont.)

Authors	*Measure name*	*Country*	*Type*	*Items/Dimensions & Response format*	*Psychometric Evidence*	*Facet of CARR*	*Sample*
Carlson et al. (2015)	Use of Technology in Relationships	US	A	5 items adapted by Schnurr, Mahatmya, and Basche (2013) from Draucker and Martsolf (2010) Question (Has partner used technology to …) 1. Embarrass you? 2. Make you feel bad? 3. Control you? 4. Monitor you? 5. Argue with you? Response format: "yes" (1) or "no" (0)	α = .54	Victimization	*N* = 138 university students (87% female) Age range = 18–25 years.
Celis-Sauce, & Rojas-Solís (2015)	Ciber-violencia en el Noviazgo [Cyberviolence in Dating]	Mexico	A	4 parallel items that assess psychological aggressions such as control, monitoring, and surveillance. Response format: 5-point Likert scale: 1 (never) – 5 (very often).	α = .74 & .43 for perpetration and victimization, respectively.	Victimization Perpetration	*N* = 149 who had had a romantic relationship for at least one month (100% male). Age range = 15–22 years.

Chaulk, & Jones (2011)	Online Obsessive Relational Intrusion	Canada	B	12 items adapted from the tactics proposed by Spitzberg & Cupach (2003). Items are focused on behaviors that take place on Facebook. 3 dimensions: Benevolent behavior (2) Potentially harmful (7) Dangerous (3) Response format: 1 (*only once*) – 4 (*more than five times*)	Victimization Perpetration	*N* = 230 Age range = 18–25 years.
Dank et al. (2014)	Cyber Dating Abuse	US	B	16 items adapted from Picard (2007) and 10 from Griezel (2007). Items assess cyber dating abuse by current or most recent partner. Response options: 0 (*never*) – 3 (*very often*).	Victimization Perpetration	*N* = 3,745 youth (52.3% women) Age range = 12–19 years
Darvell, Walsh, & White (2011)	Facebook Partner-Monitoring	Australia	A	One item describing the use of Facebook to monitor a partner's activities at least 3 times a week. Dimensions: Intention Attitude Subjective norm Perceived behavioral control	Perpetration	*N* = 244 Facebook users (78% female) Age range = 18–47 years

(Continued)

TABLE 10.1 (Cont.)

Authors	*Measure name*	*Country*	*Type*	*Items/Dimensions & Response format*	*Psychometric Evidence*	*Facet of CARR*	*Sample*
Dick et al. (2014)	Cyber Dating Abuse	US	A	7 items modified from Ybarra, Espelage, & Mitchell (2007) and Bennett et al., (2011). It includes two categories of items: sexual cyber dating abuse and nonsexual cyber dating abuse. Response format: 5 response options referring to the last three months.	EFA α = .72	Victimization	*N* = 1062 youth seeking health services (76% female) Age range = 14–19 years.
Domínguez-Mora et al. (2016)	Victimización en Redes Sociales [Victimization in Social Networks]	Mexico	A	6 items that include control behaviors Response format: 1 (never) - 4 (6 or more times).	α = .90.	Victimization	*N* = 1663 (54% female), Age range = 12–17 years
Duran, & Martínez-Pecino (2015)	Escalas de Ciberacoso contra la Pareja a través del Teléfono Móvil y de Internet [Cyber Harassment of the Partner via Cell Phone and the Internet Scales]	Spain	C	It is an adaptation to romantic relationships of the Victimization Scales (Buelga, Cava, & Musitu, 2010). Two dimensions: Cyber harassment using cell phones, Cyber harassment over the Internet Response format: 1 (*never*) – 4 (*many times*)	α = .75 for each of the perpetration scales. α = .62 - .70 for the victimization scales	Perpetration Victimization	*N* = 336 University students Age range = 18–30 years

Finn (2004)	E-mail and Instant Messa-ging Harassment	US	A	One item that describes receiving insults, threats, harassments or inappropriate materials, such as pornography, through email or instant messaging. Response format: 4 point response scale: : 1 (*never*) – 4 (*more than 5 times*)		Victimization	N = 339 (64.9% female) Mean age = 20.34 years
Fox, & Warber (2013)	Interpersonal Electronic Surveillance for Social Networking Sites via Facebook	US	A	13 items adapted from Tokunaga's questionnaire (2011) to measure partner monitoring via Face-book. Response format: 5-point Likert scale: 1 (*strongly disagree*) – 5 (*strongly agree*)	α = .96.	Perpetration	N = 328; Age range = 18–48 years
Fox et al. (2014)	Experiences of victimization	UK	D	1 item within a broader survey Think about people you have dated, and past or current boy-friends or girlfriends. Have they ever checked up on whom you have phoned or sent messages to?		Victimization perpetration	N = 1143 (50% female) Age range = 13–14 years

(*Continued*)

TABLE 10.1 (Cont.)

Authors	*Measure name*	*Country*	*Type*	*Items/Dimensions & Response format*	*Psychometric Evidence*	*Facet of CARR*	*Sample*
Jaen-Cortés et al. (2017)	Escala de Violencia de Pareja que se Expresa a través de Medios Electrónicos [Partner Violence through Electronic Tools]	Mexico	C	32 items 5 dimensions Control, intrusive monitoring and cyber surveillance (10) Verbal aggression (11) Sexual aggression (5) Sexual coercion (3) Humiliation (3) Response format: 1 (*never*) – 4 (*always*).	EFA α = .94 for the total scale α = .78 -.93 for subscales	Victimization	*N* = 878 adolescents, (47% female) Age range = 12–19 years
Korchmaros et al. (2013)	Computer-Mediated Communication-based Teen Dating Violence	US	B	4 items from Victimization in Dating Relationships Scales (Foshee, 1996) adapted to ask whether these behaviors had taken place online or by text message. 3 dimensions: Control (2) Jealousy (1) Degradation (1) Response format: 0 (*never*) – 3 (*10 or more times*).		Perpetration	*N* = 615 (50% female) Age range = 14–19

Leisring, & Giumetti (2014)	The Cyber Psychological Abuse Scale	US	C	18 parallel items 2 dimensions: minor and severe abuse Response options = 0 (*never*) – 6 (*more than 20 times*).	EFA, CFA α = .81 - .82 for the total scales. α values close to or greater than .70 for the minor and severe victimization and perpetration scales	Victimization Perpetration	*N* = 271 undergraduate students (79% female). Mean age = 19.03 years
Lyndon et al. (2011)	Facebook Survey	US	C	13 items that assess the frequency with which participants used Facebook to communicate with, monitor or harass their ex-romantic partners Covert Provocation (5) Public Harassment (5) Venting (3) Response format: four-point Likert scale: 0 (*never*) – 3 (*all of the time*)	EFA α = .79 - .88	Perpetration	*N* = 411 (64% female). Age range = 18–32 years.

(Continued)

TABLE 10.1 (Cont.)

Authors	*Measure name*	*Country*	*Type*	*Items/Dimensions & Response format*	*Psychometric Evidence*	*Facet of CARR*	*Sample*
Marcum Higgins, & Nicholson (2017)	Cyberstalking	US	A	1 item, asking whether the individual attempted to login to his/her significant other's social networking account without their knowledge. Response format: 1 (Never) – 5 (all of the time)		Perpetration	*N* = 890 undergraduate and graduate students (28% female) >18 years
Morelli et al. (2018)	The Cyber Dating Violence Inventory	Italy	C	22 parallel items adapted from items of the CADRI (Wolfe et al., 2001). 2 dimensions: Psychological cyber dating violence Relational cyber dating violence Response format: 0 (*never*) – 3 (*6 times or more*).	EFA y CFA α = .81 - .82 for the perpetration scales α = .82 for the two victimization scales	Victimization Perpetration	*N* = 1405 (65% female) Mean age = 18.17 years
Muñiz (2017)	Teen Dating Violence in Social Networks Scale	Spain	C	10 items that assess violent behaviors exhibited toward the partner and former partner over the Internet. 2 dimensions: Violent actions Controlling actions Response format: 1 (never) – 4 (always)	EFA, CFA α = .80 - .86	Victimization Perpetration	*N* = 919 (52% female) Mean age = 16.12 years

Pereira et al. (2016)	Cyber-harassment Assessment Scale	Portugal	A	18 items adapted mostly from a previous measure developed by Spitzberg and Hoobler (2002). Participants have to indicate who was the cyberaggressor (i.e., friends, intimate partners, known [e.g., relatives, neighbors] and unknown people). Response format: 0 (*Never*) – 5 (*five or more times*)	α = .90 for both victimization and perpetration	Victimization Perpetration	*N* = 627 adolescents (54.9% females). Age range = 12–16 years
Powell, & Henry (2016)	Technology-Facilitated Sexual Violence Victimization Scale	Australia	B	21 items Includes potential perpetrators other than the partner. 4 dimensions Digital sexual harassment, Image-based sexual abuse, Sexual aggression and/or coercion, Gender and/or sexuality-based hate speech	α = .93	Victimization	*N* = 2,956 (50.1% female). Age range = 18–54 years

(Continued)

TABLE 10.1 (Cont.)

Authors	*Measure name*	*Country*	*Type*	*Items/Dimensions & Response format*	*Psychometric Evidence*	*Facet of CARR*	*Sample*
Reed et al. (2016)	Digital Dating Abuse Measure	US	A	19 parallel items that assess abuse, which implies a pattern of behavior that controls, pressures, harasses, threatens or otherwise harms a dating partner, by means of cell phones, computers and Internet communications. Response format: Yes/no In case of yes, frequency was indicated from 0 (*0 times*) – 4 (*More than 5 times*)	α = .76 and .73 for victimization and perpetration, respectively	Victimization Perpetration	*N* = 321 Age range = 17–22 years
Sánchez et al. (2015)	Cyberdating Q A	Spain	D	6 dimensions, 2 of which are related with cyber dating abuse: Online Control (6 items) Online Intrusive Behaviors (4 items)	EFA and CFA α = .84 - ,85 In an Italian sample (Sánchez, Muñoz, Nocentini, Ortega-Ruiz, & Menesini, 2014): α = .72	Perpetration	*N* = 458 adolescents and young adults (46.9% female) Age range = 12–21 years
Schnurr et al. (2013)	Cyber Aggression Perpetration	US	A	5 items adapted from Draucker & Martsolf (2010) Response format: 1 (yes) or 0 (no)	α =.76 and .71 for male and female, respectively	Perpetration measured by opposite sex's report of victimization.	*N* = 148 couples Mean age = 20.17 years

Shorey et al. (2015)	Stalking in Intimate Relationships	US	D	6 items of cyberstalking in a general measure of stalking in intimate relationships. Response format: 0 (*never*) – 6 (*more than twenty times*). In the previous 6 months	α = .65 (perpetration) and .63 (victimization).	Perpetration Victimization	N = 650 (78% female). Mean age = 18.97 years
Spitzberg, & Hoobler (2002)	Cyber Obsessional Pursuit Scale	US	C	24 items regarding the frequency with which the partner has exhibited pursuit behaviors. 3 dimensions: Hyperintimacy RL-transference Threat	EFA α = .77 - .88	Victimization	N = 235 college students (55% female) Age range = 20–64 years.
Temple et al. (2016)	Cyber Abuse	US	A	13 parallel items modified and adapted from previous studies (Zweig et al. 2013; Picard 2007): Response format: Yes/no In the past year	α = .65 -.67 for perpetration α = .74 - .79 for victimization	Victimization Perpetration	N = 780 diverse group of adolescents (58 % female), Mean age = 18.09 years
Tokunaga (2011) Used and modified by Fox and Warber (2013)	Interpersonal Electronic Surveillance for Social Networking Sites	US	A	12 items describing surveillance and control behaviors on social networking sites. Response format: 7-point Likert scale	EFA and CFA α = . 97	Perpetration	N = 126 (72.2% female) Age range = 18–56.

(*Continued*)

TABLE 10.1 (Cont.)

Authors	*Measure name*	*Country*	*Type*	*Items/Dimensions & Response format*	*Psychometric Evidence*	*Facet of CARR*	*Sample*
Van Ouytsel et al. (2016)	Victimization of Digital Controlling Behaviors	Belgium	A	4 items from the Cyber Dating Abuse Questionnaire (Borrajo et al., 2015) Response format: 1 (Never) - 5 (very often)		Victimization	*N* = 466 (71.0% female). Age range = 16–22
Wolford-Clevenger et al. (2016)	The Partner Cyber Abuse Questionnaire	US	A	9 items from Hamby (2013), including harassment, monitoring, humiliation, and verbal abuse via technology, such as cell phones, social media or electronic mail, perpetrated by a current partner. Response format: 0 (*never*) - 5 (*five or more times*).	EFA α = .72	Victimization	*N* = 502 undergraduate students (65.7% female) Mean age = 18.80 years
Wright (2015)	Partner Direct Cyber-Aggression	US	C	5 items adapted from a measure on face-to-face relational aggression occurring within romantic relationships (Linder, Crick, & Collins, 2002). 2 dimensions: Cyber relational aggression (3) Privacy invasion (2) Response format: 1 (*Never*) - 5 (*All the time*)	CFA α = .82 -.91	Perpetration	*N* = 600 (54% female) Mean age = 17.53 years

Zweig et al. (2013)	Cyber Dating Abuse *Used in Spanish by Sanchez et al. 2017	US	C	16 parallel items 2 dimensions Sexual cyber abuse (4) Non-sexual cyber abuse (12) Response format: 0 (never) – 3 (very often). In the past year	α = .81 -.88 for perpetration α = .89 -.92 for victimization	Victimization Perpetration	N = 3,745 7th to 12th grade youth (52 % female)

Note: Type: A = Unidimensional, B = Unidimensional with various categories, C = Multidimensional, D = items of CDA within a broader measure, EFA= Exploratory factor analysis, CFA = Confirmatory Factor Analysis.

which was created in Spanish, have been used in Belgium (Van Ouytsel, Ponnet, & Walrave, 2016). Finally, the Cyber-harassment Assessment Scale was developed in Portuguese (Pereira, Spitzberg, & Matos, 2016), mainly from items on a previous measure developed by Spitzberg and Hoobler (2002) in a study of cyberstalking in the US. This relative lack of common measures makes cross-country comparisons difficult and serves as a major constraint on current CARR research.

As seen in Table 10.1, the nature of the measures is very diverse. Nineteen measures are unidimensional. In other words, they allow a single CARR score to be obtained, although, in five of them, the authors describe several categories of CARR within the single dimension (Barter et al., 2017; Chaulk & Jones, 2011; Dank, Lachman, Zweig, & Yahner, 2014; Korchmaros, Ybarra, Langhinrichsen-Rohling, Boyd, & Lenhart, 2013; Powell & Henry, 2016). Twelve measures (34%) include multiple dimensions, with the number of dimensions ranging from two to five. Some measures are not specific to abuse by a romantic partner (Finn, 2004; Pereira et al., 2016; Powell & Henry, 2016), but rather to general online abuse, and participants must indicate the source of the abuse (e.g., romantic partner, unknown, etc.). Some of the measures consist of one or more items, or even subscales, of CARR within a larger survey (e.g., Bennett, Guran, Ramos, & Margolin, 2011; Fox, Corr, Gadd, & Butler, 2014; Sánchez et al., 2015; Shorey, Cornelius, & Strauss, 2015). Finally, regarding the age of the participants for whom the questionnaire was developed, 18 were created for young adults, 12 for adolescents, and 5 for both adolescents and adults.

Whereas some scales include items specifically created to evaluate forms of CARR (e.g., Borrajo, Gámez-Guadix, Pereda, & Calvete, 2015; Burke, Wallen, Vail-Smith, & Knox, 2011), others tailor measures of traditional dating violence to CARR. Thus, Morelli, Bianchi, Chirumbolo, and Baiocco (2018) developed the Cyber Dating Violence Inventory from items of the Conflict in Adolescent Dating Relationships Inventory (CADRI; Wolfe et al., 2001). Likewise, Leisring and Giumetti (2014) developed the Cyber Psychological Abuse Scale from items of the psychological aggression subscale from the revised Conflict Tactics Scale (CTS2; Straus, Hamby, Boney McCoy, & Sugarman, 1996) and the Psychological Maltreatment of Women Inventory (Tolman, 1999). Finally, some measures use items adapted from questionnaires of cyberbullying or general cyber-harassment (Durán & Martínez-Pecino, 2015).

Regarding the psychometric characteristics of the questionnaires, most of them (82.9%) use a frequency response format for the items, which ranges from never to a large number of occasions (e.g., very often, 10 or more times), usually referring to the last year. Some measures use a yes/no response format (Carlson, Fripp, Cook, & Kelchner, 2015; Powell & Henry, 2016; Schnurr, Mahatmya, & Basche, 2013; Temple et al., 2016). A yes/no response format can be a limitation, because it does not allow occasional abuse to be differentiated from reiterative abuse. Finally, a few measures employ different response formats, such as the degree of agreement with the items (Fox & Warber, 2014).

Most measures provide data on the internal consistency, with Cronbach's alpha generally ranging from 0.70 to 0.97 (see exceptions in Carlson et al., 2015; Celis-Sauce, & Rojas-Solís, 2015; Shorey et al., 2015; Temple et al., 2016). In two of the measures displaying low internal consistency, the reason is probably due to the use of a dichotomous response system (yes/no; Carlson et al., 2015; Temple et al., 2016). Information about other psychometric properties is scarcer. For instance, only 37% of the measurements contribute data regarding the factor structure through exploratory and/or confirmatory factor analysis. In particular, evidence of factor analysis is provided for three of the 19 one-dimension measures and in nine of the 12 multidimensional measures. Finally, several measures provide other data concerning the validity of the measure, such as content and face validity established by expert researchers in the field (Burke et al., 2011; Jaen-Cortés et al., 2017).

One of the most relevant aspects is whether the facets of victimization and perpetration of violence are assessed. As discussed later in this chapter, there is an important reciprocity between the victimization and the perpetration of CARR, as is the case with offline forms of partner abuse (Fernández-González, Calvete, & Orue, 2017). It is, therefore, important to include both aspects in the CARR measures. Nonetheless, as shown in Table 10.1, 12 measures assess victimization, 14 assess perpetration, and only nine (25.71%) evaluate both victimization and perpetration. When the information concerning the dimensionality of the measure is combined with that of the facets of victimization and perpetration, six of the 20 unidimensional measures (30%) and six of the 12 multidimensional measures (50%) include both facets of CARR. By country, seven out of 20 (35%) of the measures developed in the US, five out of the nine developed in Europe (55.6%), and one out of the three developed in Mexico include both victimization and perpetration.

An analysis of the dimensions included indicates that, in most cases, dimensions are created according to thematic content or modalities of abuse. Moreover, some dimensions are very common and appear in many of the CARR questionnaires. In this chapter, we propose a classification of the main modalities of CARR. To obtain this classification, the content of all the questionnaires included in Table 10.1 was assessed, both at the item level and the scale level. The result is a classification consisting of five main modalities (four psychological and one sexual), which are described below.

The first modality refers to *direct verbal aggressions* in the form of phone calls or texts that seek to either denigrate or threaten the victim (e.g., Bennett et al., 2011; Borrajo, Gámez-Guadix, Pereda, & Calvete, 2015; Burke et al., 2011; Jaen-Cortés et al., 2017; Morelli et al., 2018; Muñiz, 2017; Spitzberg & Hoobler, 2002). It is a category that clearly has its equivalent in face-to-face violence and is included in most questionnaires on offline psychological intimate partner violence (e.g., Straus et al., 1996; Wolfe et al., 2001).

The second modality consists of *control/monitoring* through the technologies. This modality includes behaviors of monitoring and constantly checking the partner's behavior via the Internet. It also includes controlling the behavior of the partner on social networks, determining, for example, with whom the partner can or cannot associate. Within this category is also the use of the identity and password of the partner, often through usurpation, in order to be able to control what he/she does and with whom he/she associates. The control/monitoring modality appears in most of the questionnaires on CARR (e.g., Borrajo, Gámez-Guadix, Pereda, & Calvete, 2015; Jaen-Cortés et al., 2017; Sánchez et al., 2015; Tokunaga, 2011). In a qualitative study conducted with Mexican adolescents, almost all the participants knew the password of their partners and admitted to checking their partners' accounts without their partners knowing it. Moreover, most indicated that their partners had given them the password as a sign of trust or for sending or handling information (Alvarado-Bravo, Salinas, Heras, & Santana, 2015). Thus, sharing the password could represent in some cultures a symbol of trust in the partner.

Finally, within the control/monitoring modality, some questionnaires include more sophisticated behaviors of monitoring and surveillance, such as the use of hidden webcams or spyware to monitor a partner's behavior (Burke et al., 2011). The control of the partner is a form of abuse that also has its parallel in offline abuse, for example through behaviors such as preventing the victims from associating with their friends or family, or deciding what the victims can or cannot do (e.g., Calvete, Corral, & Estevez, 2005; Wolfe et al., 2001). Nevertheless, the manifestation of this type of abuse over the Internet gives it its own characteristics, and can contribute to an even greater extent to controlling the victim's social life.

Closely related to the previous modality, the third modality consists of *relational abuse*, which aims to exclude the victim (e.g., terminate or block electronic communication, remove the victim from a top friend list) and publicly humiliate the victim over the Internet (e.g., posting publicly texts and/or images of the victim that may be humiliating or embarrassing). The latter type of behavior is reflected in many of the CARR questionnaires (e.g., Bennett et al., 2011; Borrajo, Gámez-Guadix, Pereda, & Calvete, 2015; Jaen-Cortés et al., 2017; Leisring & Giumetti 2014; Celis-Sauce & Rojas-Solís, 2015; Zweig et al., 2013). Public humiliation of the victim is a form of abuse that also takes place in offline abuse, but the Internet can make this type of abuse even more harmful by spreading the texts and images quickly, in a way in which they sometimes become viral over the Internet.

A fourth modality of CARR, which is included in only a few measures, is *excessive communication*. This modality is described in some questionnaires as intrusive online behaviors (Sánchez et al., 2015) and excessive communication (Burke et al., 2011). It includes behaviors such as excessive cell phone calls or texts. This excessive communication can be perceived in a very threatening and invasive way on the part of the victim, especially when there has been a previous conflict with the partner or when it is the ex-partner who engages in these behaviors.

In addition to the modalities of cyber psychological abuse described above, CARR may also consist of forms of cyber sexual abuse. Cyber sexual abuse includes behaviors such as sending texts or images of a sexual nature (when the perpetrator knows that the victim does not want to receive them), publishing photos in which the victim appears naked or exhibiting positions or behaviors of a sexual nature, and pressuring or even threatening the victim to get him or her to send sexual or naked photos of him/herself to the perpetrator (Jaen-Cortés et al., 2017; Zweig et al., 2013). This is an important category that is absent in many of the questionnaires. However, this category has a relevant role in the questionnaire of Zweig et al. (2013), in which the behaviors are classified according to their sexual vs. nonsexual nature, and in the questionnaire of Powell and Henry (2016), which is specific to technology-facilitated sexual violence.

Although most of the questionnaires that include several dimensions base their classification on the type of abuse (e.g., direct verbal aggressions, control/monitoring), the criterion is different in a few cases. Thus, Leisring and Giumetti (2014) employed two dimensions of CARR, based on the severity of the abuse: minor, which includes behaviors such as insulting and abruptly stopping e-mailing, instant messaging, or text messaging during a disagreement, and severe, including behaviors such as threatening and posting inappropriate pictures or embarrassing information online to humiliate the victim. Thus, this questionnaire uses the same criteria as used in the CTS scales (Straus et al., 1996), by which it is partially inspired. This distinction between minor and severe forms of cyber abuse can help to detect those cases in which abuse is particularly problematic. Finally, the questionnaire developed by Durán and Martínez-Pecino (2015) bases its two dimensions on the tool (mobile phone vs. Internet) employed to perpetuate the abuse.

Prevalence and Sex Differences in Cyber Abuse in Romantic Relationships

The diversity of instruments created to measure the CARR phenomenon as well as the age difference amongst the samples used in the different studies could explain the great variability in the data in the incidence of this phenomenon. The 35 studies reviewed showing prevalence data are the same that had been presented in Table 10.1.Table 10.2 displays the prevalence obtained in terms of CARR perpetration and victimization. Studies conducted in Europe show victimization rates of between 2.5% and 75%, whereas perpetration rates are between 1.8% and 83.5% (e.g., Barter et al., 2017; Borrajo, Gámez-Guadix, Pereda, & Calvete, 2015; Van Ouytsel et al., 2016). In the US, between 5.1% and 93% of the respondents have been victims of CARR, and between 2.7% and 93.7% have committed some of these behaviors (e.g., Kellerman, Margolin, Borofsky, Baucom, & Iturralde, 2013; Leisring & Giumetti, 2014; Peskin et al., 2017). It should be noted that only the study by Dank et al. (2014) in the US offers data on the incidence of this phenomenon in the LGTBI (lesbian, gay, transgender,

TABLE 10.2 Prevalence and Sex Differences

Authors (Year)	*Measure Name*	*Country*	*Prevalence*
Barter et al. (2017)	Online Interpersonal Violence and Abuse	Bulgaria, Cyprus, England, Italy, Norway	Victimization: Total (40%) Controlling behavior (23–31% W; 9–36% M) Surveillance (25–38% W; 10–30% M)
Bennett et al. (2011)	Electronic Victimization Cyber Dating Abuse Questionnaire	US	Victimization: Electronic hostility (56.4% W; 60.2% M), Electronic intrusiveness (56.4% W; 66.1% M), Electronic humiliation (36.6% W; 48.3% M), Electronic exclusion (17.7% W; 34.7% M)
Borrajo, Gámez-Guadix, Pereda, & Calvete (2015)	Electronic Victimization Cyber Dating Abuse Questionnaire	Spain	Perpetration: Control (82%), Direct aggression (10.6%) Victimization: Control (75%), Direct aggression (14%)
Burke et al. (2011)	Controlling Partner Inventory	US	Victimization: Monitoring call history (63% W; 48% M) Perpetration: Monitoring Facebook profile (58% W; 41% M)
Carlson et al. (2015)	Use of Technology in Relationships	US	Victimization: Control (5.1%), Monitoring (28.3%), Argue (44.9%)
Chaulk & Jones (2011)	Online Obsessive Relational Intrusion	Canada	Using Facebook profile to obtain information about the partner (52% Perpetration; 19% Victimization) Reading the partner's wall conversations (posts and replies; 60% Perpetration; 13% Victimization)
Cutbush, Ashley, Kan, Hampton, & Hall (2010)	Electronic Dating Aggression	US	Perpetration: 29.4% Victimization: 56% (higher in women) Insults and hurtful words (35.5% victimization; 20.4% perpetration) Calls, emails, text messages to make the partner / ex-partner angry (31.4% victimization, 14.1% perpetration)
Cutbush et al. (2012)	Electronic Dating Aggression	US	Perpetration: 18.4% Victimization: 31.5%
Dank et al. (2014)	Cyber Dating Abuse	US	Victimization and perpetration: LGTB (37.2%); Heterosexual (25.7%)

(Continued)

TABLE 10.2 (Cont.)

Authors (Year)	*Measure Name*	*Country*	*Prevalence*
Dick et al. (2014)	Cyber Dating Abuse	US	Victimization: Total (41.4%), Sexual cyber dating abuse (13%), and Non-sexual cyber dating abuse (37%) More female than male respondents reported nonsexual cyber dating abuse (40% W vs. 29% M)
Domínguez-Mora et al. (2016)	Victimización en Redes Sociales [Victimization in Social Networks]	México	Women scored higher on victimization
Donoso-Vázquez et al. (2018)	Cuestionario de violencias de género 2.0 [Gender Violence Questionnaire 2.0]	Spain	Perpetration: Have controlled the partner on Facebook (26.2%) Know the partner's password to block friendships in social networks (17.4%) Monitor where the partner is by cell phone (7.7%) Take the partner's mobile phone to inspect it (6.5%) Force the partner to remove photos from Facebook or to stop connecting with someone (5.8%) Girls scored higher than boys in control behaviors (5.97% W; 5.61% M)
Durán & Martínez-Pecino (2015)	Escala de Ciberacoso con la Pareja a través del Teléfono Móvil y de Internet [Cyber Harassment of the Partner via Cell Phone and the Internet Scales]	Spain	Victimization: Mobile phone (57.2%); Internet (27.4%) Perpetration: Mobile phone (47.6%); Internet (14%) Men scored higher in victimization and perpetration
Hinduja & Patchin (2011)	Electronic Dating Violence	US	Victimization: 12% Perpetration: 7%
Jaen-Cortés et al. (2017)	Escala de Violencia de Pareja que se Expresa a través de Medios Electrónicos [Partner Violence through Electronic Tools]	México	Victimization: Control, intrusive monitoring and cyber surveillance (44.3%); Verbal aggression (15.5%); Sexual assault (11.9%); Sexual coercion (7.7%), and humiliation (6.1%) Men have higher rates of violence as compared to women
Kellerman et al. (2013)	Electronic Aggresion	US	Victimization Perpetration (71.7%) No significant sex differences

(Continued)

TABLE 10.2 (Cont.)

Authors (Year)	*Measure Name*	*Country*	*Prevalence*
Korchmaros et al. (2013)	Computer-Mediated Communication-based Teen Dating Violence	US	Perpetration: Internet (13.2%) Instant messaging (37.6%)
Leisring & Giumetti (2014)	The Cyber Psychological Abuse Scale	US	Victimization: Minor cyber abuse (93%); Severe cyber abuse (12.6%) Perpetration: Minor cyber abuse (93.7%); Severe cyber abuse (13.3%) Men presented higher rate of severe aggressions
Lyndon et al. (2011)	Facebook Survey	US	Perpetration: Covert provocation (67.3%); Public harassment (18%); Venting (18%)
Lucio-López, & Prieto-Quezada (2014)	Not provided	México	Perpetration: Try to gain access to their partner's social network account (42.7%); Has been posing as a friend to test the partner (39.5%)
Martinez-Lanz et al. (2016)	Partner Violence on Social Media	México	Victimization: Low level of partner violence on social media (59.9% M; 70.1% W); high level (37.4% M; 25.2% W) and severe level (2.7% M; 4.7% W).
Martin Montilla et al. (2016)	Not provided	Spain	Use of email to harass (1.8% Perpetration; 2.5% Victimization); Usurpation of email addresses of their partners (7.1% Perpetration; 11% Victimization); Sending smear messages (12% Perpetration; 15.4% Victimization); Sending threatening messages (6.2% Perpetration; 11.2% Victimization)
Melander (2010)	Cyber Aggression	US	Victimization: 75% (Men presented higher prevalence on reviewing online accounts and posting negative information without permission) Perpetration: 71% (Women presented higher prevalence in control behaviors)
Peskin et al. (2017)	Cyber Dating Abuse (Adapted from Zweig et al., 2013)	US	Perpetration: 15% No sex differences
Pereira et al. (2016)	Cyber Harassment Assessment Scale	Portugal	Double involvement as both cyber-victim and cyber-aggressor (66.1%) By intimate partners (2.9%)

(Continued)

TABLE 10.2 (Cont.)

Authors (Year)	*Measure Name*	*Country*	*Prevalence*
Powell & Henry (2016)	Technology-Facilitated Sexual Violence Victimization Scale	Australia	Victimization: Accessed their emails and online accounts without permission (16%) Checked up on them multiple times a day to find out where they were, who they were with or what they were doing (23.3%)
Reed et al. (2016)	Digital Dating Abuse Measure	US	Victimization: 74.1% Perpetration: 69.5% No significant differences in total scores Men: Higher scores on threatening to distribute embarrassing information about their partner using the Internet or mobile phone and pressure the partner to take naked photos or videos
Sánchez et al. (2015)	Cyberdating QA	Spain	Perpetration: Online control (83.5%), online jealousy (86.9%), online intrusive behavior (75.3%), online intimacy (97.7%), emotional communication strategies (97.1%) and cyberdating practices (93.7%) Men: Higher scores on intrusive behavior and cyberdating practices
Sánchez et al. (2014)	Cyberdating QA	Spain, Italy	Perpetration of intrusiveness: (54.2% Spain; 48.5% Italy)
Shorey et al. (2015)	Stalking in Intimate Relationships	US	Perpetration: Calling the partner when he/she didn't want you to (34.8 %) Attempting to obtain information about the partner without his/her knowledge (34.9 %) Monitor partner's behavior and/or activities by checking his/her social networking sites (38.2 %). Similar prevalence rates were found for victimization
Temple et al. (2016)	Cyber Abuse	US	Victimization: 24.01% Perpetration: 12.22%
Tompson, Benz, & Agiesta (2013)	Digital Dating Abuse	US	Victimization: Total (40%) Control the partner to know where he/she is and with whom (22%) Read messages without permission (21%)
Van Ouytsel et al. (2016)	Victimization of Digital Controlling Behaviors	Belgium	65.0% of respondents had experienced at least one of the four controlling behaviors

(Continued)

TABLE 10.2 (Cont.)

Authors (Year)	*Measure Name*	*Country*	*Prevalence*
Wolford-Clevenger et al., (2016)	The Partner Cyber Abuse Questionnaire	US	Perpetration: Sending angry or insulting text messages to the partner (30.6%) Victimization: Their partner checked the email or text messages without their permission (20.4%) No sex differences
Zweig et al. (2013)	Cyber Dating Abuse *Used in Spanish by Sánchez et al. (2017)	US	Victimization: Total (26.3%); Sexual cyber abuse (11.2%); Non-sexual cyber abuse (22.2%). Girls scored higher Perpetration: Total (11.8%); Sexual cyber abuse (2.7%); Non-sexual cyber abuse (10.5%). Girls scored higher on non-sexual. Boys scored higher on sexual cyber abuse

Note: W = Women; M = Men.

bisexual, and intersexual) group (37.2%), comparing it to the heterosexual group (25.7%). Therefore, this would be an important aspect to examine in future research on CARR.

The prevalence rates of behaviors related to *direct verbal aggressions*, such as the sending of threatening or harmful messages or the publication of information with the intention of humiliating or damaging the partner, show great variability. For example, the prevalence of perpetration and victimization harassment ranges from 1.8% (Martin Montilla, Pazos Gomez, Montilla Coronado, & Romero Oliva, 2016) to 18% (Lyndon, Bonds-Raacke, & Cratty, 2011). The victimization by means of these behaviors ranges between 2.5% (Martin Montilla et al., 2016) and 56.4% (Bennett et al., 2011; electronic hostility dimension). The behaviors related to the *control/monitoring* dimension of the partner present prevalence rates of between 1.8% (Wolford-Clevenger et al., 2016) and 75% (Borrajo, Gámez-Guadix, Pereda, & Calvete, 2015) for victimization, and between 3.2% (Donoso Vázquez, Rubio Hurtado, & Vilà Baños, 2018) and 83.5% (Sánchez et al., 2015) for perpetration. Interestingly, the rates of victimization for control/monitoring seem to be higher in Spain and Mexico (e.g., 80%, Borrajo, Gámez-Guadix, Pereda, & Calvete, 2015; and 60%, Lucio-López & Prieto-Quezada, 2014) as compared to other European countries or the US, where they do not exceed 50% (Burke et al., 2011).

Although data on the prevalence of other modalities of CARR are scarce compared to the previous two, the available data suggest that the incidence of *relational abuse* victimization ranges from 10% (Hinduja & Patchin, 2011) to 34.7% (Bennett et al., 2011; electronic exclusion dimension), and that *excessive communication* can be very frequent in Spain, reaching 80% (Sánchez et al., 2015). Finally, the prevalence of sexual cyber-abuse victimization ranges between 2% (Melander, 2010) and 13% (Dick et al., 2014), and the prevalence of perpetration is about 2% (see Zweig et al., 2013).

An important aspect that has been examined in a large number of studies is sex differences in CARR. Five of the 19 studies that provide data on sex differences in CARR have found no significant differences in either victimization or perpetration (Kellerman et al., 2013; Peskin et al., 2017; Reed, Tolman, & Ward, 2016). However, the vast majority have found differences between men and women. Regarding victimization, the results are mixed, since some research has found that it is boys who present higher scores, especially in studies conducted in the US (e.g., Barter et al., 2017; Bennett et al., 2011) and Mexico (Jaen-Cortés et al., 2014). In contrast, other studies conducted in Mexico and Europe indicate that girls score higher than boys (e.g., Domínguez-Mora, Vargas-Jiménez, Castro-Castañeda, & Nuñez-Fadda, 2016; Durán & Martínez-Pecino, 2015).

Regarding sex differences in perpetration, fewer studies have found differences. For instance, one study conducted in Spain (Durán & Martínez-Pecino, 2015) and one in the US (Zweig et al., 2013) found that girls presented higher scores. In this latter study, the exception was sexual cyber abuse, in which men scored higher. Therefore, there are no conclusive results regarding sex differences in CARR.

Reciprocity of Cyber Abuse in Romantic Relationships

Numerous studies have shown a relationship between victimization and the perpetration of offline aggression in dating relationships (Capaldi, Kim, & Shortt, 2007; Fernández-González et al., 2017). The empirical evidence regarding the reciprocity of CARR is scarcer, although available data show that this reciprocity also exists online. In most instances, the magnitude of the relationship between victimization and perpetration has been high according to the criteria of Cohen (1992), who suggested that correlations of 0.10, 0.30, and 0.50 are considered small, medium, and large, respectively. Given the high correlations, further information regarding discriminant validity between perpetration and victimization is needed, which could be assessed through the use of CFA (comparing an unconstrained model and a constrained model) or analyzing the distinctive correlates for each one separately (see, for example, Shaffer, DeGeest, & Li, 2016). In a Mexican sample, Celis-Sauce and Rojas-Solís (2015) found a correlation of 0.76 between victimization and perpetration in CARR, using a measure consisting of control, monitoring, and surveillance in romantic relationships. In a Spanish sample of young people, Borrajo, Gámez-Guadix, Pereda, and Calvete (2015) reported that the correlation between perpetration and victimization was 0.67 for direct verbal aggressions that seek to either denigrate or threaten the victim and 0.69 for control/monitoring. Also in a Spanish sample, Durán and Martínez-Pecino (2015) found a relationship between victimization and perpetration both via Internet (.47) and via cell phone (.57), using a measure of cyber abuse focused on cyber harassment. In addition, it was found that, when victimization was low, there were no sex differences in the level of perpetration; however, when victimization was high, men tended to perpetrate more abusive behaviors against the partner than women did. According to Durán and Martínez-Pecino (2015), these results may indicate a different way of reacting to CARR between men and women: men would tend to carry out more cyber abuse behaviors in response to previous victimization, whereas women would tend to ignore victimization and not respond with more aggression (Durán & Martínez-Pecino, 2015).

The reciprocity of cyber abuse in dating relationships has been also documented in samples from the US. Leisring and Giumetti (2014) found a relationship of 0.90 for minor forms of psychological cyber abuse victimization and perpetration. An identical correlation was found for severe forms of psychological cyber abuse victimization and perpetration. However, relationships were weaker between minor and severe forms of cyber abuse: the relationship between minor perpetration and severe perpetration was 0.21, whereas the correlation between severe perpetration and minor victimization was 0.14. Similarly, in the study by Reed et al. (2016), associations between different indicators of perpetration and victimization (ever, past year, frequency) ranged from 0.62 to 0.73.

Longitudinal research on CARR is scarce. However, some longitudinal evidence exists for the reciprocity of cyber dating abuse. Temple et al. (2016) found that cyber perpetration predicted victimization over a year, whereas cyber victimization did not significantly predict perpetration over the following year when controlling for all demographic variables and previous traditional and cyber dating abuse.

Cultural factors could contribute to the reciprocity of cyber abuse. Attitudes that justify violence have been found to be important in offline dating violence (e.g., Ali, Swahn, & Hamburger, 2011), and may play an important role in cyber abuse in romantic relationships. The justification for violence has been found to be related to CARR (Borrajo, Gámez-Guadix, & Calvete, 2015a), although more cross-cultural research is needed. Moreover, adherence to traditional gender-role beliefs and stereotypes increases offline dating violence victimization and perpetration in different cultural contexts (Morelli, Bianchi, Baiocco, Pezzuti, & Chirumbolo, 2016; Shen, Chiu, & Gao, 2012). It is an empirical question whether traditional gender roles also increased the relationship between perpetration and victimization of CARR. Additional related variables, such as gender inequality or dominance, vary across cultural contexts (e.g., Straus, 2008, 2009) and could be associated with mutuality of cyber dating violence.

In addition, more specific cultural variables, such as *machismo* (i.e., the stereotype in Latin culture that associates masculinity with being strong and virile, showing emotional restraint, and assuming duty as the decision-maker), could also make aggression more likely in response to victimization. In this sense, as previously mentioned, it has been found in Spanish samples that, when cyber victimization is high, men are more likely than women to respond with online perpetration against the partner (Durán & Martínez-Pecino, 2015). It is reasonable to think that in a culture characterized by *machismo,* men might feel more empowered to assault women in response to aggression than vice versa. However, as mentioned above, research on cross-cultural influences in cyber dating abuse has been scarce and future studies should address this issue.

Findings of reciprocity between victimization and perpetration have implications for prevention. First, preventive efforts should focus on the factors favoring reciprocity between perpetration and victimization. In this sense, it is necessary that preventive programs provide strategies to learn how to handle specific situations that could facilitate the appearance of these behaviors. Jealousy or anger appear to be important precursors in the onset of online abuse (Borrajo, Gámez-Guadix, & Calvete, 2015b), so it is important to detect these situations and favor strategies to interpret and manage them optimally. Second, prevention programs should avoid labeling youth who perpetrate cyber abuse (e.g., "the abuser"). Given that perpetration and victimization are often reciprocal, the use of stigmatizing terms could be counterproductive (Borrajo, Gámez-Guadix, Pereda, & Calvete, 2015). Rather, from an educational perspective, we recommend identifying the inappropriate behaviors that need to be corrected. Third, it is necessary to promote protective factors that include self-esteem, empathy, assertiveness, and adequate conflict resolution strategies, which, in turn, will favor the prevention of perpetration and victimization.

Conclusions and Recommendations

From the above review, the following conclusions and recommendations can be derived.

Regarding the measurement of CARR, the review reveals several limitations in the available measures that provide excellent opportunities for new studies. First, not all the questionnaires developed to assess CARR provide data on psychometric properties such as internal consistency and the study of the dimensionality through exploratory and confirmatory factor analyses. However, these aspects are crucial to guarantee the validity and reliability of the findings obtained. Second, it is important to include facets of both victimization and perpetration, given the reciprocity between the two in dating violence. Third, there is a paucity of cross-validations of measures across different languages and cultures. This implies an important limitation to approaching cyber abuse in romantic relationships from an international perspective. Future research should adapt the same measures in multiple languages so that cross-cultural studies can be carried out. The comparison between countries would allow for a better identification of risk factors that can be universal and others that can be specific to some cultures. Fourth, very few measures include the sexual dimension of cyber dating abuse. This type of abuse should be assessed to capture a complete view of the forms that cyber abuse can adopt in romantic relationships. Finally, new technologies and the internet are changing and developing rapidly so the measures should adapt continuously. Accordingly, some of the questionnaires reviewed in this chapter differentiated between behaviors through the cell phone and over the Internet (Durán & Martínez-Pecino, 2015). However, this distinction does not make much sense, given that people currently access the Internet using cell phones. Moreover, some of the questionnaires reviewed are based on behaviors that took place in a Facebook context (e.g., Chaulk & Jones, 2011; Fox & Warber, 2014; Lyndon et al., 2011). However, there are currently other environments and Internet applications (e.g., WhatsApp, Instagram, etc.) that are widespread and in which abuse in romantic relationships is manifested. This requires a continuous effort to adapt the measures of cyber dating abuse to these new environments and forms of communication.

The current development of research on CARR also requires future methodological improvements. With very few exceptions (Temple et al., 2016), there is a striking scarcity of longitudinal studies. Longitudinal evidence is essential to continue advancing the knowledge about this problem. It would be useful, for example, to examine long-term consequences of different types of CARR victimization. In addition, much more research is required on aspects of criterion validity (e.g., predictive power). For example, it would be important to examine the extent to which CARR measures predict dyadic adjustment or breakups of the couple's relationship in the future. Finally, cross-cultural studies should be conducted to identify both universal and culturally specific factors (e.g., level of equality between men and women; traditional gender roles, etc.) associated with CARR. This would inform the design of interventions.

References

Ali, B., Swahn, M., & Hamburger, M. (2011). Attitudes affecting physical dating violence perpetration and victimization: Findings from adolescents in a high-risk urban community. *Violence and Victims*, *26*(5), 669–683. doi:10.1891/0886-6708.26.5.669

Alvarado-Bravo, B. G., Salinas, S. G., Heras, J. A. V., & Santana, J. E. T. (2015). Repercusiones de la tecnología en las relaciones de pareja. In A. Gutiérrez Cedeño, J. A. Vírseda Heras, & J. M. Serrano García (Eds.), *Por una Psicología sin fronteras* (pp. 161–174). Toluca (México): Universidad Autónoma del Estado de México.

Barter, C., Stanley, N., Wood, M., Lanau, A., Aghtaie, N., Larkins, C., & Øverlien, C. (2017). Young people's online and face-to-face experiences of interpersonal violence and abuse and their subjective impact across five European countries. *Psychology of Violence*, 7(3), 375–384. doi:10.1037/vio0000096

Bennett, D. C., Guran, E. L., Ramos, M. C., & Margolin, G. (2011). College students' electronic victimization in friendships and dating relationships: Anticipated distress and associations with risky behaviors. *Violence and Victims*, *26*(4), 410–429. doi:10.1891/0886-6708.26.4.410

Borrajo, E., Gámez-Guadix, M., & Calvete, E. (2015a). Justification beliefs of violence, myths about love and cyber dating abuse. *Psicothema, 27*, 327–333. doi:10.7334/psicothema2015.59

Borrajo, E., Gámez-Guadix, M., & Calvete, E. (2015b). Cyber dating abuse: Prevalence, context, and relationship with offline dating aggression. *Psychological Reports, 116*(2), 565–585. doi:10.2466/21.16.PR0.116k22w4

Borrajo, E., Gámez-Guadix, M., Pereda, N., & Calvete, E. (2015). The development and validation of the cyber dating abuse questionnaire among young couples. *Computers in Human Behavior, 48*, 358–365. doi:10.1016/j.chb.2015.01.063

Buelga, S., Cava, M.J. & Musitu, G. (2010). Cyberbullying: Victimización entre adolescentes a través del teléfono móvil y de Internet. *Psicothema, 22*, 784–789.

Burke, S. C., Wallen, M., Vail-Smith, K., & Knox, D. (2011). Using technology to control intimate partners: An exploratory study of college undergraduates. *Computers in Human Behavior, 27*(3), 1162–1167. doi:10.1016/j.chb.2010.12.010

Calvete, E., Corral, S., & Estévez, A. (2005). Desarrollo de un inventario para evaluar el abuso psicológico en las relaciones de pareja. *Clínica y Salud, 16*(3), 203–221.

Capaldi, D. M., Kim, H. K., & Shortt, J. W. (2007). Observed initiation and reciprocity of physical aggression in young, at-risk couples. *Journal of Family Violence, 22*(2), 101–111. doi:10.1007/s10896–10007–9067–9061

Carlson, R. G., Fripp, J., Cook, C., & Kelchner, V. (2015). Examining intimate partner violence, stress and technology use among young adults. *The Professional Counselor, 5*(3), 365–378. doi:10.15241/rgc.5. 3. 365

Celis-Sauce, A., & Rojas-Solís, J. (2015). Violencia en el noviazgo desde la perspectiva de varones adolescentes. *Informes Psicológicos, 15*(1), 83–104. doi:doi:10.18566/infpsicv15n1a05

Chaulk, K., & Jones, T. (2011). Online obsessive relational intrusion: Further concerns about Facebook. *Journal of Family Violence, 26*(4), 245–254. doi:10.1007/s10896–10011-

Cohen, J. (1992). A power primer. *Psychological Bulletin, 112*(1), 155–159. doi:0033–2909/92/S3–00

Cutbush, S., Ashley, O.S., Kan, M.L., Hampton, J., & Hall, D. M. (2010, November). *Electronic aggression among adolescent dating partner: Demographic correlates and associations with other types of violence*. Poster presented at the 138th American Public Health Association Annual Meeting, Denver, CO. Retrieved from: http://www.rti.org/pubs/apha10_cutbush_poster.pdf

Cutbush, S., Williams, J., Miller, S., Gibbs, D., & Clinton-Sherrod, M. (2012, October). *Electronic dating aggression among middle school students: Demographic correlates and associations with other types of violence*. Poster presented at the 140th American Public Health Association, annual meeting, San Francisco, CA. Retrieved from: http://www.rti.org/pubs/apha12_cutbush_poster.pdf

Dank, M., Lachman, P., Zweig, J. M., & Yahner, J. (2014). Dating violence experiences of lesbian, gay, bisexual, and transgender youth. *Journal of Youth and Adolescence, 43*(5), 846–857. doi:10.1007/s10964–10013–9975–9978

Darvell, M. J., Walsh, S. P., & White, K. M. (2011). Facebook tells me so: Applying the theory of planned behavior to understand partner-monitoring behavior on Facebook. *Cyberpsychology, Behavior, and Social Networking, 14*(12), 717–722. doi:10.1089/cyber.2011.0035

Dick, R. N., McCauley, H. L., Jones, K. A., Tancredi, D. J., Goldstein, S., Blackburn, S., … & Miller, E. (2014). Cyber dating abuse among teens using school-based health centers. *Pediatrics, 134*(6), e1560–e1567. doi:10.1542/peds.2014-0537d

Domínguez-Mora, R., Vargas-Jiménez, E., Castro-Castañeda, R., & Nuñez-Fadda, S. M. (2016). Impacto de la comunicación familiar en la victimización por internet en parejas adolescentes. *Opción, 32*(13), 979–1000.

Donoso Vázquez, T., Rubio Hurtado, M. J., & Vilà Baños, R. (2018). La adolescencia ante la violencia de género 2.0: Concepciones, conductas y experiencias. *Educación, 21*, 109–134. doi:10.5944/educxx1.20180

Draucker, C. B., & Martsolf, D. S. (2010). The role of electronic communication technology in adolescent dating violence. *Journal of Child and Adolescent Psychiatric Nursing, 23*(3), 133–142. doi:10.1111/j.1744–6171.2010.00235.x

Durán, M., & Martínez-Pecino, R. (2015). Ciberacoso mediante teléfono móvil e Internet en las relaciones de noviazgo entre jóvenes. *Comunicar, 22*(44), 159–167. doi:10.3916/C44-2015-17

Fernández-González, L., Calvete, E., & Orue, I. (2017). Adolescent dating violence stability and mutuality: A 4-year longitudinal study. *Journal of Interpersonal Violence, 10*. doi:10.1177/0886260517699953

Finn, J. (2004). A survey of online harassment at a university campus. *Journal of Interpersonal Violence, 19*(4), 468–483. doi:10.1177/0886260503262083

Foshee, V. A. (1996). Gender differences in adolescent dating abuse prevalence, types and injuries. *Health Education Research, 11*(3), 275–286. doi:10.1006/pmed.2000.0793

Fox, C. L., Corr, M. L., Gadd, D., & Butler, I. (2014). Young teenagers' experiences of domestic abuse. *Journal of Youth Studies, 17*(4), 510–526. doi:10.1080/13676261.2013.780125

Fox, C.L., & Warber, K. (2014). Social networking sites in romantic relationships: Attachment, uncertainty, and partner surveillance on Facebook. *Cyberpsychology, Behavior, and Social Networking*, 7(1), 3–7. doi:10.1089/cyber.2012.0667

Gámez-Guadix, M., Almendros, C., Borrajo, E., & Calvete, E. (2015). Prevalence and association of sexting and online sexual victimization among Spanish adults. *Sexuality Research and Social Policy, 12*, 145–154. doi:10.1007/s13178–13015–0186–0189

Griezel, L. (2007). *Out of the schoolyard and into cyber space: Elucidating the nature and psychosocial consequences of traditional and cyber bullying for Australian secondary students.* Unpublished honours thesis, University of Western Sydney, Sydney

Hamby, S. (2013, March). *The Partner Cyber Abuse Questionnaire: Preliminary psychometrics of technology-based intimate partner violence.* Paper presented at the annual convention of the Southeastern Psychological Association, Atlanta, GA.

Hinduja, S., & Patchin, J. W. (2011). *Electronic dating violence: A brief for educators and parents.* Cyberbullying Research Center. Retrieved from: www.cyberbullying.us

Jaen-Cortés, C. I., Rivera-Aragón, S., Reidl-Martínez, L. M., & García-Méndez, M. (2017). Violencia de pareja a través de medios electrónicos en adolescentes mexicanos. *Acta de Investigación Psicológica*, 7, 2593–2605. doi:10.1016/j.aipprr.2017.01.001

Kellerman, I., Margolin, G., Borofsky, L., Baucom, B., & Iturralde, E. (2013). Electronic aggression among emerging adults: Motivations and contextual factors. *Emerging Adulthood, 1*, 293–304. doi:10.1177/2167696813490159

Korchmaros, J. D., Ybarra, M. L., Langhinrichsen-Rohling, J., Boyd, D., & Lenhart, A. (2013). Perpetration of teen dating violence in a networked society. *Cyberpsychology, Behavior, and Social Networking, 16*, 561–567. doi:10.1089/cyber.2012.0627

Leisring, P. A., & Giumetti, G. W. (2014). Sticks and stones may break my bones, but abusive text messages also hurt: Development and validation of the Cyber Psychological Abuse scale. *Partner Abuse, 5*(3), 323–341. doi:10.1891/1946-6560.5.3.323

Linder, J. R., Crick, N. R., & Collins, W. A. (2002). Relational aggression and victimization in young adults' romantic relationships: Associations with perceptions of parent, peer, and romantic relationship quality. *Social Development, 11*(1), 69–86. doi:10.1111/1467-9507.00187

Lucio-López, L. A., & Prieto-Quezada, M. (2014). Violencia en el ciberespacio en las relaciones de noviazgo adolescente. Un estudio exploratorio en estudiantes mexicanos de escuelas preparatorias. *Revista de Educación y Desarrollo, 31*, 61–72. Retrieved from http://www.seg.guanajuato.gob.mx/Ceducativa/CDocumental/Doctos/2014/Octubre/Violenciaciberespacio.pdf

Lyndon, A., Bonds-Raacke, J., & Cratty, A. D. (2011). College students' Facebook stalking of ex-partners. *Cyberpsychology, Behavior, and Social Networking, 14*(12), 711–716. doi:10.1089/cyber.2010.0588

Marcum, C. D., Higgins, G. E., & Nicholson, J. (2017). I'm watching you: Cyberstalking behaviors of university students in romantic relationships. *American Journal of Criminal Justice, 42*, 373–388. doi:10.1007/s12103-016-9358-2.

Martinez-Lanz, P., Cazares, P. A., Kuri, N. A., Huerta, M. D., Araiza, A. L. P., & Valdez, P. H. (2016). Inmate partner violence through social networks. *European Scientific Journal, 12*(29), 95–111. doi:10.19044/esj.2016.v12n29p95

Martin Montilla, A.; Pazos Gomez, M.; Montilla Coronado, M. V. C. & Romero Oliva, C. (2016). Una modalidad actual de violencia de género en parejas de jovenes: Las redes sociales. *Educación XX1, 19*(2), 405–429, doi:10.5944/educXX1.13934

Melander, L.A. (2010). *Explaining college partner violence in the digital age: An instrumental design mixed methods study* (Unpublished doctoral dissertation). Department of Psychology, University of Nebraska at Lincoln, Nebraska, United States. Retrieved from: http://digitalcommons.unl.edu/cgi/viewcontent.cgi?article=1000&context=sociologydiss.

Morelli, M., Bianchi, D., Baiocco, R., Pezzuti, L., & Chirumbolo, A. (2016). Not-allowed sharing of sexts and dating violence from the perpetrator's perspective: The moderation role of sexism. *Computers in Human Behavior, 56*, 163–169. doi:10.1016/j.chb.2015.11.047

Morelli, M., Bianchi, D., Chirumbolo, A., & Baiocco, R. (2018). The cyber dating violence inventory. Validation of a new scale for online perpetration and victimization among dating partners. *European Journal of Developmental Psychology, 15*(4), 464-471. doi:10.1080/17405629.2017.1305885

Muñiz, M. (2017). Online teen dating violence, family and school climate from a gender perspective/Violencia de pareja online en la adolescencia, clima familiar y escolar desde la perspectiva de género. *Infancia y Aprendizaje, 40*(17), 572-598. doi:10.1080/02103702.2017.1341101

Pereira, F., Spitzberg, B. H., & Matos, M. (2016). Cyber-harassment victimization in Portugal: Prevalence, fear and help-seeking among adolescents. *Computers in Human Behavior, 62*, 136–146. doi:10.1016/j.chb.2016.03.039

Peskin, M. F., Markham, C. M., Shegog, R., Temple, J. R., Baumler, E. R., Addy, R. C., … Emery, S. T. (2017). Prevalence and correlates of the perpetration of cyber dating abuse among early adolescents. *Journal of Youth and Adolescence, 46*(2), 358–375. doi:10.1007/s10964-016-0568-1

Picard, P. (2007). *Tech abuse in teen relationships*. Chicago, IL: Teen Research Unlimited. Retrieved from: www.loveisrespect.org/wp-content/uploads/2009/03/liz-claiborne-2007-tech-relationship-abuse.pdf.

Powell, A., & Henry, N. (2016). Technology-facilitated sexual violence victimization: results from an online survey of Australian adults. *Journal of Interpersonal Violence*, 1–29. Advance online publication. doi:10.1177/0886260516672055

Reed, L.A., Tolman, R.M., & Ward, L.M. (2016). Snooping and sexting: Digital media as a context for dating aggression and abuse among college students. *Violence Against Women, 22,* 1556–1576. doi:10.1177/1077801216630143

Sánchez, V., Muñoz, N., Nocentini, A., Ortega-Ruiz, R., & Menesini, E. (2014). Online intrusiveness, online jealousy and dating aggression in young adults: A cross-national study (Spain-Italy). *Maltrattamento e Abuso all'infanzia, 16,* 47–65. doi:10.3280/MAL2014-003004

Sánchez, V., Muñoz-Fernández, N., & Ortega-Ruíz, R. (2015). "Cyberdating Q_A": An instrument to assess the quality of adolescent dating relationships in social networks. *Computers in Human Behavior, 48,* 78–86. doi:10.1016/j.chb.2015.01.006

Sánchez, V., Muñoz-Fernández, N., & Vega-Gea, E. (2017). Peer sexual cybervictimization in adolescents: Development and validation of a scale. *International Journal of Clinical and Health Psychology, 17,* 171–179. doi:10.1016/j.ijchp.2017.04.001

Schnurr, M. P., Mahatmya, D., & Basche, R. A., III. (2013). The role of dominance, cyber aggression perpetration, and gender on emerging adults' perpetration of intimate partner violence. *Psychology of Violence, 3,* 70–83. doi:10.1037/a0030601

Shaffer, J. A., DeGeest, D., & Li, A. (2016). Tackling the problem of construct proliferation: A guide to assessing the discriminant validity of conceptually related constructs. *Organizational Research Methods, 19*(1), 80–110. doi:10.1177/1094428115598239

Shen, A. C. T., Chiu, M. Y. L., & Gao, J. (2012). Predictors of dating violence among Chinese adolescents: The role of gender-role beliefs and justification of violence. *Journal of Interpersonal Violence, 27*(6), 1066–1089. doi:10.1177/0886260511424497

Shorey, R. C., Cornelius, T. L., & Strauss, C. (2015). Stalking in college student dating relationships: A descriptive investigation. *Journal of Family Violence, 30*(7), 935–942. doi:10.1007/s10896-015-9717-7

Smith, P. K. (2012). Cyberbullying and cyber aggression. In A. B. N. S.R. Jimerson, M. J. Mayer, & M. J. Furlong (Eds.), *Handbook of school violence and school safety: International research and practice* (2nd ed; pp. 93–103). New York: Routledge.

Spitzberg, B. H., & Cupach, W. R. (2003). What mad pursuit? Obsessive relational intrusion and stalking related phenomena. *Aggression and Violent Behavior, 8*(4), 345–375. doi:10.1016/S1359-1789(02)00068-X

Spitzberg, B. H., & Hoobler, G. (2002). Cyberstalking and the technologies of interpersonal terrorism. *New Media & Society, 4,* 71–92. doi:10.1177/14614440222226271

Stonard, K. E., Bowen, E., Lawrence, T. R., & Price, S. A. (2014). The relevance of technology to the nature, prevalence and impact of adolescent dating violence and abuse: A research synthesis. *Aggression and Violent Behavior, 19*(4), 390–417. doi:10.1016/j.avb.2014.06.005

Straus, M. A. (2008). Dominance and symmetry in partner violence by male and female university students in 32 nations. *Children and Youth Services Review, 30*(3), 252–275. doi:10.1016/j.childyouth.2007.doi:10.004

Straus, M. A. (2009). The national context effect: An empirical test of the validity of cross-national research using unrepresentative samples. *Cross-Cultural Research, 43*(3), 183–205. doi:10.1177/1069397109335770

Straus, M. A., Hamby, S. L., Boney-McCoy, S., & Sugarman, D. B. (1996). The revised conflict tactics scale (CTS2): Development and preliminary psychometric data. *Journal of Family Issues, 17,* 283–316. doi:10.1177/019251396017003001

Temple, J. R., Choi, H. J., Brem, M., Wolford-Clevenger, C., Stuart, G. L., Peskin, M. F., & Elmquist, J. (2016). The temporal association between traditional and cyber dating abuse among adolescents. *Journal of Youth and Adolescence, 45*, 340–349. doi:10.1007/s10964-015-0380-3

Tokunaga, R. S. (2011). Social networking site or social surveillance site? Understanding the use of interpersonal electronic surveillance in romantic relationships. *Computers in Human Behavior, 27*(2), 705–713. doi:10.1016/j.chb.2010.08.doi:014

Tolman, R. M. (1999). The validation of the psychological maltreatment of women inventory. *Violence and Victims, 14*(1), 25–35. doi:10.1891/0886-6708.doi:14.1.25

Tompson, T., Benz, J., & Agiesta, J. (2013). *The digital abuse study: Experiences of teens and young adults*. Chicago, IL: Associated Press-NORC Center/MTV.

Van Ouytsel, J., Ponnet, K., & Walrave, M. (2016). Cyber dating abuse victimization among secondary school students from a lifestyle-routine activities theory perspective. *Journal of Interpersonal Violence, 145*, 147–151 doi:10.1177/0886260516629390

Wolfe, D. A., Scott, K., Reitzel-Jaffe, D., Wekerle, C., Grasley, C., & Straatman, A.-L. (2001). Development and validation of the Conflict in Adolescent Dating Relationships Inventory. *Psychological Assessment, 13*, 277–293. doi:10.1037//1040-3590.13.doi:2.277

Wolford-Clevenger, C., Zapor, H., Brasfield, H., Febres, J., Elmquist, J., Brem, M., … Stuart, G. L. (2016). An examination of the partner cyber abuse questionnaire in a college student sample. *Psychology of Violence, 6*, 156–162. doi:10.1037/a0039442

Wright, M. F. (2015). Cyber aggression within adolescents' romantic relationships: Linkages to parental and partner attachment. *Journal of Youth and Adolescence, 44*(1), 37–47. doi:10.1007/s10964-014-0147-2

Ybarra, M.L., Espelage, D.L., & Mitchell, K.J. (2007). The co-occurrence of Internet harassment and unwanted sexual solicitation victimization and perpetration: associations with psychosocial indicators. *Journal of Adolescence Health, 41*(6), 31–41. doi:10.1016/j.jadohealth.2007.09.010

Zweig, J. M., Dank, M., Yahner, J., & Lachman, P. (2013). The rate of cyber dating abuse among teens and how it relates to other forms of teen dating violence. *Journal of Youth and Adolescence, 42*, 1063–1077. doi:10.1007/s10964-013-9922

11

CYBERBULLYING IN ROMANTIC RELATIONSHIPS

Developmental Perspectives

Diana C. Bennett and Michelle C. Ramos

Both adolescence and emerging adulthood are transitional periods and the development of romantic relationships is central to each of these time points. As electronic media use becomes more prevalent in youths' lives, digital platforms increasingly become an arena for conflict with romantic partners, and the potential for electronic dating aggression (EDA) also emerges. Understanding how EDA functions as a part of young people's relationships is important in drawing connections from earlier life experiences to later relationship outcomes and psychological functioning. This chapter reviews the prevalence of electronic media use and EDA through adolescence and emerging adulthood, followed by attention focused on developmental tasks and context in which to understand EDA in these age groups. Next, we review gender differences and psychological and behavioral correlates of EDA in both adolescence and emerging adulthood. Finally, suggestions for prevention and intervention efforts are made.

Prevalence of Electronic Media Use in Adolescence and Emerging Adulthood

National estimates suggest that over 75% of adolescents ages 12–17 have cellular phones and the vast majority (93%) used the internet (Lenhart, Purcell, Smith, & Zickuhr, 2010; see also Chapter 2, this volume). More recent estimates, as expected, demonstrate that the rates only seem to be increasing (e.g., Lenhart, 2015). Nearly 95% of youth and adolescents were estimated to access the internet, with an average of about an hour and a half of internet use per day, much of this taking place in a youth's own bedroom or on a personal computer or mobile phone (CHILDWISE, 2013). Youth spend an average of as many as 11 hours per day in total exposed to electronic media (Kaiser Family Foundation, 2010), suggesting that much of this internet use is being done with a level of independence from direct parental monitoring. Among emerging adults, a recent survey suggested that 88% of 18–29-year-olds use some form of social media and engage across a variety of platforms (Pew Research Center, 2018). For example, over 80% of Snapchat and Instagram users ages 18–24 use the platforms daily, with 71% and 55%, respectively, reporting that they visit the platform multiple times a day. Approximately half of young adult social media users say it would be difficult to give up social media sites. In terms of text-messaging and emailing, one study indicated that over 80% of college men and women reported daily use, with the majority using these methods multiple times per day (Bennett, Guran, Ramos, & Margolin, 2011). Overall, electronic media use is seemingly ubiquitous for adolescents and emerging adults, although a number of challenges make accurate estimates difficult to ascertain. Research on the pervasiveness of electronic media use must be frequently updated as technology changes. In addition, what is being measured (types of media, frequency/duration of use) is not consistent across studies, and self-report estimates of media use may not always be accurate.

Electronic Media Use and Adolescent Development

Adolescence is a period full of transition, characterized by several developmental tasks including youths' pursuit of identity, autonomy, sexuality, and intimacy (Hill, 1983). As electronic media usage among adolescents becomes ubiquitous (e.g., Lenhart, 2015), increasing attention has been paid to the ways in which electronic media relate to meeting these developmental goals. With regard to identity development, electronic media may help adolescents construct their identity through self-disclosure and self-presentation (Subrahmanyam & Greenfield, 2008). This self-disclosure via social media can facilitate belongingness (Davis, 2012), and may also enhance autonomy as adolescents are free to choose what to present about themselves (Shapiro & Margolin, 2014). Online self-disclosure may be a "rehearsal" for later offline disclosure, as adolescents may essentially "test the water" with online communication to gain comfort in face-to-face disclosure at a later time (Valkenburg, Sumter, & Peter, 2011).

Online interactions also allow adolescents the ability to connect with like others and enhance affiliation. Through electronic media, adolescents can expand their social circles (Subrahmanyam & Greenfield, 2008) and enhance existing relationships (Lenhart, Rainie, & Lewis, 2001). Cross-sectional studies generally indicate that young people use social networking as an extension of their existing face-to-face networks, and much more rarely to meet new people (see Shapiro & Margolin, 2014, for a review). Through electronic media, adolescents are able to join groups with others which may be especially valuable for youth with limited offline friendships. However, electronic social interactions may place some youth at risk for negative consequences. For example, youth who have poorer social skills may receive more negative feedback from peers online or compare themselves negatively to others (Shapiro & Margolin, 2014). Electronic media may also amplify adolescent egocentrism, the heightened self-consciousness that adolescents experience (Elkind, 1976), in particular the aspect of the imaginary audience. Imaginary audience, which occurs when an individual believes their actions, appearance, or behavior are being closely monitored by family, peers, and even strangers, influences one's actions and how they interpret otherwise ambiguous cues in their social interactions. As a result, adolescents may overestimate how peers are perceiving them online and may misconstrue feedback as being more negative in nature.

Electronic media also intersect with one of the central tasks of adolescence: the development of autonomy, primarily from parents and family of origin. Although adolescents are generally living with their family of origin, electronic media allow for the formation of new relationships outside of the family and the extension of existing relationships with peers or romantic partners. Electronic media use may also play a role in separating adolescents from their parents, as young people tend to be more well versed than their parents in the modes and methods of electronic communication (Lenhart, 2015). Although parents may use electronic media to improve communication with adolescents, and as a tool to monitor their interactions, tech-savvy youth may be able to work around attempts at parental monitoring (Subrahmanyam & Greenfield, 2008). For instance, youth can create multiple profiles on a social networking site, or screen calls and messages from parents, placing adolescents in greater control over their electronic communication. There is some evidence that media use in adolescence impacts existing parent-child relationships, as parents report that electronic media use interferes with family life and that they are concerned about their children's media use (Rosen, Cheever, & Carrier, 2008). Estimates suggest that as many as 90% of adolescents have not disclosed negative online interactions to parents (Juvonen & Gross, 2008).

Electronic media also play a key role in the development and maintenance of adolescent romantic relationships (Stonard, Bowen, Walker, & Price, 2017). Electronic platforms often are involved in the establishment of the relationship, in facilitating daily communication, and can be arenas for conflict and resolution following conflict (Draucker & Martsolf, 2010). Sexual and romantic exploration can take place through media without real-life contact, including use of sexual dialog (Mishna, McLuckie, & Saini, 2009) or through sexting with partners who may or may not be known to the youth in a face-to-face context (de Bruijn, Burrie, & vanWel, 2006). There is also some evidence that media usage provides a safer space for adolescent girls to initiate romantic relationships (Subrahmanyan & Greenfield, 2008), as well as for sexual minority (i.e., LGBTQ) youth to expand their dating pool (Russell, Franz, & Driscoll, 2001). Coupled with less oversight from parents in relationships and communication taking place through electronic media, and the potential for increased contact with either new partners or existing face-to-face contacts, electronic media plays a central role in adolescents' romantic relationships. However, electronic tools also allow for harassment, monitoring, and controlling behaviors in adolescent dating relationships (Stonard et al., 2017). The prevalence, risk factors, and correlates of EDA during adolescence will be discussed later in this chapter.

Electronic Media Use and Development in Emerging Adulthood

Emerging adulthood is a developmental period distinct from adolescence, characterized by change and exploration for youth in their late teens through twenties (~18 to 25; Arnett, 2000; 2004). Emerging adults are concerned with identity exploration, particularly in the domains of love, intimacy, education, and work; their lives often reflect instability as they explore the range of possibilities available to them (Arnett, 2000; Erikson, 1959; Schulenberg, Sameroff, & Cicchetti, 2004). As youth transition through emerging adulthood, individual differences become more pronounced based on the timing of achievement of developmental tasks, and opportunities for achievement or failure in new roles and social contexts can potentially influence the development of psychopathology (see Schulenberg, Bryant, & O'Malley, 2004, for a review). Along with the changes that come with expanding social, occupational, and educational opportunities, there is potential for youth who were struggling during adolescence to thrive, or for those who were functioning well in adolescence to encounter more difficulties. Indeed, emerging adulthood is the period in which many psychiatric disorders onset. Emerging adulthood is also a developmental period associated with risky behavior as young people have increasing autonomy and exploration. Thus, dating aggression can occur as part of a broader constellation of risky behaviors.

Traditional dating abuse in adolescence and emerging adulthood has been associated with a host of risky behaviors, including risky sexual behavior and substance use (Decker, Silverman, & Raj, 2005; Eaton, Davis, Barrios, Brener, & Noonan, 2007; Pallitto, Campbell & O'Campo, 2005; Shorey, Stuart, & Cornelius, 2011; Sullivan, Farrell, & Kliewer, 2006; Teitelman, Ratcliffe, Morales-Aleman, & Sullivan, 2008), and EDA in adolescence and emerging adulthood has been associated with behavioral problems and risky behaviors such as carrying a weapon, substance abuse, and risky sexual behavior (Bennett et al., 2011; Wolak, Mitchell, & Finkelhor, 2007; Ybarra, Diener-West, & Leaf, 2007). How young people navigate the developmental tasks in the transitional period of emerging adulthood is related to well-being in later years (Schulenberg, Bryant, & O'Malley, 2004), indicating that, like adolescence, this developmental period is quite salient as a transition in one's life.

As emerging adults' use of electronic media continues to expand as compared to adolescence, with even less parental or school oversight (Kowalski, Giumetti, Schroeder, & Lattanner, 2014) and increased autonomy, so too does the potential for electronic media use to be both an asset and a vulnerability for negative outcomes. For young adults moving away from home, electronic media use allows for continued contact with friends and family living far away with whom face-to-face contact is limited. Newer features such as video chat may help to maintain bonds to parents and friends that highly resemble face-to-face interactions. Electronic media can help young adults forge new relationships in their new environments, for example, in "checking out" people they have met through college classes or campus housing to investigate the potential for friendships or dating relationships (Lampe, Ellison, & Steinfield, 2006). However, having weaker support systems in their lives may also place them at risk for deleterious effects when electronic communication is negative in nature.

Although overall rates of interpersonal violence decline from high school to college (Forke, Myers, Catallozzi, & Schwarz, 2008), college students still report high rates of victimization in dating relationships (Hines & Saudino, 2003; Straus, 2004). As young adults increasingly focus on establishing intimacy in this stage of development and romantic relationships become more salient than in adolescence, dating aggression can be even more likely via the use of electronic media. Next, we will discuss EDA among adolescents and emerging adults.

Definition and Prevalence of EDA among Adolescents and Emerging Adults

EDA involves using mobile and online platforms to perpetrate hostile (e.g., threats), intrusive (e.g., monitoring activities), and humiliating (e.g., posting inappropriate pictures) behaviors against a romantic partner (Bennett, et al., 2011). EDA falls within the umbrella of intimate partner violence, but is especially pernicious due to continuous access available via electronic media and the potentially public and permanent nature of digital communication between dating partners. Various labels for hurtful electronic behaviors between romantic partners include electronic dating aggression, cyberbullying, cyber-victimization, cyber dating aggression, digital dating abuse, and online harassment. We specifically use the term *EDA* because we conceptualize these behaviors as extensions of psychological aggression within the context of a romantic relationship, rather than characteristically cyberbullying behaviors that constitute repeated behaviors with intent to harm, and that often involve a power-differential among peers or acquaintances rather than dating partners (Tokunaga, 2010).

Prevalence of EDA among Adolescents

For both adolescents and young adults, prevalence estimates of EDA are difficult to ascertain for a number of reasons (Stonard, Bowen, Lawrence, & Price 2014). Studies vary considerably in the time frame being sampled (e.g., past month, past year, lifetime) and in the detail of measurement (e.g., single-item versus a range of specific behaviors). Additionally, the platforms of electronic media are constantly evolving, such that in the time it takes from study development to data collection to ultimate publication, technology has generally advanced beyond the scope and relevance of what was studied. In addition, the burgeoning research on EDA has relied primarily on self-reports, which are prone to social desirability bias. At the time of our review, there were no known EDA studies using objective measurements of real time social media communication or experimental methods. Finally, much of the early literature examining youths' electronic aggression failed to differentiate aggression between strangers and peers from aggression with dating partners.

Given these caveats, the extant research on EDA indicates that aggression between romantic partners through electronic media is present from a relatively young age. Nearly one-third of 7th grade students (M_{age}=12.3 years) reported being a victim of EDA (Cutbush, Williams, Miller, Gibbs, & Clinton-Sherrod, 2012), and by 9th grade (M_{age}=14.3 years), estimates increase to 56% (Cutbush, Ashley, Kan, Hampton, & Hall 2010). A study of over 500 adolescents ages 13–18 from across the United States provided estimates of the prevalence of a variety of EDA experiences (Picard, 2007). The authors found that one quarter of youth reported having been harassed or called names by a partner through cell phone or text message. Slightly fewer (22%) reported having received an unwanted sexual proposition via phone or internet. Nearly 1 in 5 participants reported rumors being spread by a partner via cell phone or internet or being harassed via social network site by a partner. Seventeen percent felt afraid of potential retribution from a partner should they not respond to electronic communication. Finally, about 10% had had a partner share embarrassing images or video of them through electronic media or been physically threatened through electronic media. In another large-scale study of over 5600 youth in 7th to 12th grade (90% in high school), 26% of adolescents endorsed past-year electronic victimization from a dating partner, with the most common aggressive acts including intrusion (use of social networking account without permission) and sexual solicitation/pressure (Zweig, Dank, Yahner, & Lachman, 2013). Rates of EDA among adolescents are comparable to reported rates of physical dating violence, more common than sexual coercion, and about half as prevalent as traditional psychological aggression (Zweig et al., 2013).

Gender also may be an important factor to consider in adolescent EDA. Findings on the prevalence and impact of EDA suggest that adolescent females are at increased risk compared to adolescent males. There is some evidence that females experience higher rates of electronic dating victimization compared to adolescent males (Zweig, Lachman, Yahner, & Dank, 2014; Zweig et al., 2013), and that males are likely to perpetrate sexual EDA against female partners (Zweig et al., 2013). Zweig et al. (2013) found that females experienced significantly more EDA (29%) than males (23%), particularly sexual EDA victimization (15% females vs. 7% males). Females also perpetrated higher levels of non-sexual EDA (14% females vs. 9% males); however, adolescent males perpetrated more sexual EDA (4%) than females (2%).

Gender differences in EDA victimization rates were also found in a clinic-based sample, with notably higher rates, where 45% of adolescent females endorsed EDA victimization during the past three months compared to 31% of males (Dick et al., 2014). Even in studies that demonstrate similar rates of EDA among adolescent females and males (Reed, Tolman, & Ward, 2017), females reported being more upset and expressing more negative emotional responses related to EDA than males. Taken together, the literature suggests that adolescent girls may be particularly vulnerable to the impact of EDA, even if rates of exposure are similar to that of males.

Prevalence of EDA among Emerging Adults

Far fewer studies have examined the prevalence of EDA among college students and emerging adults. In one study of past-year EDA among college students, over half of the sample reported acts of hostility (56.4% of women, 60.2% of men; such as being sent a mean or threatening text message) and intrusion (56.4% of women, 66.1% of men; such as excessive monitoring or accessing one's email or social networking profile) (Bennett et al., 2011). Nearly half of participants reported humiliation (36.6% of women, 48.3% of men; such as posting an embarrassing photo online), and fewer endorsed exclusion (17.7% of women, 34.7% of men; such as being blocked on a social networking site). College men, compared to women, reported significantly more electronic dating victimization (Bennett et al., 2011). Less data are available on rates of electronic dating perpetration among college students and emerging adults. Leisring and Giumetti (2014) identified that 93% of college students endorsed having perpetrated at least a minor form of electronic aggression toward a dating partner, whereas 13% endorsed perpetrating a more severe form, such as being threatened or intentionally humiliated. In another study, one in five participants (21.7%) endorsed having bullied a dating partner through text message, nearly half (56.9%) had sent a mean or hurtful text message, 39.4% had intrusively called or texted a dating partner to check up on them, and about one third (29.6%) had tried to make a partner jealous by posting on someone else's internet profile, all in the past year (Kellerman, Margolin, Borofsky, Baucom, & Iturralde, 2013).

Similar to adolescents, gender appears to be an important factor in emerging adults' electronic dating aggression. Although many studies found that overall rates of electronic dating victimization do not differ by gender (Borrajo, Gámez-Guadix, & Calvete, 2015; Reed, Tolman, Ward, & Safyer, 2016; Wolford-Clevenger et al., 2016), females compared to males reported more anticipated negative reactions to electronically aggressive behaviors, particularly sexual electronic messaging (Reed, Tolman, & Ward, 2016). With regards to electronic perpetration, the data are inconsistent. One study found no gender differences in rates of electronic intrusion against dating partners (Reed, Tolman, & Safyer, 2015), while another study showed women reported higher electronically aggressive acts toward dating partners than men (Bennett et al., 2011), and another showed that college men reported both more victimization and perpetration toward partners than women (Leisring & Giumetti, 2014). Gender differences have also been identified in motives for college students' electronic perpetration against both friends and dating partners, including humor or misplaced goodwill (more common among men), privacy or self-protection (more common among women), and jealousy/insecurity being the most commonly endorsed motivation (also more common among women) (Kellerman et al., 2013).

Correlates of Electronic Dating Aggression

Given the prevalence of EDA described above, researchers have turned attention toward examining potential risk factors and consequences of exposure to EDA. The literature is limited in that most studies are cross-sectional, making causal statements impossible. Thus, we refer to the findings of these studies as correlates of EDA given the limitation in temporal precedence.

Adolescence

Adolescents who experience EDA are at increased risk for concurrent physical, sexual, and psychological dating violence (Dick et al., 2014; Yahner, Dank, Zweig, & Lachman, 2015; Zweig et al., 2013) as well as cyberbullying more generally (Yahner et al. 2015). Over half of adolescents (54%) who experienced EDA victimization were also victims of physical dating aggression, and 86% were victims of psychological aggression (Zweig et al., 2013). In particular, engaging in sexual EDA increased risk for sexual coercion. Adolescents who received sexual EDA from dating partners were seven times more likely to be victims of sexual coercion (55%) compared to non-victims (8%). Adolescents who perpetrated sexual EDA were 17 times more likely to have also perpetrated sexual coercion (34%) than non-perpetrators (2%). For females, increased rates of EDA were associated with non-use of contraception and reproductive coercion (Dick et al., 2014).

Additional factors associated with adolescent electronic dating victimization include perpetrating delinquent behaviors, reporting higher levels of depressive symptoms, higher levels of anger and hostility, and having a previous history of sexual activity (Zweig et al., 2014). Insecure attachment is also related to EDA. Adolescents with insecure maternal attachment reported higher levels of perpetrating electronic dating aggression one year later (Wright, 2015). Anxious and avoidant romantic partner attachment predicted electronically intrusive behaviors against dating partners concurrently (Reed, Tolman, Ward, & Safyer, 2016) and in the following year (Wright, 2015).

A limitation of the existing EDA literature is the dearth of longitudinal studies. Such investigations are necessary to determine whether these negative associations are found beyond adolescence. Available evidence from adolescent cyberbullying studies (not limited to that which is perpetrated by dating partners) suggests risks carry over into emerging adulthood: adolescents who experienced cyberbullying in high school were over three times more likely to both receive and perpetrate cyber aggression in college compared to those who did not experience cyber-bullying (Beran, Rinaldi, Bickham, & Rich, 2012).

Emerging Adulthood

The literature on correlates of emerging adults' EDA demonstrates some of the same patterns found for adolescents. Most notably, emerging adults who experience EDA with romantic partners are likely to experience concomitant psychological, physical, and sexual dating violence (Bennett et al., 2011; Borrajo et al., 2015; Reed, Tolman, & Ward, 2016). Like adolescents, emerging adults' insecure attachment to dating partners is related to perpetrating EDA. Anxious attachment was associated with higher levels of electronically intrusive behaviors. For females, avoidant attachment predicted less EDA against partners (Reed et al., 2015).

Emerging adults' EDA is also concurrently associated with a range of negative factors and contexts. For instance, college students reported higher levels of anticipated distress for EDA victimization than by electronic victimization from peers (Bennett et al., 2011). Notably, however, there is also some indication that not all behaviors that fall under the umbrella of EDA are considered upsetting by the victim (Bennett et al., 2011), suggesting that there are likely a number of important moderating variables. EDA victimization was related to higher levels of alcohol use, substance use, and engagement in risky sex, with the effect of alcohol still significant after controlling for non-electronic types of dating victimization (Bennett et al., 2011). Additionally, the role of jealousy in emerging adults' EDA has been consistently demonstrated (Borrajo et al., 2015, Kellerman, et al., 2013, Wright, 2017). Studies found that common motivations for perpetrating EDA were in retaliation for hurtful behaviors (Kellerman et al., 2013) or to control dating partners in the context of jealousy (Borrajo et al., 2015). Moreover, jealousy mediated the association between emerging adults' anxious romantic attachment style and electronically intrusive behaviors against partners (Wright, 2017). Finally, family-of-origin aggression (Ramos, Miller, Moss, & Margolin, 2017) and risky family contexts (i.e., environments characterized by neglect, conflict, chaos, and parental substance use) are also associated with increased EDA (Kellerman, et al., 2013), providing support for the intergenerational transmission of aggression within the electronic domain. Furthermore, perspective-taking and empathy both buffered the link between family aggression during childhood and perpetrating EDA in emerging adulthood (Ramos et al., 2017).

As with the literature on adolescent EDA, there is a need to move beyond documenting prevalence rates and correlates of emerging adult EDA to examining predictors and potential mediators and moderators of effects. Relatedly, longitudinal, multi-informant investigations are necessary in order to clarify direction of effects, determine whether associations are time-limited or long-term, and minimize recall bias. Future work should also incorporate innovative alternative methods such as ecological momentary assessment and accessing social media and text message logs to capture EDA in real time, and identify precursors and consequences.

Given that the extant literature clearly demonstrates that both adolescents and emerging adults who experience EDA are vulnerable to other types of dating violence with known sequelae, it is critical that future research elucidate potential targets for EDA prevention and intervention.

Directions for Prevention and Intervention Efforts

Meta-analytic research suggests that the most successful prevention programs for electronic aggression include multiple levels of intervention at the individual, family, school, peer, and broader social context levels (Guo, 2016). To our knowledge, no research has yet focused on EDA specifically, and thus the following suggestions are drawn from studies aimed at reducing electronic aggression generally, with the expectation that recommendations might generalize to EDA given the use of the same electronic platforms. Among adolescents, parents can monitor and place limits on youths' usage of electronic media (Rosen et al., 2008). Generally, parental involvement has been shown to affect media use. Parents making recommendations about websites, and not simply setting restrictions on internet use generally, resulted in changes to the types of sites children were visiting (Li, 2006; Mnet, 2001). Additionally, locating a home computer in a shared family space rather than in the youth's bedroom resulted in less internet usage (Livingstone, 2007). There is also some evidence that parental monitoring of online activities resulted in less disclosure of personally identifying information online (Rosen et al., 2008), and disclosure of personal information has been associated with greater chances of electronic victimization (Mesch, 2009). As adolescents are increasing autonomy and using self-disclosure through electronic media to gain affiliation and aid in identity development, this is an important finding in which the developmental goals of adolescence may actually be a risk factor for victimization.

Using a representative sample of the U.S. population, Mesch (2009) identified that youth who had not been electronically victimized were more likely to have parents who set rules about the types of websites they were allowed to visit and the amount of time they were allowed to be online, as well as more likely to have a filter restricting online activity and to have their computer located in a shared family space. Despite these associations, Mesch concluded that only the existence of restrictions as to the type of sites visited online was significantly related to less likelihood of victimization, and this may be more true for boys than girls. He asserts that parental monitoring may be limited in effectiveness by youths' ability to work around parental controls, or that electronic aggression may occur in contexts parents deem safe, and thus parental monitoring is missing potential areas for risk. However, he recommends that discussion about the nature of different websites and possible risks of types of media use may be protective.

Parental discussions with youth about EDA, in addition to attempts to monitor media usage, may be helpful interventions at home. For traditional dating violence, one study indicated that Latino adolescents' levels of perceived parent caring were protective against physical and sexual dating violence, and a high level of communication with parents was associated with less dating victimization (Kast, Eisenberg, & Sieving, 2016), suggesting that parental involvement may play a key role in preventing dating violence more generally. When having discussions with youth about dating relationships, parents should be sure to include discussion of the potential role of electronic media. Among young adults living outside the home, parental monitoring is less useful. However, parents and loved ones can maintain open lines of communication with college students and young adults about their relationships with others, and inquire about potential dating aggression, as well as monitoring for signs that an individual might be in need of mental health care. Adolescents and young adults would also benefit from education about safe media use, including instructions for how to manage privacy settings on social media and how to block unwanted electronic contact (Ramos & Bennett, 2016).

Additionally, given that electronic victimization is often an extension of offline relationships and aggression, there is room for intervention and prevention efforts at school for middle school, high school, and college-aged students. School-level interventions may be most effective when students are trained to respond, and leaders of campus organizations may benefit from being educated about identifying potential victims of any type of dating abuse, including EDA. Peer leaders may be uniquely situated to identify and intervene in these cases and can help direct peers to appropriate mental health resources when needed (Ramos & Bennett, 2016). EDA is increasingly viewed as a public health problem, and primary or secondary prevention programs addressing peer aggression in general have begun to show effectiveness in addressing cyberbullying and cyber-victimization as well (e.g., Gradinger, Yanagida, Strohmeier, & Spiel, 2015). Social media literacy may also help raise adolescents' awareness of EDA victimization, perpetration, and consequences. Education might include how electronic platforms might be used for dating aggression, the types of behaviors that constitute EDA, and a broader discussion of healthy versus unhealthy dating behaviors (see Ramos & Bennett, 2016). Adolescence may be a prime time to provide social skills training to young people with a focus on empathy and appropriate electronic interactions. Research identifying perspective-taking and empathy as inversely linked to perpetrating EDA (Ramos et al., 2017) suggests that programs aimed at strengthening cognitive and affective empathy to decrease anger and in-person aggression (e.g., Reddy et al., 2013) may also effectively reduce aggression in the electronic domain.

Traditional adolescent dating violence prevention programs targeting perpetration and victimization can be effective, particularly if they are of longer duration, delivered across multiple settings (e.g., school and community), and involve important individuals in youths' environments (see De Koker, Mathews, Zuch, Bastien, & Mason-Jones, 2014, for a review). Existing dating violence prevention and intervention efforts should include components to address electronic media as an arena for dating aggression and further research is needed to understand the short- and long-term impact of these programs on EDA.

At the college level, student feedback suggests that, from the time students are oriented to campus, universities can make policies about electronic aggression and resources for victims clearly available to students, and classes with online components can include information about respectful online communication in the course syllabus (Reed et al., 2015). These same recommendations can be made for middle and high schools, as having clear policies in place and plans for response and resources that students are aware of will increase the odds of compliance and increase the likelihood that students will seek help when needed. At all levels of the educational system, this includes clear statements in student codes of conduct, having a clear channel for reporting offenses, and clearly identified disciplinary steps (Ramos & Bennett, 2016). Other school-level interventions may be easier to achieve with younger students, for example, blocking of certain sites on school computers and regulations around personal cell phone use on middle or high school campuses, which may be less easily achieved at the college level.

Healthcare providers can also play a role in prevention and intervention efforts. Pediatricians and providers serving youth might consider including screeners for dating aggression that include electronic means in intake paperwork alongside questions about depression or anxiety that may be more commonly asked. School counselors should stay informed of the types of electronic media youth are currently using, and educate themselves on things such as privacy settings in order to be able to speak with students at their school about potentially risky electronic communication. Similarly, college counseling centers should include items about electronic aggression when screening for dating violence, and be prepared to work with college students who may be affected.

Conclusions

EDA is prevalent across adolescence and emerging adulthood, often coinciding with other types of more traditional aggression. Estimates of prevalence and correlates are difficult to ascertain, as the nature of media use is constantly changing, and methodological differences in research studies also limit generalizability and comparison across studies. Additional research is needed to better understand the factors that aid in predicting who will perpetrate or be the victim of EDA, as well as to better understand the ways in which, above and beyond or in conjunction with traditional dating aggression, EDA impacts young people in both the short and long term. EDA is likely part of a constellation of risky behaviors that emerge during adolescence and emerging adulthood, in part due to the developmental tasks of seeking autonomy, identity, intimacy, and affiliation. Parents, schools, and health care providers should be cognizant of the role of electronic media use in adolescents' and young adults' romantic relationships, and guide efforts at prevention and intervention of dating aggression generally to include electronic communication.

References

Arnett, J. J. (2000). Emerging adulthood: A theory of development from the late teens through the twenties. *American Psychologist, 55*, 469–480. doi:10.1037/0003-066X.55.5469

Arnett, J. J. (2004). *Emerging adulthood: The winding road from the late teens through the twenties.* London: Oxford University Press.

Bennett, D. C., Guran, E. L., Ramos, M. C., & Margolin, G. (2011). College students' electronic victimization in friendships and dating relationships: Anticipated distress and associations with risky behaviors. *Violence & Victims, 26*, 410–429. doi:10.1891/0886-6708.26.4.410

Beran, T. N., Rinaldi, C., Bickham, D. S., & Rich, M. (2012). Evidence for the need to support adolescents dealing with harassment and cyber-harassment: Prevalence, progression, and impact. *School Psychology International, 33*, 562–576. doi:10.1177/0143034312446976

Borrajo, E., Gámez-Guadix, M., & Calvete, E. (2015). Cyber dating abuse: Prevalence, context, and relationship with offline dating aggression. *Psychological Reports, 116*, 565–585. doi:10.2466/21doi:16.PR0.116k22w4

CHILDWISE. (2013). *The Monitor Trends Report 2013: Trends data from the CHILDWISE Monitor Report 1997–2012.* Retrieved from www.childwise.co.uk/childwisepublished-research-detail.asp?PUBLISH=53

Cutbush, S., Williams, J., Miller, S., Gibbs, D., & Clinton-Sherrod, M., (2012, October). *Electronic dating aggression among middle school students: Demographic correlates and associations with other types of violence.* Poster presented at the American Public Health Association annual meeting, San Francisco, CA. Retrieved from https://www.rti.org/sites/default/files/resources/apha12_cutbush_poster.pdf

Cutbush, S., Ashley, O.S., Kan, M.L., Hampton, J. & Hall, D.M. (2010, November). *Electronic aggression among adolescent dating partners: Demographic correlates and associations with other types of violence.* Poster presented at the American Public Health Association annual meeting, Denver, CO. Retrieved from https://www.rti.org/sites/default/files/resources/apha10_cutbush_poster.pdf

Davis, K. (2012). Friendship 2.0: Adolescents' experiences of belonging and self-disclosure online. *Journal of Adolescence, 35*, 1527–1536. doi:10.1016/j.adolescence.2012.02.013

de Bruijn, P., Burrie, I., & vanWel, F. (2006). A risky boundary: Unwanted sexual behavior among youth. *Journal of Sexual Aggression, 12*, 81–96. doi:10.1080/13552600600841631

De Koker, P., Mathews, C., Zuch, M., Bastien, S., & Mason-Jones, A. J. (2014). A systematic review of interventions for preventing adolescent intimate partner violence. *Journal of Adolescent Health, 54*(1), 3–13. doi:10.1080/15388220.2014.963231

Decker, M. R., Silverman, J. G., & Raj, A. (2005). Dating violence and sexually transmitted disease/HIV testing and diagnosis among adolescent females. *Pediatrics, 116*, e272–e276. doi:10.1542/peds.2005-0194

Dick, R. N., McCauley, H. L., Jones, K. A., Tancredi, D. J., Goldstein, S., Blackburn, S., … & Miller, E. (2014). Cyber dating abuse among teens using school-based health centers. *Pediatrics, 134*, e1560–e1567. doi:10.1542/peds.2014-0537

Draucker, C. B., & Martsolf, D. S. (2010). The role of electronic communication technology in adolescent dating violence. *Journal of Child and Adolescent Psychiatric Nursing, 23*, 133–142. doi:10.1111/j.1744-6171.2010.00235.x

Eaton, D. K., Davis, K. S., Barrios, L., Brener, N. D., & Noonan, R. K. (2007). Associations of dating violence victimization with lifetime participation, co-occurrence, and early initiation of risk behaviors among U.S. high school students. *Journal of Interpersonal Violence, 22*, 585–602. doi:10.1177/0886260506298831

Elkind, D. (1976). *Child development and education: A Piagetian perspective*. New York: Oxford University Press.

Erikson, E. (1959). *Identity and the life cycle*. New York: W. W. Norton.

Forke, C. M., Myers, R. K., Catallozzi, M., & Schwarz, D. F. (2008). Relationship violence among female and male college undergraduate students. *Archives of Pediatrics & Adolescent Medicine, 162*, 634–641. doi:10.1001/archpedi.162.7.634

Gradinger, P., Yanagida, T., Strohmeier, D., & Spiel, C. (2015). Prevention of cyberbullying and cyber victimization: Evaluation of the ViSC Social Competence Program. *Journal of School Violence, 14*, 87–110. doi:10.1080/15388220.2014.963231

Guo, S. (2016). A meta-analysis of the predictors of cyberbullying perpetration and victimization. *Psychology in The Schools, 53*(4), 432–453. doi:10.1002/pits.21914

Hill, J. (1983). Early adolescence: A framework. *Journal of Early Adolescence, 3*, 1–21. doi:10.1177/027243168331002

Hines, D. A., & Saudino, K. J. (2003). Gender differences in psychological, physical, and sexual aggression among college students using the Revised Conflict Tactics Scales. *Violence and Victims, 18*, 197. doi:10.1891/vivi.2003.18.2.197

Juvonen, J., & Gross, E. F. (2008). Extending the school grounds?—Bullying experiences in cyberspace. *Journal of School Health, 78*, 496–505. doi:10.1111/j.1746-1561.2008.00335.x

Kaiser Family Foundation (2010). *Total media exposure, by age*. Media and health. Retrieved from: http://facts.kff.org/chart.aspx?ch=1368

Kast, N. R., Eisenberg, M. E., & Sieving, R. E. (2016). The role of parent communication and connectedness in dating violence victimization among Latino adolescents. *Journal of Interpersonal Violence, 31*, 1932–1955. doi:10.1177/0886260515570750

Kellerman, I., Margolin, G., Borofsky, L. A., Baucom, B. R., & Iturralde, E. (2013). Electronic aggression among emerging adults: Motivations and contextual factors. *Emerging Adulthood, 1*, 293–304. doi:10.1177/2167696813490159.

Kowalski, R. M., Giumetti, G. W., Schroeder, A. N., & Lattanner, M. R. (2014). Bullying in the digital age: A critical review and meta-analysis of cyberbullying research among youth. *Psychological Bulletin, 140*, 1073–1137. doi:10.1037/a0035618

Lampe, C., Ellison, N., & Steinfield, C. (2006, November). A Face (book) in the crowd: Social searching vs. social browsing. In *Proceedings of the 2006 20th anniversary conference on computer supported cooperative work* (pp. 167–170). New York: ACM.

Leisring, P. A., & Giumetti, G. W. (2014). Sticks and stones may break my bones, but abusive text messages can also hurt: Development and validation of the Cyber

Psychological Abuse (CPA) Scale. *Partner Abuse, 5*(3), 323–341. doi:10.1891/1946-6560.5.3.323

Lenhart, A., Purcell, K., Smith, A., & Zickuhr, K. (2010). *Social media and mobile Internet use among teens and young adults*. Pew and American Life Project. PEW Research Centre. Retrieved from www.pewinternet.org/~/media/Files/Reports/2010/PIP_Social_Media_and_Young_Adults_Report_Final_with_toplines.pdf

Lenhart, A., Rainie, L., & Lewis, O. (2001). *Teenage life online: The rise of the instant-message generation and the internet's impact on friendships and family relationships*. Pew Research Center. Retrieved from www.pewinternet.org/pdfs/PIP_Teens_Report.pdf

Lenhart, A. (2015). *Teen, social media and technology overview 2015*. Pew Research Center. Retrieved from http://assets.pewresearch.org/wp-content/uploads/sites/14/2015/04/PI_TeensandTech_Update2015_0409151.pdf

Li, Q. (2006). Cyberbullying in schools: A research of gender differences. *School Psychology International, 27*, 157–170. doi:10.1177/0143034306064547

Livingstone, S. (2007). From family television to bedroom culture: Young people's media at home. In E. Devereux (Ed.), *Media studies: Key issues and debates* (pp 303–321). London, UK: SAGE Publications.

Mesch, G. S. (2009). Parental mediation, online activities, and cyberbullying. *CyberPsychology & Behavior, 12*, 387–393. doi:10.1089/cpb.2009.0068

Mishna, F., McLuckie, A., & Saini, M. (2009). Real-world dangers in an online reality: A qualitative study examining online relationships and cyber abuse. *Social Work Research, 33*, 107–118. doi:10.1093/swr/33.2.107

Mnet. (2001). *Young Canadians in a Wired World*. Retrieved from http://www.media-awareness.ca/english/special_initiatives/surveys/index.cfm

Pallitto, C. C., Campbell, J. C., & O'Campo, P. (2005). Is intimate partner violence associated with unintended pregnancy? A review of the literature. *Trauma, Violence, & Abuse, 6*, 217–235. doi:10.1177/1524838005277441

Pew Research Center. (2018). *Social media use in 2018*. Retrieved from http://assets.pewresearch.org/wp-content/uploads/sites/14/2018/03/01105133/PI_2018.03.01_Social-Media_FINAL.pdf

Picard, P. (2007). *Tech abuse in teen relationships*. Chicago, IL: Teen Research Unlimited. Retrieved from http://www.loveisrespect.org/wp-content/uploads/2009/03/liz-claiborne-2007-tech-relationship-abuse.pdf.

Ramos, M. C., & Bennett, D. C. (2016). Cyberbullying: Who hurts, and why. *Psychiatric Times, 33*, 20–25. Retrieved from http://www.psychiatrictimes.com/special-reports/cyberbullying-who-hurts-and-why

Ramos, M. C., Miller, K. F., Moss, I. K., & Margolin, G. (2017). Perspective-taking and empathy mitigate family-of-origin risk for electronic aggression perpetration toward dating partners: A brief report. *Journal of Interpersonal Violence*. Advance online publication. doi:10.1177/0886260517747605

Reddy, S. D., Negi, L. T., Dodson-Lavelle, B., Ozawa-de Silva, B., Pace, T. W., Cole, S. P., … Craighead, L. W. (2013). Cognitive-based compassion training: A promising prevention strategy for at-risk adolescents. *Journal of Child and Family Studies, 22*, 219–230. doi:10.1007/s10826-012-95717

Reed, L. A., Tolman, R. M., & Safyer, P. (2015). Too close for comfort: Attachment insecurity and electronic intrusion in college students' dating relationships. *Computers in Human Behavior, 50*, 431–438. doi:10.1016/j.chb.2015.03.050

Reed, L.A., Tolman, R.M., Ward, L. M., & Safyer, P. (2016) Keeping tabs: Attachment anxiety and electronic intrusion in high school dating relationships. *Computers in Human Behavior, 58*, 259–268. doi:10.1016/j.chb.2015.12.019

Reed, L.A., Tolman, R.M., & Ward, L.M. (2016). Snooping and sexting: Digital media as a context for dating aggression and abuse among college students. *Violence Against Women, 22*, 1556–1576. doi:10.1177/1077801216630143

Reed, L. A., Tolman, R. M., & Ward, L. M. (2017). Gender matters: Experiences and consequences of digital dating abuse victimization in adolescent dating relationships. *Journal of Adolescence, 59*, 79–89. doi:10.1016/j.adolescence.2017.05.015

Rosen, L. D., Cheever, N. A., & Carrier, L. M. (2008). The association of parenting style and child age with parental limit setting and adolescent MySpace behavior. *Journal of Applied Developmental Psychology, 29*, 459–471. doi:10.1016/j.appdev.2008.07.005

Russell, S. T., Franz, B. T., & Driscoll, A. K. (2001). Same-sex romantic attraction and experiences of violence in adolescence. *American Journal of Public Health, 91*, 903–906.

Schulenberg, J. E., Bryant, A. L., & O'Malley, P. M. (2004). Taking hold of some kind of life: How developmental tasks relate to trajectories of well-being during the transition to adulthood. *Development and Psychopathology, 16*, 1119–1140. doi:10.1017/S0954579404040167

Schulenberg, J. E., Sameroff, A. J., & Cicchetti, D. (2004). The transition to adulthood as a critical juncture in the course of psychopathology and mental health. *Development and Psychopathology, 16*, 799–806. doi:10.1017/S0954579404040015

Shapiro, L. A. S., & Margolin, G. (2014). Growing up wired: Social networking sites and adolescent psychosocial development. *Clinical Child and Family Psychology Review, 17*, 1–18. doi:10.1007/s10567-013-0135-1

Shorey, R. C., Stuart, G. L., & Cornelius, T. L. (2011). Dating violence and substance use in college students: A review of the literature. *Aggression and Violent Behavior, 16*, 541–550. doi:10.1016/j.avb.2011.08.003

Stonard, K. E., Bowen, E.Lawrence, T. R., & Price, S. A. (2014). The relevance of technology to the nature, prevalence and impact of adolescent dating violence and abuse: A research synthesis. *Aggression and Violent Behavior, 19*, 390–417. doi:10.1016/j.avb.2014.06.005

Stonard, K. E., Bowen, E., Walker, K., & Price, S. A. (2017). "They'll always find a way to get to you": Technology use in adolescent romantic relationships and its role in dating violence and abuse. *Journal of Interpersonal Violence, 32*, 2083–2117. doi:10.1177/0886260515590787

Straus, M. A. (2004). Prevalence of violence against dating partners by male and female university students worldwide. *Violence Against Women, 10*, 790–811. doi:10.1177/1077801204265552

Subrahmanyam, K., & Greenfield, P. (2008). Online communication and adolescent relationships. *The Future of Children, 18*, 119–146. doi:10.1353/foc.0.0006

Sullivan, T. N., Farrell, A. D., & Kliewer, W. (2006). Peer victimization in early adolescence Association between physical and relation victimization and drug use, aggression, and delinquent behaviors among urban middle school students. *Development and Psychopathology, 18*, 119–137. doi:10.1017/S095457940606007X

Teitelman, A. M., Ratcliffe, S. J., Morales-Aleman, M. M., & Sullivan, C. M. (2008). Sexual relationship power, intimate partner violence, and condom use among minority urban girls. *Journal of Interpersonal Violence, 23*, 1694–1712. doi:10.1177/0886260508314331

Tokunaga, R. S. (2010). Following you home from school: A critical review and synthesis of research on cyberbullying victimization. *Computers in Human Behavior, 26*, 277–287. doi:10.1016/j.chb.2009.11.014

Valkenburg, P. M., Sumter, S. R., & Peter, J. (2011). Gender differences in online and offline self- disclosure in pre-adolescence and adolescence. *British Journal of Developmental Psychology, 29*, 253–269. doi:10.1348/2044-835X.002001.

Wolak, J., Mitchell, K. J, & Finkelhor, D. (2007). Does online harassment constitute bullying? An exploration of online harassment by known peers and online-only contacts. *Journal of Adolescent Health, 41*, S51–S58. doi:10.1016/j.jadohealth.2007.08.019

Wolford-Clevenger, C., Zapor, H., Brasfield, H., Febres, J., Elmquist, J., Brem, M., … & Stuart, G. L. (2016). An examination of the Partner Cyber Abuse Questionnaire in a college student sample. *Psychology of Violence, 6*, 156–162. doi:10.1037/a0039442

Wright, M. F. (2015). Cyber aggression within adolescents' romantic relationships: Linkages to parental and partner attachment. *Journal of Youth and Adolescence, 44*, 37–47. doi:10.1007/s10964-014-0147-2

Wright, M. F. (2017). Intimate partner aggression and adult attachment insecurity: The mediation of jealousy and anger. *Evolutionary Behavioral Sciences, 11*, 187–198. doi:10.1037/ebs0000097

Yahner, J., Dank, M., Zweig, J. M., & Lachman, P. (2015). The co-occurrence of physical and cyber dating violence and bullying among teens. *Journal of Interpersonal Violence, 30*, 1079–1089. doi:10.1177/0886260514540324

Ybarra, M. L., Diener-West, M., & Leaf, P. J. (2007). Examining the overlap in Internet harassment and school bullying: Implications for school intervention. *Journal of Adolescent Health, 41*, S42–S50. doi:10.1016/j.jadohealth.2007.09.004

Zweig, J. M., Dank, M., Yahner, J., & Lachman, P. (2013). The rate of cyber dating abuse among teens and how it relates to other forms of teen dating violence. *Journal of Youth and Adolescence, 42*, 1063–1077. doi:10.1007/s10964-013-9922-8

Zweig, J. M., Lachman, P., Yahner, J., & Dank, M. (2014). Correlates of cyber dating abuse among teens. *Journal of Youth and Adolescence, 43*, 1306–1321. doi:10.1007/s10964-013-0047-x

12

CYBERBULLYING IN SCHOOLS, WORKPLACES, AND ROMANTIC RELATIONSHIPS

Summary and Future Research

Gary W. Giumetti and Robin M. Kowalski

Across the chapters in this edited volume, authors have painted a picture of the prevalence, measurement, and correlates of involvement with cyberbullying across three contexts (schools, workplaces, and romantic relationships) and from multiple lenses (cross-cultural and developmental). From these chapters, we can see that cyberbullying is a prevalent phenomenon among school-aged children, romantic relationship partners, and employees in the workforce. It is also clear that cyberbullying is linked with a host of negative outcomes for school-aged children, romantic relationship partners, and working adults. We are also able to understand the global nature of this phenomenon and the challenges of conducting cross-cultural research on cyberbullying. In addition, we can begin to see how the developmental changes in individuals across the lifespan might be related to cyberbullying victimization and perpetration.

In the current chapter, we summarize the key themes that emerged in the preceding chapters related to cyberbullying in schools, the workplace, and in romantic relationships. We also discuss similarities and differences in the research findings across contexts, age groups, and cultures. Then, we outline a series of future research directions related to cyberbullying in schools, in the workplace, and in romantic relationships. Finally, we highlight the need for more cross-contextual, longitudinal research on cyberbullying to help us better understand the many lenses and perspectives of electronic mistreatment. We start by examining the themes that emerged from the three chapters focusing on cyberbullying across cultures (Smith, Görzig, & Robinson, Chapter 4, this volume; Richard, Walsh, & Zhou, Chapter 7, this volume; Calvete, Gámez-Guadix, & Borrajo, Chapter 10, this volume).

Key Themes in Cross-Cultural Research Across Contexts

In their chapter on cyberbullying in schools: cross-cultural issues, Smith et al. (Chapter 4, this volume) reviewed two large-scale cross-national survey studies that examined cyberbullying (the EU Kids Online survey, Livingstone, Haddon, Görzig, & Ólafsson, 2011; and the Health Behavior of School-aged Children survey, Inchley et al., 2016). They report a surprising lack of agreement across these two large-scale surveys in terms of cross-country differences in rates of cyberbullying victimization. Smith and colleagues highlight a number of possible reasons why there may be a lack of agreement between these two large-scale surveys. Several of these reasons also emerged as themes in the other cross-cultural chapters in this book. We review these themes below.

Differences in What the Term for Cyberbullying Means

Smith et al. (Chapter 4, this volume) and Richard et al. (Chapter 7, this volume) both highlight how a major challenge for cross-cultural research on bullying or cyberbullying is differences in the label used for bullying or how it is defined in a given culture. For example, Smith et al. (Chapter 4, this volume) note that the translation of the word cyberbullying to other languages may not be as precise or have the same meaning, which could impact the prevalence rates across countries (see also Smith, Cowie, Olafsson, & Liefooghe, 2002). Additionally, Smith et al. (Chapter 4, this volume) point out that there are differences in whether the main elements of cyberbullying, specifically power imbalance, were present in the two cross-national studies, which could give rise to differences in prevalence rates. Richard et al. (Chapter 7, this volume) highlight a study by Escartín, Zapf, Arrieta, and Rodríguez-Carballeira (2011) that identified differences in how bullying is defined by employees from Central America vs. Southern Europe. For example, Central American employees included both physical and psychological behaviors in their definition of bullying, whereas Southern European employees included only psychological behaviors. Given these challenges in labeling cyberbullying, cross-cultural researchers need to take extra care to ensure that participants understand the meaning and the key components of the term cyberbullying.

Differences in Cultural Values

Smith et al. (Chapter 4, this volume), Richard et al. (Chapter 7, this volume), and Calvete et al. (Chapter 10, this volume) all underscore the role of cultural values (e.g., Hofstede, 1980) in understanding cross-cultural differences in cyberbullying prevalence rates. Smith et al. (Chapter 4, this volume) reviewed research that predicted cyberbullying prevalence rates would be higher in individualistic cultures (e.g., Ji, Zhang, & Jones, 2016). However, Migliaccio and Rauskauskas (2015) found the opposite – bullying was lower in individualistic countries than collectivist countries, which Smith and colleagues predict is due to greater regulatory frameworks in highly individualistic societies. Smith and colleagues also predict that Hofstede's (1980) dimensions, other than individualism/collectivism, such as power distance, masculinity-femininity, and uncertainty avoidance might influence cyberbullying prevalence rates.

Richard and colleagues (Chapter 7, this volume) also highlight the possible role that Hofstede's (1980) cultural values may play in looking at cross-cultural differences in workplace cyberbullying by presenting evidence from the traditional workplace bullying literature. They highlight findings from D'Cruz, Paull, Omari, and Guneri-Cangarli (2016) that found higher rates of supervisor bullying in Turkey and India (higher power-distance countries) than Australia (lower power-distance country). Richard et al. also note the predictions by Jacobson, Hood, and Van Buren (2014) that covert bullying (such as cyberbullying) might be more common in cultures low on assertiveness, high on in-group collectivism, or low on power distance. Lastly, Richard et al. also highlight that cultural differences in the variables of context (e.g., high context vs. low context cultures) and face (i.e., honor, respectability, or dignity) may influence the perceptions of cyberbullying. For example, individuals in high context cultures (such as Japan, Korea, or China) rely heavily on contextual cues and non-verbal behavioral displays. As such, individuals in high context cultures may have more difficulty understanding the meaning behind email messages (as a lean form of communication, which lack many contextual cues) than individuals in low context cultures. Thus, misunderstandings during email exchanges may be more common in these cultures.

In the romantic relationships context, Calvete et al. (Chapter 10, this volume) focus on slightly different cultural variables, including justification for violence and machismo. They note that differences in justification for violence are linked with cyber abuse in romantic relationships, as well as adherence to traditional gender role beliefs and stereotypes. Additionally, differences in machismo (which is a Latin culture-based stereotype that equates masculinity with being tough and macho) might make retaliatory cyber abusive behaviors more likely (Durán & Martínez-Pecino, 2015).

Taken together, the three chapters exploring cyberbullying across cultures provide us with a number of important considerations when designing future research studies that span national borders and cultural backgrounds. We will describe a number of these ideas in the future research directions at the end of this chapter. In the next section, we will describe some of the key themes that emerged from the three chapters focusing on developmental perspectives on cyberbullying (Englander, Chapter 5, this volume; Mowry & Giumetti, Chapter 8, this volume; Bennett & Ramos, Chapter 11, this volume).

Key Themes in Developmental Perspectives Across Contexts

As individuals move from childhood to adolescence to adulthood, they move through at least three different contexts: school, romantic relationships, and the workplace. Within each of these developmental periods, researchers have attempted to describe age-related changes in prevalence and outcomes of cyberbullying. In this section, we now look across these three contexts and explore themes that emerge related to how the prevalence and outcomes of cyberbullying might change across the lifespan. Three major themes that emerged from the chapters focusing on developmental perspectives include access and use of technology, cognitive changes, and social changes in individuals across the lifespan.

Developmental Differences in Access and Use of Technology

As noted in Chapter 2, access to and use of technology changes as individuals age, and this may impact the prevalence and outcomes of cyberbullying. As Englander (Chapter 5, this volume) highlights, younger children are less likely to have their own smartphone or tablet, whereas almost all adolescents have their own smartphone (Anderson & Jiang, 2018; Englander, 2017). This alone might help to explain the relatively lower prevalence of cyberbullying experiences among younger as compared to older school-aged children. If an individual is not online, he/she cannot physically be involved with cyberbullying.

Among working adults, Mowry and Giumetti (Chapter 8, this volume) highlight that younger employees (i.e., young adults) are more likely to access and use different information and communication technologies (ICTs) than older employees. Thus, it is not surprising that younger adults are more likely to experience cyberbullying than older adults (Center for the Digital Future, 2017; Duggan, 2017). Looking across the lifespan, then, we might expect to see an inverted-U shaped relationship between age and cyberbullying involvement. That is, younger children and older adults might experience the least amount of cyberbullying, and adolescents and young adults might experience the greatest amount of cyberbullying.

Bennett and Ramos (Chapter 11, this volume) point out that adolescents and young adults in romantic relationships are equally as likely to own smartphones and spend time on social media. For example, the Pew Research Center indicates that 94% of young adults (age 18–29) own a smartphone (Pew Research Center, 2018), as compared to 95% of adolescents (Anderson & Jiang, 2018). Thus, technology access and use alone may not be as useful for explaining differences in cyberbullying prevalence between these two age groups. Thus, next, we will explore two other factors that emerged as themes across these three contexts that may help us understand developmental differences in cyberbullying.

Cognitive Changes across the Lifespan

Beyond access and use of technology, individuals also experience changes in cognitive development as they age, and these changes may be associated with involvement in cyberbullying across contexts. As Englander (Chapter 5, this volume) highlights, younger children are still at Piaget's concrete-operational stage of cognitive development, and thus might not understand abstract concepts. Thus, they may be more likely to incorrectly interpret vague online communications (Kota, Schoohs, Benson, & Moreno, 2014) or even misunderstand what the term cyberbullying means, as compared to older children and adolescents (Englander, 2017).

During adolescence, the ability to reflect on one's own thoughts improves, and so teens tend to think more about themselves during this stage (Berk, 2018). This self-concern, as Bennett and Ramos (Chapter 11, this volume) point out, is related to greater self-consciousness and perceptions that there is an imaginary audience watching them at all times. During this age, adolescents may be more likely to misinterpret vague cues in their online interactions and view feedback as more negative than intended. This may make adolescents more likely to perceive cyberbullying. During emerging adulthood, planning, reasoning, and decision making improve and thinking becomes more abstract (Berk, 2018). However, as Bennett and Ramos (Chapter 11, this volume) highlight, increased autonomy and exploration during this age may be linked with increased risky behaviors, including electronic dating abuse. Thus, researchers have linked different aspects of cognitive development with cyberbullying in romantic relationships for adolescents and emerging adults.

Mowry and Giumetti (Chapter 8, this volume) highlight that older adults experience a number of mental and physical changes (such as slower processing of information, decreased memory, and reduced ability to inhibit impulses, Berk, 2018) as they age, and these changes may be linked with decreased coping abilities. As a result, Mowry and Giumetti speculate that one way that age and cyberbullying may interact to predict outcomes is that older workers may be more negatively impacted by interpersonal mistreatment such as cyberbullying than younger workers. Thus, looking across the three contexts, researchers have described how possible changes in cognitive development at different ages may be related to different experiences with cyberbullying.

Social Changes across the Lifespan

In addition to cognitive changes, individuals also experience changes in their social development and social goals as they grow from childhood to adulthood. Developmental researchers note that prosocial behavior tends to increase among children 6 to 11 years old and physically aggressive behaviors tend to decrease (Berk, 2018). However, children at this age are also beginning to concern themselves with peer groups and social acceptance (Berk, 2018). Among school-aged children, Englander (Chapter 5, this volume) notes that younger children may be more likely to make social errors such as underestimating the emotional impact of an online message (Englander, 2015). Younger children may also be less well informed about cyberbullying, as education about cyberbullying is less common in elementary school than in middle and high school (Eden, Heiman, & Olenik-Shemush, 2013).

Among romantic couples, Bennett and Ramos (Chapter 11, this volume) note that adolescence is a time when individuals are pursuing many social goals, including several in the areas of identity and intimacy. As such, they may be more likely to establish and maintain a romantic relationship using technology. This increased time spent online with a romantic partner may put them at increased risk for cyber dating abuse victimization (Stonard, Bowen, Walker, & Price, 2017). Bennett and Ramos note that emerging adulthood is also a time for identity exploration, and that young adults often experience instability as they try out different experiences in life. Additionally, emerging adults typically experience less supervision from parents or school officials, and so they may be more vulnerable to the negative outcomes of cyberbullying.

Mowry and Giumetti (Chapter 8, this volume) state that older adults may place more value on social interactions and goals than younger adults (e.g., see Carstensen, Isaacowitz, & Charles, 1999), which could mean that older adults are more negatively impacted by cyberbullying than younger adults are. Another possibility is that older workers will be less negatively impacted by cyberbullying than younger workers, due to becoming more emotionally stable, more emotionally competent, and more effectively using coping resources (e.g., see Shirom, Gilboa, Fried, & Cooper, 2008). These possibilities are recommended as avenues for future research. In the next section, we will discuss a number of other possible directions for future research. First, we will describe themes that emerged across the chapters as future research directions. Then, we will describe future research directions that could be pursued across contexts.

Future Research Directions

Research on cyberbullying is still in its relative infancy, with the first papers on the topic of online harassment emerging in 2000 (Finkelhor, Mitchell, & Wolak, 2000). A recent search of PsycINFO (in September, 2018) reveals that at least 2,000 published studies have been performed on cyberbullying to date, and the number of studies published each month continues to rise. Given the amount of media and research attention on the topic, we hope to offer several possible avenues for future research that will help to push the field toward a better understanding of cyberbullying across cultures, developmental stages, and contexts. In the first section below, we provide a summary of the themes that emerged from the chapters in this volume regarding future research. Then, we describe some additional directions for research that span contexts.

Themes for Future Research

Across Chapters 2 through 11 of this book, experts have offered many possible directions for future research. We have identified the following six themes that were mentioned across multiple chapters as future research recommendations: 1) more longitudinal research; 2) more sophisticated research designs; 3) examining other predictors and outcomes of cyberbullying; 4) more work on younger and older individuals and their experiences with cyberbullying; 5) more work that develops and tests the efficacy of prevention or intervention efforts; and, 6) more work to explore the role of cultural variables and how they relate to differences in cyberbullying across countries and contexts. We will summarize these directions for future research below.

More longitudinal research. Nearly every chapter in this book has recommended that future researchers use longitudinal research designs to study cyberbullying in the future. For example, Leisring (Chapter 9, this volume) recommends that future researchers use longitudinal designs to understand whether cyberbullying in romantic relationships precedes or comes after other forms of relationship abuse. Additionally, Richard et al. (Chapter 7, this volume) recommend that researchers conduct longitudinal studies to explore the cross-level relationships between cultural values and reactions to or perceptions of cyberbullying. Across contexts, much of our understanding of cyberbullying is based on studies involving cross-sectional designs (that is, designs where each variable was measured at only one point in time). This type of design can provide only one of the three forms of information needed to establish causality, namely covariance. That is, cross-sectional designs can only tell us that a set of variables is related, but little else. Two other forms of information are needed to establish causality, namely temporal precedence and ruling out third variable explanations. Examining the patterns of relationships among predictors, cyberbullying experiences, and outcomes at different measurement occasions can begin to help us understand the temporal ordering of these phenomena.

However, as Ployhart and Vandenberg (2010) reported, two waves of data collection are not sufficient for understanding dynamic relationships among variables. Thus, researchers wishing to conduct longitudinal studies of cyberbullying should collect data on the hypothesized variables during three or more waves of measurement. To meet the last criterion to support causal claims, researchers should take care to identify and control for possible confounding variables in their studies (see Spector & Brannick, 2011; and Carlson & Wu, 2012, for a list of recommended practices when dealing with control variables).

More sophisticated research designs. Beyond longitudinal research designs, several chapters also called for researchers to explore other, more sophisticated research designs. For example, Scisco (Chapter 6, this volume) recommends that researchers use laboratory experiments with mock work situations or vignettes. As with the recommendation above for more longitudinal research, using experimental designs (with control groups, random assignment, and other experimental controls) will also help to provide evidence for causal linkages between predictors, cyberbullying experiences, and outcomes.

Additionally, both Scisco (Chapter 6, this volume) and Bauman and Meter (Chapter 3, this volume) recommend examining models of cyberbullying that involve mediation and moderation (such as the Emotion Reaction Model of Vranjes, Baillien, Vandebosch, Erreygers, & De Witte, 2017). Examining cyberbullying in a more comprehensive framework will help us better understand the "how and for whom" behind cyberbullying. That is, testing assumed mediation models will uncover the mechanisms for how cyberbullying relates to outcomes. For example, when an individual experiences cyberbullying as a victim, what impact does this have on his/her cognitive and affective state, and how does this subsequently relate to appraisal of the situation and later outcomes (cf. Kowalski, Giumetti, Schroeder, & Lattanner, 2014)? Researchers interested in testing mediation models should ensure that their studies follow the recommendations for adequately testing assumed mediation models (e.g., see Stone-Romero & Rosopa, 2008, 2011), including the use of randomized experimental designs where the predictor and mediator are manipulated, and the outcome is measured.

Additionally, testing models that involve individual difference variables (such as age, gender, race/ethnicity, personality, intelligence, resilience) as moderators may reveal for whom cyberbullying has a greater impact. For example, are individuals with higher levels of trait anger more likely to react with cyberbullying perpetration in response to receiving a series of aggressive text messages than individuals with lower trait anger? Aspects of the situation may also serve as moderators of predictor → cyberbullying relationships or cyberbullying → outcome relationships. For example, past research has found that greater parental monitoring weakens the relationship between being a cyberbullying victim and subsequent retaliation with cyberbullying perpetration (Hood & Duffy, 2018). Researchers should explore the moderating role of other situational factors such as social support, school climate, and perceived anonymity in future research.

Examine other predictors and outcomes. A number of chapter authors in this volume recommended that future researchers explore other possible predictors and outcomes of cyberbullying. In terms of predictors, authors have recommended examining variables at three levels of analysis: micro (individual or psychological variables), meso (social or group-level variables), and macro (society or cultural level variables). At the micro level, authors in this volume recommend that future research explore demographic variables (such as SES, gender, age, sexual orientation) and individual differences (such as coping styles, disability status, academic achievement, moral disengagement, and personality traits such as anger, narcissism, psychopathy, Machiavellianism, and emotional intelligence) as predictors of cyberbullying involvement. At the group, social, or meso level, authors in this volume recommend examining the links between cyberbullying and a number of variables, such as parental involvement, peer influences, school climate, workplace policies, social support, family-to-work conflict, high work demands, poor leadership, and climate for organizational justice. Finally, at the macro or societal level, authors in this volume recommend that researchers explore how cyberbullying is influenced by such variables as socio-economic stratification, regulatory frameworks, technological infrastructure, education systems, and cultural values (cf. EU Kids Online model, Chapter 4, this volume).

In terms of outcomes, chapter authors recommended that future researchers explore how cyberbullying relates to a number of possible effects or sequelae of cyberbullying. These include examining linkages between workplace cyberbullying and physical health or psychophysiology, symptoms of post-traumatic stress disorder, organizational commitment, sickness absence, job dissatisfaction, and counterproductive workplace behaviors (Scisco, Chapter 6, this volume). Additionally, authors recommended exploring how cyberbullying in romantic relationships links with relationship outcomes, such as dyadic adjustment or relationship dissolution (Calvete et al., Chapter 10, this volume).

More work on younger and older individuals. As Englander (Chapter 5, this volume) and Mowry and Giumetti (Chapter 9, this volume) note, there is more research needed that examines the cyberbullying experiences of younger individuals (that is, children in elementary school) and older adults. Englander describes how parents today are more likely to allow their children to use a tablet or smartphone to play social games or watch online videos. With this increased time spent online and in possible contact with others, younger children may be at risk for cyberbullying victimization. However, very little research has attempted to study children in elementary school or younger. Given the increasing use of technology among young children and the growing adoption of technology by older adults, studies should aim to uncover the prevalence of cyberbullying among these age groups as well as the possible negative outcomes of experiencing cyberbullying. As technology use becomes more and more prevalent across all age groups, longitudinal research would help to demonstrate the stability of the predicted U-shaped relationship between age and cyberbullying involvement. With the passage of time, one might expect the U-shaped function to lose some of its curve.

Testing the efficacy of prevention or intervention efforts. Whereas there are many programs being developed by schools, communities, states, and national governments to tackle the problem of bullying and cyberbullying, there are relatively few published studies that evaluate the effectiveness of these prevention or intervention efforts. Chapter authors from this volume made a number of useful recommendations for future studies on prevention and intervention efforts. Specifically, Bauman and Meter (Chapter 3, this volume) recommend that the target population for the intervention (e.g., children in school) be involved in developing the features of such interventions so that the programs are more interesting and relevant to the individuals who will be the focus of the intervention. Bennett and Ramos (Chapter 11, this volume) recommend that intervention programs be of a longer duration and involve multiple levels of support (e.g., individual, peer, family, and school) in order to be the most effective (De Koker, Mathews, Zuch,

Bastien, & Mason-Jones, 2014; Guo, 2016). Additionally, Scisco (Chapter 6, this volume) highlights the fact that no existing research has examined the efficacy of workplace cyberbullying prevention or intervention approaches. She also mentions that future research on interventions needs to understand the racial/ethnic and cultural contexts in which cyberbullying interventions are taking place. After establishing effective cyberbullying interventions, we hope that the rate of cyberbullying perpetration will decrease and the quality of life for victims of cyberbullying will be improved in schools, workplaces, and romantic relationships.

Further exploring the role of cultural variables. Researchers across the globe have been studying cyberbullying and the evidence to date suggests that this phenomenon occurs in most of the world where humans interact with technology. As the authors of the cross-cultural chapters have highlighted, considerably more research is needed to help us better understand cross-cultural differences in the prevalence of cyberbullying as well as the predictors and outcomes of cyberbullying. For example, Smith et al. (Chapter 4, this volume) recommend that future cross-cultural studies build comprehensive models that account for country-level predictors of cyberbullying involvement, including socio-economic stratification and cultural values. With regard to specific cultural values, Richard and colleagues (Chapter 7, this volume) provide a host of research directions to explore related to specific cultural values from the Hofstede (1980) framework and how these might impact the sender, the message, and the receiver of cyberbullying communications. In addition, these authors recommend examining how other cultural variables such as face and context might influence how messages are constructed and perceived.

Additionally, Scisco (Chapter 6, this volume), Richard et al. (Chapter 7, this volume), and Calvete et al. (Chapter 10, this volume) recommend that future cross-cultural research translate existing measures of cyberbullying into other languages and demonstrate their validity. Additionally, researchers who conduct cyberbullying studies in different countries should use the same measure and procedures across cultures, as this will enable cross-cultural comparisons in prevalence rates that are based on the same measure, response scale, reporting time window, and procedures (Smith et al., Chapter 4, this volume). Without consistent definitions and measurement of cyberbullying, meaningful cross-cultural comparisons will not be possible.

Additional Directions for Future Research

In addition to the themes that emerged from the first 11 chapters of this book, we have several additional directions that future research might take. These include longitudinal cross-contextual research and multi-contextual research. We will describe each of these directions further below.

Longitudinal cross-contextual research. The majority of the research to date has examined one group of individuals in a single context (e.g., only at school) and at a single time point. In addition to the recommendations above for more longitudinal research, we also think that more research is needed that examines the phenomenon of cyberbullying across a longer timeframe and across contexts. Specifically, researchers should explore how cyberbullying experiences change as an individual changes contexts, such as when a child moves from middle school to high school, or from high school to college, or from college to the workforce. Multi-year prospective studies of cyberbullying are rare (for exceptions, see Hemphill et al., 2012; van den Eijnden, Vermulst, van Rooij, Scholte, & van de Mheen, 2014). If researchers were able to follow the same individuals across schools or from schools to the workforce, there are a number of possible research questions to explore. For example, how do experiences with cyberbullying change or stay the same as one moves into new schools or workplace environments? That is, are victims in middle school also likely to be victims in high school and college? In one of the few multi-year prospective studies of cyberbullying, Festl, Vogelgesang, Scharkow, and Quandt (2017) examined adolescents over a three-year period (including the transition from middle school to high school) and found that involvement with cyberbullying (e.g., not involved, involved) remained stable for many, but not all of these adolescents. How might this differ when students transition from high school to college or from college to the workforce? What are the variables that predict consistent involvement in cyberbullying from one setting to another across time?

In addition, researchers could explore the temporal stability of cyberbullying perpetration. That is, do students who perpetrate cyberbullying in high school or college also tend to perpetrate cyberbullying or engage in other counterproductive workplace behaviors once they enter the working world? Research on aggressive behavior suggests that this would be the case, as researchers have found a high degree of stability in aggression (Olweus, 1979). That is, individuals who are aggressive as children also tend to be aggressive as adults. Additionally, other research suggests that aggressiveness as a young child is linked with adult violence and adjustment problems (Farrington, 1991).

Another direction for longitudinal cross-contextual research is to examine the extent to which cyberbullying victimization at an early age (such as in middle school) is linked with negative outcomes at later life stages (e.g., college or the workforce) and how it fits into the broader social experiences of the individual. A review of the research on the long-term outcomes of childhood peer victimization by McDougall and Vaillancourt (2015) suggests that victimization in elementary school is linked with a number of later life outcomes, including heavy smoking in late adolescence (Niemelä et al., 2011) as well as problematic social relationships and lower educational achievement (Wolke, Copeland, Angold, & Costello, 2013), among others. Future research is needed that examines whether or not online victimization (perhaps on its own or in conjunction with traditional bullying) is linked with later life outcomes.

Multi-contextual research. In addition to exploring how experiences with cyberbullying change or stay the same for individuals across the lifespan, it would also be interesting to explore how cyberbullying experiences in one context (e.g., at school or work) might relate to cyberbullying experiences in another context (e.g., in a romantic relationship). Existing workplace research suggests that interpersonal mistreatment received at work spills over to the home life, leading to the mistreatment of one's partner at home. For example, Meier and Cho (2018) found that individuals who experienced workplace incivility were more likely to socially undermine their romantic partner at home, and this was partially explained by a lack of detachment from work as well as an increase in negative affect. Researchers who pursue this line of research could determine which predictors might relate to the spill-over of cyberbullying across contexts. Additionally, it would be important to examine whether individuals who experience cyberbullying across contexts are at greater risk of negative outcomes, and if so, to target intervention efforts to these individuals.

Conclusion

In the past 15 to 20 years, there has been a rapid proliferation of research on cyberbullying. However, there has been a lack of consensus among researchers on how cyberbullying should be defined, how it should be measured, how often cyberbullying occurs, which risk and protective factors are most closely tied to cyberbullying, and whether there are developmental and cultural variations in cyberbullying involvement. By focusing on the contexts (school, workplace, romantic relationships) and lenses (cross-cultural and developmental) through which research on cyberbullying can be examined, the current book evolved to bring clarity to some of these issues and to offer directions for future research that might shed light on others.

Examined as a whole, the current chapters point to the need for cyberbullying researchers to step back and take a broader look at the field as they conduct their research. For example, in defining cyberbullying for a particular study, investigators need to thoroughly examine how cyberbullying is conceptualized across cultures. Similarly, rather than continuing to often associate cyberbullying with middle school, a lifespan developmental approach that examines continuity (or the lack thereof) in cyberbullying involvement across developmental stages is more suitable. This not only allows us to more closely examine patterns in cyberbullying involvement, but also provides more information about risk and protective factors. Clearly, there is much still to be learned in this area, but the number of articles published monthly on the topic suggests that researchers are eager to do so.

References

Anderson, M., & Jiang, J. (2018, May 31). *Teens, social media, and technology 2018*. Retrieved from www.pewinternet.org/2018/05/31/teens-social-media-technology-2018/

Berk, L. E. (2018). *Development through the lifespan* (7th ed.). Hoboken, NJ: Pearson.

Carlson, K. D., & Wu, J. (2012). The illusion of statistical control: Control variable practice in management research. *Organizational Research Methods, 15*(3), 413–435. doi:10.1177/1094428111428817

Carstensen, L. L., Isaacowitz, D. M., & Charles, S. T. (1999). Taking time seriously: A theory of socioemotional selectivity. *American Psychologist, 54*(3), 165–181. doi:10.1037/0003-066X.54.3.doi:165

Center for the Digital Future. (2017). *The 2017 digital future report*. Retrieved from www.digitalcenter.org/wp-content/uploads/2018/04/2017-Digital-Future-Report-2.pdf

D'Cruz, P., Paull, M., Omari, M., & Guneri-Cangarli, B. (2016). Target experiences of workplace bullying: Insights from Australia, India and Turkey. *Employee Relations, 38*(5), 805–823. doi:10.1108/ER-06-2015-0116

De Koker, P., Mathews, C., Zuch, M., Bastien, S., & Mason-Jones, A. J. (2014). A systematic review of interventions for preventing adolescent intimate partner violence. *Journal of Adolescent Health, 54*(1), 3–13. doi:10.1080/15388220.2014.963231

Duggan, M. (2017). *Online harassment 2017*. Pew Research Center. Retrieved from www.pewinternet.org/2017/07/11/online-harassment-2017/

Durán, M., & Martínez-Pecino, R. (2015). Ciberacoso mediante teléfono móvil e Internet en las relaciones de noviazgo entre jóvenes. *Comunicar, 22*(44), 159–167. doi:10.3916/C44-2015-17

Eden, S., Heiman, T., & Olenik-Shemesh, D. (2013). Teachers' perceptions, beliefs and concerns about cyberbullying: Teachers' perceptions about cyberbullying. *British Journal of Educational Technology, 44*(6), 1036–1052. doi:10.1111/j.1467-8535.2012.01363.x

Englander, E. (2015). Section IV: It's not all cyberbullying: Different problem behaviors and perceptual factors online. In *Cyberbullying: Current & future research & directions: A White Paper submitted to the Institute of Child Development and Digital Media*. New York: Institute of Child Development and Digital Media.

Englander, E. (2017). Risky business. *Child & Adolescent Psychiatric Clinics of North America, 27*, 287–305.

Escartín, J., Zapf, D., Arrieta, C., & Rodríguez-Carballeira, Á. (2011). Workers' perception of workplace bullying: A cross-cultural study. *European Journal of Work and Organizational Psychology, 20*(2), 178–205. doi:10.1080/13594320903395652

Farrington, D. P. (1991). Childhood aggression and adult violence: Early precursors and later-life outcomes. In D. J. Pepler, K. H. Rubin (Eds.), *The development and treatment of childhood aggression* (pp. 5–29). Hillsdale, NJ: Lawrence Erlbaum Associates, Inc.

Festl, R., Vogelgesang, J., Scharkow, M., & Quandt, T. (2017). Longitudinal patterns of involvement in cyberbullying: Results from a latent transition analysis. *Computers in Human Behavior, 66*, 7–15. doi:10.1016/j.chb.2016. 09. 02doi:7

Finkelhor, D., Mitchell, K.J., & Wolak, J. (2000). *Online victimization: A report on the nation's youth*. Alexandria, VA: National Center for Missing and Exploited Children.

Guo, S. (2016). A meta-analysis of the predictors of cyberbullying perpetration and victimization. *Psychology in the Schools, 53*(4), 432–453. doi:10.1002/pits.21914

Hemphill, S. A., Kotevski, A., Tollit, M., Smith, R., Herrenkohl, T. I., Toumbourou, J. W., & Catalano, R. F. (2012). Longitudinal predictors of cyber and traditional bullying perpetration in Australian secondary school students. *Journal of Adolescent Health, 51*(1), 59–65. doi:10.1016/j.jadohealth.2011.11doi:019

Hofstede, G. (1980). *Culture's consequences: International differences in work-related values.* Newbury Park, CA: Sage Publications.

Hood, M., & Duffy, A. L. (2018). Understanding the relationship between cyber-victimisation and cyber-bullying on social network sites: The role of moderating factors. *Personality and Individual Differences, 133,* 103–108. doi:10.1016/j.paid.2017.doi:04.004

Inchley, J., Currie, D., Young, T., Samdal, O., Torsheim, T., Augustson, L., … Barnekow, V. (Eds.) (2016). *Growing up unequal: gender and socioeconomic differences in young people's health and well-being: Health Behaviour in School-aged Children (HBSC) study: International report from the 2013/2014 survey.* Copenhagen: WHO Regional Office for Europe.

Jacobson, K. J. L., Hood, J. N., & Van Buren, H. J., III. (2014). Workplace bullying across cultures: A research agenda. *International Journal of Cross Cultural Management, 14*(1), 47–65. doi:10.1177/1470595813494192

Ji, L., Zhang, W. & Jones, K. (2016). Children's experience of and attitudes towards bullying and victimization: A cross-cultural comparison between China and England. In P.K. Smith, K. Kwak & Y. Toda (Eds.), *School bullying in different cultures: Eastern and western perspectives* (pp. 170–188). Cambridge: Cambridge University Press.

Kota, R., Schoohs, S., Benson, M., & Moreno, M. (2014). Characterizing cyberbullying among college students: Hacking, dirty laundry, and mocking. *Societies, 4*(4), 549–560. doi:10.3390/soc4040549

Kowalski, R. M., Giumetti, G. W., Schroeder, A. N., & Lattanner, M. R. (2014). Bullying in the digital age: A critical review and meta-analysis of cyberbullying research among youth. *Psychological Bulletin, 140*(4), 1073–1137. doi:10.1037/a0035618

Livingstone, S., Haddon, L. G., Görzig, A., & Olafsson, K. (2011). *Technical Report and User Guide: The 2010 EU Kids Online Survey.* London, UK: London School of Economics and Political Science.

McDougall, P., & Vaillancourt, T. (2015). Long-term adult outcomes of peer victimization in childhood and adolescence: Pathways to adjustment and maladjustment. *American Psychologist, 70*(4), 300–310. doi:10.1037/a0039174

Meier, L. L., & Cho, E. (2018). Work stressors and partner social undermining: Comparing negative affect and psychological detachment as mechanisms. *Journal of Occupational Health Psychology.* Advance online publication. doi:10.1037/ocp0000120

Migliaccio, T. & Rauskauskas, J. (2015). *Bullying as a social experience: Social factors, prevention and intervention.* London: Routledge.

Niemelä, S., Brunstein-Klomek, A., Sillanmäki, L., Helenius, H., Piha, J., Kumpulainen, K.,…Sourander, A. (2011). Childhood bullying behaviors at age eight and substance use at age 18 among males. A nationwide prospective study. *Addictive Behaviors, 36,* 256–260. doi:10.1016/j.addbeh.2010.10.012

Olweus, D. (1979). Stability of aggressive reaction patterns in males: A review. *Psychological Bulletin, 86*(4), 852–875. doi:10.1037/0033-2909.86.4.852

Pew Research Center. (2018, February 5). *Mobile fact sheet.* Retrieved from http://www.pewinternet.org/fact-sheet/mobile/

Ployhart, R. E., & Vandenberg, R. J. (2010). Longitudinal research: The theory, design, and analysis of change. *Journal of Management, 36*(1), 94–120. doi:10.1177/0149206309352110

Shirom, A., Gilboa, S. S., Fried, Y., & Cooper, C. L. (2008). Gender, age and tenure as moderators of work-related stressors' relationships with job performance: A meta-analysis. *Human Relations*, *61*(10), 1371–1398. doi:10.1177/0018726708095708

Smith, P. K., Cowie, H., Olafsson, R. & Liefooghe, A. (2002). Definitions of bullying: a comparison of terms used, and age and sex differences, in a 14-country international comparison. *Child Development*, *73*, 1119–1133.

Spector, P. E., & Brannick, M. T. (2011). Methodological urban legends: The misuse of statistical control variables. *Organizational Research Methods*, *14*(2), 287–305. doi:10.1177/1094428110369842

Stonard, K. E., Bowen, E., Walker, K., & Price, S. A. (2017). "They'll always find a way to get to you": Technology use in adolescent romantic relationships and its role in dating violence and abuse. *Journal of Interpersonal Violence*, *32*, 2083–2117. doi:10.1177/0886260515590787

Stone-Romero, E. F., & Rosopa, P. J. (2008). The relative validity of inferences about mediation as a function of research design characteristics. *Organizational Research Methods*, *11*(2), 326–352. doi:10.1177/1094428107300342

Stone-Romero, E. F., & Rosopa, P. J. (2011). Experimental tests of mediation models: Prospects, problems, and some solutions. *Organizational Research Methods*, *14*(4), 631–646. doi:10.1177/1094428110372673

van den Eijnden, R., Vermulst, A., van Rooij, A. J., Scholte, R., & van de Mheen, D. (2014). The bidirectional relationships between online victimization and psychosocial problems in adolescents: A comparison with real-life victimization. *Journal of Youth and Adolescence*, *43*(5), 790–802. doi:10.1007/s10964-013-0003-9

Vranjes, I., Baillien, E., Vandebosch, H., Erreygers, S. & De Witte, H. (2017). The dark side of working online: Towards a definition and an Emotion Reaction model of workplace cyberbullying. *Computers in Human Behavior*, *69*, 324–334. doi:10.1016/j.chb.2016.12.055

Wolke, D., Copeland, W. E., Angold, A., & Costello, E. J. (2013). Impact of bullying in childhood on adult health, wealth, crime, and social outcomes. *Psychological Science*, *24*, 1958–1970. doi:10.1177/0956797613481608

CONTRIBUTORS

Sheri Bauman is a professor of counseling at the University of Arizona, Tucson, AZ. She earned her Bachelor's degree at City College of New York, and Master's Degrees at the University of Northern Colorado and Colorado State University. She earned her PhD in Counseling Psychology from New Mexico State University.

Diana C. Bennett is a staff psychologist at the New Mexico VA in the outpatient PTSD program. She holds a PhD in Clinical Psychology from the University of Utah. Her research interests include trauma exposure across the lifetime, particularly the effects of different trauma types and cumulative trauma exposure on outcomes such as PTSD symptom clusters and treatment engagement.

Erika Borrajo is a researcher and teaching assistant at the Faculty of Psychology and Education of University of Deusto. Her research interests include intimate partner violence and problematic internet use.

Esther Calvete is an assistant professor of psychology at University of Deusto in Bilbao (Spain). Her research focuses on psychological problems in adolescents, including several forms of aggressive behavior.

Hayden Cox recently completed his undergraduate studies with a BA in Psychology and English from Furman University in Greenville, SC. He currently works as a Cross Country and Track & Field Coach at Elon University.

Elizabeth Englander is the founder and Executive Director of the Massachusetts Aggression Reduction Center at Bridgewater State University, delivering programs, resources, and research nationwide. She is a nationally recognized researcher and expert in the area of bullying and cyberbullying, childhood causes of aggression and abuse, and children's use of technology.

Manuel Gámez-Guadix is a teaching assistant at the Autonomous University of Madrid, Spain. His research focuses on different risk behaviors through Information and Communication Technologies, including cyberbullying, problematic Internet use, and online child grooming.

Gary W. Giumetti is an associate professor of psychology at Quinnipiac University in Hamden, CT. Gary holds Bachelor's and Master's degrees in Psychology from Villanova University and a PhD in Industrial-Organizational Psychology from Clemson University. His research focuses on fairness and employee well-being in the 21st century workplace.

Anke Görzig is Senior Lecturer in Psychology at the University of West London and member of the EU Kids Online network's UK team at the London School of Economics and Political Science. Anke holds an MSc (Diplom) in Psychology from the Technical University of Berlin and a PhD in Social Psychology (Dr. rer. soc.) from the University of Mannheim. Her research interests focus around children's risks and opportunities on the internet with an emphasis on cyberbullying and disadvantaged groups.

Robin M. Kowalski is a Trevillian professor of psychology at Clemson University. She obtained her PhD in social psychology from the University of North Carolina at Greensboro. Her research interests focus primarily on aversive interpersonal behaviors, most notably complaining, teasing, and bullying, with a particular focus on cyberbullying.

Penny A. Leisring is Professor of Psychology at Quinnipiac University in Hamden, CT. She earned BA degrees in psychology and child development from Connecticut College and a PhD in clinical psychology from the State University of New York at Stony Brook. Her research examines intimate partner violence.

Diana Meter is Assistant Professor of Human Development and Family Studies at Utah State University. She earned her BA in Psychology from the University of North Carolina Asheville and her MS and PhD in Family Studies and Human Development from The University of Arizona.

Nicole L. Mowry is an undergraduate student studying psychology at Quinnipiac University in Hamden, CT. After she graduates in 2019, she plans to pursue a Masters Degree in Industrial-Organizational Psychology. Nicole is interested in researching topics such as relationships in the workplace, job satisfaction, and motivation.

Michelle C. Ramos is an assistant professor of Child and Adolescent Studies at California State University, Fullerton. Michelle holds a PhD in Clinical Psychology from the University of Southern California. Her research focuses on intergenerational transmission of family aggression, with a focus on youths' relationship and health outcomes.

Erin M. Richard, PhD, is an Assistant Professor in the School of Leadership and Human Resource Development at Louisiana State University. Her research focuses on mood and emotion regulation in the workplace, affective influences on work motivation, and the role of computer-mediated communication at work.

Susanne Robinson has a BSc in Psychology and an MSc in Applied Psychology Research Methods from the University of Greenwich. She has been involved in research projects at Goldsmiths, University of London, on cyberbullying, developmental origins, and interventions. Her current research focus is the evaluation of cultural differences in aggression among young people.

Jenna L. Scisco is Assistant Professor of Psychological Science at Eastern Connecticut State University in Willimantic, CT. Jenna holds a Bachelor's degree in Psychology from The College of New Jersey, a Master's Degree in Applied Psychology from Clemson University, and a PhD in Human Factors Psychology from Clemson University. Her interdisciplinary research focuses on stress and health.

Peter K. Smith is Emeritus Professor of Psychology, Goldsmiths, University of London, UK. His most extensive research has been on bullying and violence in schools. He was the Chair of COST ACTION IS0801 on cyberbullying from 2008–2012, and was PI of a project Bullying, Cyberbullying, and Pupil Safety and Wellbeing, financed by the Indian-European Research Networking in the Social Sciences (2012–2015). He is author of *Understanding School Bullying: Its Nature and Prevention Strategies* (Sage, 2014).

Julianna J. Walsh is a PhD Candidate in Industrial-Organizational Psychology at the Florida Institute of Technology. Julianna holds Bachelor's degrees in Psychology and Anthropology from Southern Methodist University and a Master's in Industrial-Organizational Psychology from the Florida Institute of Technology. Her research interests include global leadership and emotions in the workplace.

Zhiqing E. Zhou is Assistant Professor in Industrial and Organizational Psychology at Baruch College, City University of New York. Dr. Zhou obtained his BA from Peking University, China, and his PhD from University of South Florida. His research interests include workplace mistreatment, and employee health and well-being.

INDEX

Page numbers in **bold** refer to figures, page numbers in *italic* refer to tables.